Pesticide and
Venom Neurotoxicity

Pesticide and Venom Neurotoxicity

Edited by

D. L. Shankland
Mississippi State University
Mississippi State, Mississippi

R. M. Hollingworth
Purdue University
West Lafayette, Indiana

and

T. Smyth, Jr.
Pennsylvania State University
University Park, Pennsylvania

Plenum Press · New York and London

Library of Congress Cataloging in Publication Data

Main entry under title:

Pesticide and venom neurotoxicity.

Includex index.
   1. Insecticides—Physiological effect—Congresses. 2. Neurotoxic agents—
Physiological effect—Congresses. 3. Nervous system—Insects—Congresses.
4. Miticides—Physiological effect—Congresses. 5. Nervous system—Mites—
Congresses. 7. Insects—Physiology—Congresses. 8. Mites—Physiology—
Congresses. I. Shankland, Daniel Leslie, 1924-
SB951.5.P47   632'.951   77-25006
ISBN-13: 978-1-4615-8836-8   e-ISBN-13: 978-1-4615-8834-4
DOI: 10. 1007/978-1-4615-8834-4

Selected papers from the Fifteenth International
Congress of Entomology held in Washington, D.C.,
August 19-27, 1976

© 1978 Plenum Press, New York
Softcover reprint of the hardcover 1st edition 1978
A Division of Plenum Publishing Corporation
227 West 17th Street, New York, N.Y. 10011

Preface

The development of the modern organic insecticides has contributed a major chapter to the history of neurotoxicants. From their roots in the organochlorines and organophosphates discovered prior to and during the Second World War, to the carbamates developed in the 1950's, and most recently to the extremely potent and promising synthetic pyrethroids, the most important organic insecticides have been those whose wite of action lies within the nervous system. In this regard, man is only mimicking nature in attacking the nervous system with lethal intent since potent neurotoxins are common components of the venoms with which animals of all types defend themselves and subdue their prey.

This central role of the nervous sytem as a broad target for pesticides may also be projected into the future – a prediction to which this volume is devoted. The nervous system in its diversity is likely to be of central concern to those charged with discovering novel pesticides whether they be modifications of familiar chemical groups or structurally novel neurotoxicants such as the nitromethylene insecticides described here. On a second front, the ability to influence insect behavior through the nervous system will become increasingly important in pest management. Pheromones represent one obvious example of this; recent work described in this volume indicates that the formamidine pesticides may represent another.

It is unfortunate but true that we cannot yet hope to design pesticidal molecules ab initio, but there is an increasing interest in developing a more rational basis for pesticide discovery than has been typical in the past. Such a rational approach depends in part on the investigation of possible critical sites and modes of action for chemicals in the nervous system, including comparative aspects which can lead to more selective and safer compounds; study of the mode of action and structure–activity relations of known neurotoxicants; and development of model assay systems for screening purposes. These are the major topics addressed in this book.

Perhaps a word of justification is needed concerning the inclusion here of papers on arthropod venoms. In addition to their very real ecological, medical, and evolutionary interest, venoms and toxins have potential as chemical models for novel control agents as witnessed by the development of the insecticide cartap from the marine annelid toxin, nereistoxin. Even more significantly, they are vital aids for the exploration of the biochemistry and physiology of nervous function upon which rational development and the future understanding of the actions of neurotoxicants depends. Thus, for example, the observation presented here by Piek and Spanjer regarding the presynaptic blockade of neuromuscular transmission in insects by certain wasp venoms provides a challenging model for insecticide development in addition to its intrinsic significance for insect biology and neurophysiology.

With these themes in mind, several symposia were arranged for the 15th International Congress of Entomology held in August, 1976, in Washington, D.C. Many of the world's leaders in the study of pesticide and venom neurotoxicity participated. It is from these presentations that the current volume is drawn.

We were fortunate to persuade Dr. Clyde W. Kearns to introduce both our symposium on insecticide neurotoxicity and this volume. We would like to dedicate the book to him in recognition of the key role which he has played in the study of organic insecticides and their activity as neurotoxicants.

D. L. Shankland
R. M. Hollingworth
T. Smyth, Jr.

Contents

SECTION II
NEUROTOXIC ACTIONS OF SYNTHETIC
INSECTICIDES AND ACARICIDES

SECTION III
NEUROTOXIC ACTIONS OF ARTHROPOD VENOMS

GENERAL INTRODUCTION

C. W. Kearns

Shell Research Ltd. U.K.

The need for a better understanding of the neurotoxic action of pesticides and arthropod venoms has been apparent for many years. This publication presents clear evidence that the general subject is today being given some of the attention which it has long deserved. It presents a representative sample of some of the most interesting research which is being undertaken by workers in various parts of the world. The diversity of the subject matter is a reflection of the many different approaches which may be taken to contribute to a better understanding of the functioning of the arthropod nervous system.

It has long been known that the conduction processes of the arthropod nervous system could not be fully equated in terms of vertebrate neuropharmacology. Recognition of the fact that neuroactive pesticides may be useful tools for the elucidation of the arthropod nervous system is evident in these chapters.

The probability seems eminent that a component of arthropod venom will be isolated which will prove to have the specific property of irreversibly inhibiting the cholinergic receptor of arthropods. The advent of this discovery will most certainly lead to an inspired investigation of the nature and properties of this vital process which would appear to be different from that of the vertebrates.

Highly discriminating electrophysiological techniques and novel biochemical approaches reported in these chapters is assurance that efforts to understand the mode of action of pesticides will become increasingly more precise. Hopefully, this in turn will reduce our dependence upon the empirical approaches to the discovery of novel and useful pesticides.

   The side effects of neuroactive pesticides have not been dis-
regarded. The fact that such agents may induce the untimely release of neurohormones and other compartmentalized biogenic agents
has been clearly demonstrated. The relevance of these findings
remains to be discovered.

Section I

Sites of Neurotoxic Action in Insects

SITES OF NEUROTOXIC ACTION IN INSECTS

INTRODUCTION

D. L. Shankland

Mississippi State University

Mississippi State, Mississippi   39762

Insect nervous systems are relatively simple compared with those in higher animals. Nevertheless, they contain tens of thousands of cells in exquisitely integrated communication networks which insure functional integrity in every activity. Motor activity is of course under direct control, but through the secretion of neuroendocrine products the regulatory role of the nervous system is extended to growth and development, diapause, digestion, metabolism, excretion, reproduction, and other processes. Normal nervous function depends on a great variety of precisely timed events, and alterations in any one of them may so disrupt nervous integrity as to have lethal consequences. Many natural and synthetic poisons owe their effects to interference with one or more of these events. Some effects have unknown bases, while others can be ascribed to discrete action on biochemical entities such as receptor or enzyme molecules.

DDT, pyrethrins, tetrodotoxin, saxitoxin, and batrachotoxin, for example, interfere by unknown mechanisms with important transient changes in Na^+ permeability of axonal membrane. In so doing they produce aberrant axonal activity or block transmission entirely. On the other hand, the organophosphate and carbamate insecticides act primarily, if not solely, to inhibit acetylcholinesterase. In the same vein, nicotine mimics the action of acetylcholine on the acetylcholine receptor, while nereistoxin and the related synthetic insecticide cartap block the same receptor. Receptors of other kinds, transmitter synthesis and release, presynaptic vesicle formation,and various electrogenic processes are potential or actual targets for natural and synthetic

5

neurotoxicants.

The first of the following chapters discusses the structure, penetrability and normal function of the insect central nervous system to provide a basis of understanding for detailed discussions of selected targets and specific kinds of neurotoxic action in this and other sections of the book. In this first series of chapters, the detailed treatment of several cholinergic elements reflects the importance of that system. However, important secondary effects of neurotoxic action mediated through the neuroendocrine system are also considered, and these may well relate more directly than the primary lesion to the cause of death. Finally in this section, a chapter is devoted to neuromuscular transmission as a potential insecticide target, with an examination of the current status of the debate on glutamate as an excitatory transmitter.

THE INSECT CENTRAL NERVOUS SYSTEM AS A SITE

OF ACTION OF NEUROTOXICANTS

D. B. SATTELLE

A.R.C. Unit of Invertebrate Chemistry and Physiology
Dept. of Zoology, Cambridge University, Downing St.
Cambridge CB2 3EJ

INTRODUCTION

For safe and efficient progress in the development of chemicals for the control of insect pests it is essential to improve our understanding of the cellular and molecular mechanisms of action of these compounds. Most insecticides are potent central nervous toxins (O'Brien, 1967; Corbett, 1974). A prerequisite to the identification of the central sites of action of insecticides is a detailed knowledge of the normal function of the major cell types which constitute the central nervous system. Recent advances in neuroanatomy, neurophysiology and neurochemistry have led to the notion of the insect central nervous system as a target organ for insecticide action within which there are several potential target sites. In this chapter some of the fundamental aspects of central nervous function are discussed in order to provide a basis for interpretation of the central actions of insecticides which will be described in later chapters.

The insect central nervous system consists of paired connectives linking paired segmentally arranged ganglia. A ganglion (Fig. 1) consists of an outer connective tissue envelope (the neural lamella) overlying a modified glial layer, the perineurium. Intercellular channels can be seen between adjacent perineurial cells but towards their inner ends they are at least partially occluded by tight junctions. Beneath the perineurium is located an outer rind of nerve cell bodies. Glial cells are also prevalent in this region. Processes from the cell bodies pass into the neuropile. This region which forms the central core of the ganglion contains numerous axons (the conducting elements of the nerve cells) some glial cells and many synapses - the points at which nerve cells make functional

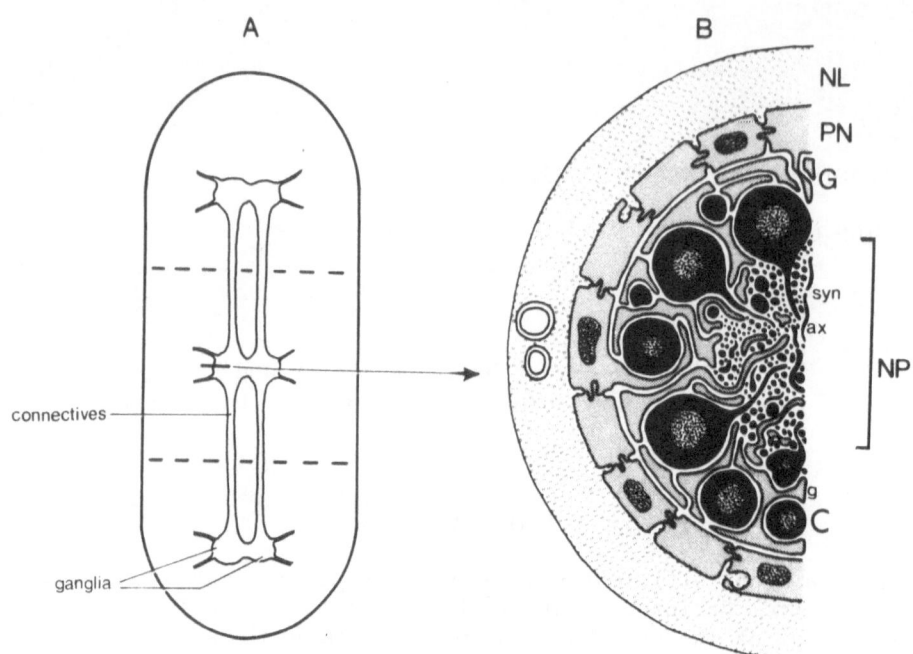

Fig. 1. The insect central nervous system. A. Generalized central
nervous system consisting of segmentally arranged ganglia and
connectives. B. Schematic hemisection of an insect ganglion
showing (not to scale) neural lamella (NL), perineurium (PN),
glia (G), nerve cell bodies (C) and the neuropile (NP). Within
the neuropile axons (ax) synapses (syn) and glial processes (g)
are shown.

connections. In this survey particular attention will be given to
synaptic function in view of the fact that many of the current
generation of insecticides are anticholinesterases.

BLOOD—BRAIN BARRIER

It is well established that neurons in the central nervous
system of insects are relatively insensitive to ions and molecules
applied to the fluid bathing the surfaces of the tissue. Early
studies established that insect central nervous tissue contained a
diffusion barrier or barriers that discriminated against large size,
positive charge and polarity (Treherne, 1966; O'Brien, 1967; Pitman
1971). In this section we shall examine recent evidence pertaining
to the location of the barrier(s).

A. The Neural Fat Body

Parts of the ganglia and connectives of the central nervous system are surrounded by patches of fat body tissue. Examples of this are reported from Periplaneta americana (Smith & Treherne, 1963; Boulton & Rowell, 1968) and Manduca sexta (Pichon et al., 1972). In the stick insect Carausius morosus the fat body cells form a complete sheath around the ventral nerve cord (Maddrell & Treherne, 1966; Lane & Treherne, 1971; Huddart, 1972). It has been suggested that this fat body sheath regulates the level of sodium ions in the fluid space between the fat body sheath and the surfaces of the central nervous system (Weidler & Diecke, 1969, 1970), However, electrophysiological studies indicate that the neural fat body sheath of Carausius is leaky to ions (Treherne, 1972). This accords with the demonstration that the exogeneous tracer molecule macroperoxidase (MW 40,000) penetrates from the haemolymph into the extraneural space (Lane & Treherne, 1971). It therefore appears that the neural fat body sheath does not constitute a major site of restriction of ion movements between the haemolymph and the neurons within the central nervous system.

B. The Neural Lamella

The neural lamella is the connective tissue layer surrounding both peripheral and central nervous systems. It contains tracheae and tracheoles and in some cases fibroblast-like cells. Neutral mucopolysaccharides and mucoproteins (Ashhurst, 1968; Ashhurst & Costin, 1971a,b) form the ground substance in which collagen-like fibres are embedded (Smith & Treherne, 1963; Locke & Huie, 1972). A number of studies have been performed on the permeability of the insect neural lamella. Electrophysiological studies reveal a rapid access of potassium ions in the bathing medium to the outer membranes of the perineurium (Treherne et al., 1970; Pichon & Treherne, 1970; Pichon et al., 1972). Histological studies have demonstrated that the neural lamella surrounding the nervous system of Periplaneta americana is permeable to water soluble dye molecules (Wigglesworth, 1960; Eldefrawi et al., 1968). Recently molecules as large as macroperoxidase (MW 40,000) have been shown to penetrate the neural lamella and enter the underlying perineurial clefts in Periplaneta americana, Carausius morosus and Manduca sexta (see Lane, 1974). Microperoxidase and colloidal lanthanum penetrate the neural lamella of Periplaneta americana (Lane & Treherne, 1972). It can therefore be concluded that the neural lamella offers no significant restriction to the access of small water soluble molecules to the underlying cellular layer, the perineurium.

C. The Perineurium

The cells forming a continuous layer immediately underlying the
neural lamella constitute the perineurium and are considered to be
modified glial cells (Wigglesworth, 1959). Cells in this layer
often contain fat globules and abundant glycogen granules (Wigglesworth, 1950; Smith & Treherne, 1963) suggesting a trophic role for
this cell layer. Perineurial cells are separated at their lateral
borders by convoluted extracellular channels and between adjacent
plasma membranes, septate desmosomes, gap and tight junctions occur
(see Lane, 1974). These cells also exhibit an increased surface
area at their inner margins, produced by long inwardly projecting
cytoplasmic flanges. In this way the fine-structure of the perineurium closely resembles that of fluid-secreting epithelia as
found in the rectal papillae of the blowfly Calliphora (Berridge &
Gupta, 1967). Fig. 2 shows an EM section through the periphery of
a connective from the ventral nerve cord of Manduca sexta.

The exogenous tracer molecule microperoxidase (MW 1,900)
penetrates the intercellular clefts of the perineurium but shows
only limited penetration of septate desmosomes and no invasion of
the underlying extracellular spaces (Lane & Treherne, 1972). These
authors also show that colloidal and ionic lanthanum penetrates
both septate desmosomes and gap junctions and the restricted
access of this substance to the extracellular system of the central
nervous system could therefore be attributed to the presence of
perineurial tight junctions.

Microsurgical removal of the outer tissue layers of the insect
central nervous system (desheathing) greatly enhances the rate of
decline of action potentials in preparations exposed to reduced
external sodium concentrations in Periplaneta americana (Treherne
et al., 1970), Carausius morosus (Treherne, 1965) and Manduca sexta
(Pichon et al., 1972). Using the known potassium sensitivity of
neurons in the central nervous systems of insects and other invertebrates, it is possible to assess the rate of change of potassium ion
concentration in the fluid bathing the neuronal surfaces (Treherne
et al., 1970; Sattelle & Howes, 1975). The effect of desheathing
on the rate of change of potassium ions at the axonal surfaces in
the central nervous system of Manduca sexta is illustrated (Fig. 3).
Although in unoperated unstretched connectives changes in the
external ionic concentration have only delayed effects on the amplitude of axonal resting and action potentials, extremely rapid D.C.
potentials have nevertheless been recorded in these preparations
from Periplaneta (Treherne et al., 1970) and Manduca (Pichon et al.,
1972). These potential changes (Fig. 4) must be located, not at the
axonal level, but rather between some part of the extracellular
system and the bathing medium. The relative potency of a series of
cations in inducing these extraneuronal potential changes is found

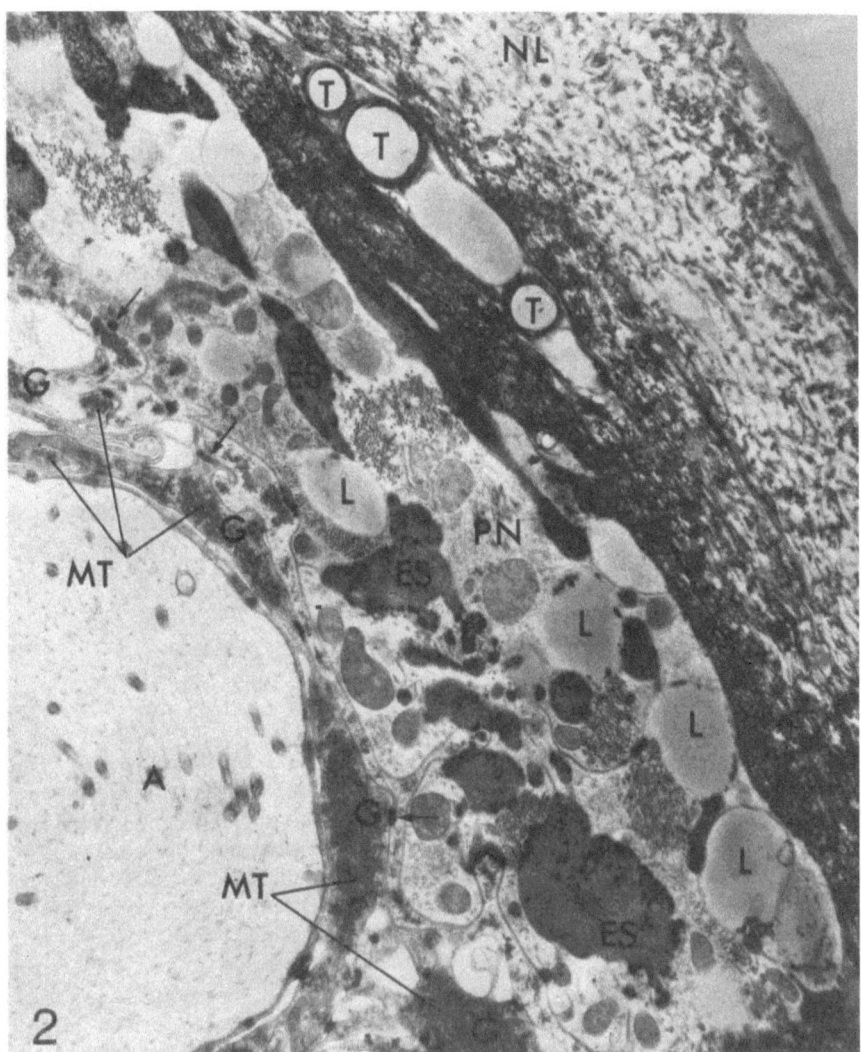

Fig. 2. An electron micrograph through the peripheral regions of a transversely sectioned connective from the ventral nerve cord of Manduca sexta. This region is near the latero-dorsal edge of the connective near where the neural lamella (NL) begins to become extended into the dorsal mass. The perineurium (PN) possesses many microtubules and lipid globules (L); between adjacent cells lie extracellular spaces (ES) containing dense material. Desmosomes (arrows) attach these perineurial cells to the underlying glia (G) whose microtubule-laden (MT) processes ensheath the axons (A). Tracheoles (T) are shown. (X13,300) (from Pichon, Sattelle & Lane, 1972).

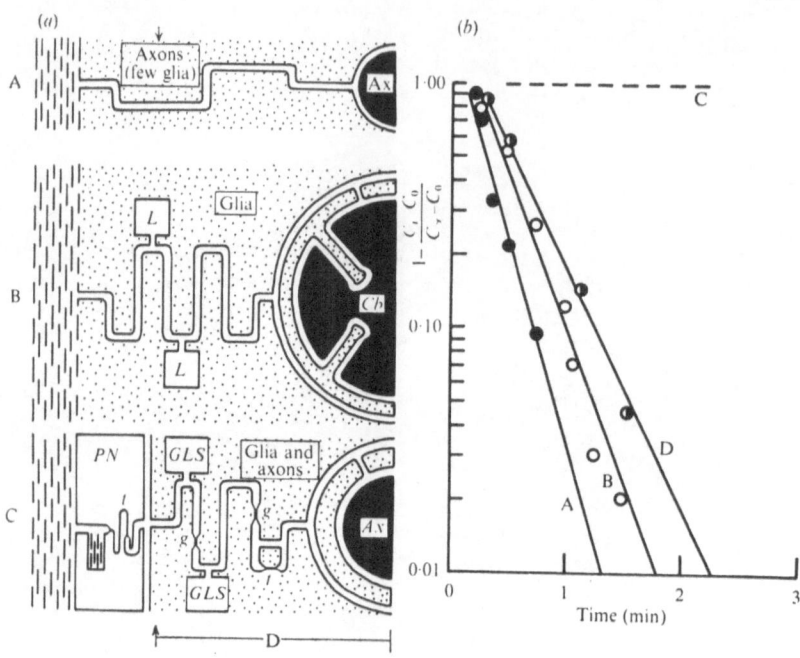

Fig. 3. (a) Schematic representation of the main features of the extracellular pathways in the central nervous systems of (A) Anodonta cygnea (connective), (B) Limnaea stagnalis (ganglion) and (C) Manduca sexta (connective). (D) represents the desheathed connective of Manduca. Tissues to the left of the arrows are removed in desheathing. Abbreviations: Ax, axons; Cb, cell body; g, gap junctions; GLS, glial lacuna system; L, lacuna; PN, perineurium; t, tight junction. These simplified models are based on electron microscopical studies on the central nervous tissues of these invertebrate organisms. In addition to data reported here, information from the following publications has been used: Limnaea (Sattelle & Lane, 1972; Sattelle, 1973, 1974) and Manduca (Lane, 1972, Pichon, Sattelle & Lane, 1972).

(b) Plots of the rate of change of potassium concentration in the extracellular spaces of various invertebrate central nervous tissues: A, intact cerebro-visceral connective of Anodonta cygnea (Sattelle & Howes,1975); B, intact parietal ganglion of Limnaea stagnalis (data from Sattelle, 1973b); C, desheathed connective of Manduca sexta (data from Pichon et al. (1972) and Sattelle (unpublished observations)); D, intact connective of Manduca sexta (inferred from data in Pichon et al., 1972). (From Sattelle & Howes, 1975).

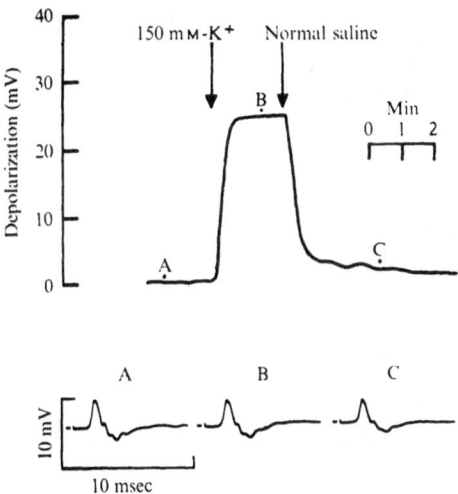

Fig. 4. Rapid 'extraneural' depolarization recorded from intact connective of <u>Manduca sexta</u> in response to an increase in the external potassium concentration from 3 mM to 150 mM. Associated action potentials are also shown (sucrose-gap recordings). (from Pichon, Sattelle & Lane, 1972).

to be as follows (Pichon <u>et al</u>., 1971):

$$K^+ > Rb^+ > Cs^+ > TEA^+ > Na^+ > Li^+ > choline^+ > tris^+$$

corresponding to scheme IV of the system devised by Diamond & Wright (1969) to describe the relative potencies of alkali cations in biological systems. These electrophysiological findings together with ultrastructural observations have led to the following interpretation (Pichon <u>et al</u>., 1971, 1972). With elevated concentrations of potassium, for example, the accessibility of the outwardly facing membranes of the perineurial cells would result in a rapid depolarization of this membrane. Depolarization of the inner surfaces of the perineurial cells could, however, be substantially prevented by the presence of the tight junctions at the base of the perineurial clefts. This restricted access of potassium ions to the inner surfaces of the perineurial cells could acocunt for the rapid D.C. (extraneuronal) potential changes (Fig. 4). The insect perineurium

resembles the frog skin in that changes in external ion concentration affect only one of the two membrane surfaces. It remains to
attempt to correlate with the above findings the results of experiments using radioisotopes to study exchange of ions between the
haemolymph and central nervous tissues. Tucker & Pichon (1972a,b)
have related the efflux curves for $^{22}Na^+$ to the electrical characteristics of connectives from the ventral nerve cord of Periplaneta
americana. These authors detect an initial 'fast' (extracellular)
component of the efflux which shows a strong correlation with the
size of the extraneuronal potential. Even in the presence of
maximal potassium-induced extraneuronal potentials, relatively
rapid exchanges of $^{22}Na^+$ occur, suggesting that at least part of
the 'fast' component is of glial origin.

In a recent study of the permeability of the insect blood-brain
barrier to various aliphatic alcohols, Thomas (1976a,b) has shown that
for intact connectives with substantial extraneuronal potentials there
is a rapid exchange of these radiolabelled lipo-soluble molecules
between the bathing medium and the central nervous tissues.

D.   Glial Cells and the Extracellular System

Having traversed the perineurium, ions and water-soluble
molecules may reach the axonal and synaptic surfaces in the neuropile either by diffusing along the narrow (200 A) extracellular
channels or by transport within the glial cell system. Attempts
to assess the relative importance of these pathways have been made
using variously manipulated preparations. For example, in intact
connectives showing minimal extraneuronal potentials access is
largely mediated by extracellular diffusion. In desheathed
preparations on the other hand ion movements to the fluid bathing
axon surfaces is primarily achieved by intracellular glial
diffusion pathways (Treherne et al., 1970). Although these
surgically manipulated preparations facilitate the separation of
various routes for ion exchange within the central nervous system
it is difficult to distinguish their relative importance in the
intact unoperated connective.

The glial cells may also provide a 'metabolic barrier' to
penetration of certain molecules into the central nervous system.
For example, a relatively rapid exchange of ^{14}C-labelled acetylcholine has been shown to occur between the bathing medium and the
intact central nervous system of Periplaneta americana (Treherne
& Smith, 1965; Eldefrawi & O'Brien, 1967). However, the amount of
acetylcholine present in the extracellular spaces after 30 minutes
in 10^{-2} M acetylcholine is found to be reduced to 8.1×10^{-5} M.
Peripheral sites of cholinesterase activity which have been
localized histochemically to glial cell membranes flanking the
extracellular channels would undoubtedly constitute an effective

barrier to the penetration of extraneously applied acetylcholine
(Smith & Treherne, 1965).

AXONAL CONDUCTION IN THE CENTRAL NERVOUS SYSTEM

Interneurons and motorneurons of insects consist of the soma
(cell body) located at the periphery of the ganglion (Fig. 1), a
proximal segment which is a single process passing into the neuropile, an integrating segment giving rise to many dendritic processes
and a distal segment, the axon. Excitation and conduction in the
insect axons studied to date (Narahashi, 1963; Pichon, 1974) appear
to be mediated by ionic mechanisms which closely resemble those
postulated for the classical nerve axon preparation, the squid giant
axon (Hodgkin, 1951). The axonal membrane of insects does not,
however, correspond to an ideal potassium electrode. For example,
axons of Periplaneta americana (Yamasaka & Narahashi, 1958, 1959;
Treherne et al., 1970) and Manduca sexta (Pichon et al., 1972)
exhibit a 42-43 mV slope and the cell bodies of Carausius morosus
(Treherne & Maddrell, 1967a) a 37 mV slope for a decade change in
external potassium ion concentration (Fig. 5).

When the axon membrane is depolarized by a brief current pulse
action potentials can be evoked. At their peak the membrane potential is inverted, the inside of the axon becoming positive with
respect to the outside. The overshoot potential is usually +20 to
+60 mV (Pichon, 1974). Yamasaki & Narahashi (1959) have shown that
the slope of the curve relating the overshoot potential does not
differ appreciably from the 59 mV slope predicted for a ten-fold
change in the external sodium concentration. In this property the
insect axon closely resembles the squid axon. Pharmacological
similarities also exist. For example tetrodotoxin (TTX) the poison
extracted from the puffer fish which blocks the sodium current in
squid giant axons (Moore et al., 1967) blocks the excitability of
the giant axon of Periplaneta americana without significantly
affecting the resting potential (Narahashi, 1965). Conduction is
also blocked by TTX in axons of the ventral nerve cord of Manduca
sexta (Pichon et al., 1972) and Carausius morosus (Treherne &
Maddrell, 1967b). Extensive voltage clamp studies on the giant
axon of Periplaneta americana have shown directly that the peak
inward current resulting from a depolarizing pulse is carried
largely by sodium ions whereas the subsequent outward current is
carried by potassium ions (Pichon, 1969).

SYNAPTIC TRANSMISSION IN THE CENTRAL NERVOUS SYSTEM

Few detailed neuropharmacological studies have been performed
on the insect central nervous system and although a range of putative transmitter substances have been applied to insect neurones it
is only in the case of acetylcholine that a substantial body of

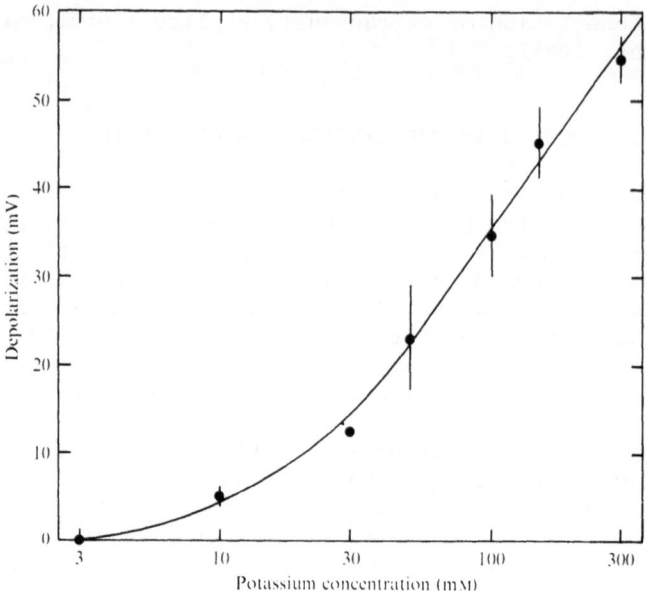

Fig. 5. Relation between the changes in resting potential (sucrose-gap recordings) and the external potassium concentration for axons in the ventral nerve cord of <u>Manduca sexta</u>. The vertical bars represent twice the standard errors of the mean. (from Pichon, Sattelle & Lane, 1972).

evidence has been accumulated. This discussion will be confined to some of the better documented insect preparations where acetylcholine is a likely neurotransmitter candidate. In establishing any neurotransmitter pathway two important criteria must be satisfied (see Werman, 1966; Gerschenfeld, 1973):
a) the release of the putative transmitter in adequate amounts from the presynaptic nerve terminal.
b) the identity of action in all respects of the applied putative transmitter and the natural transmitter.

These criteria are most closely fulfilled for the intensively studied actions of acetylcholine at the vertebrate skeletal neuromuscular junction which has become the prototype synapse for neurobiologists (see Hall, Hildebrand & Kravitz, 1974). In addition to these criteria, other properties are characteristic of synaptic transmission:
  i) a presynaptic synthetic pathway,
 ii) presynaptic presence of the transmitter and a storage mechanism,
iii) the presence of a specific transmitter release mechanism,
 iv) postsynaptically located specific receptors,
  v) a specific mechanism to terminate transmitter action.

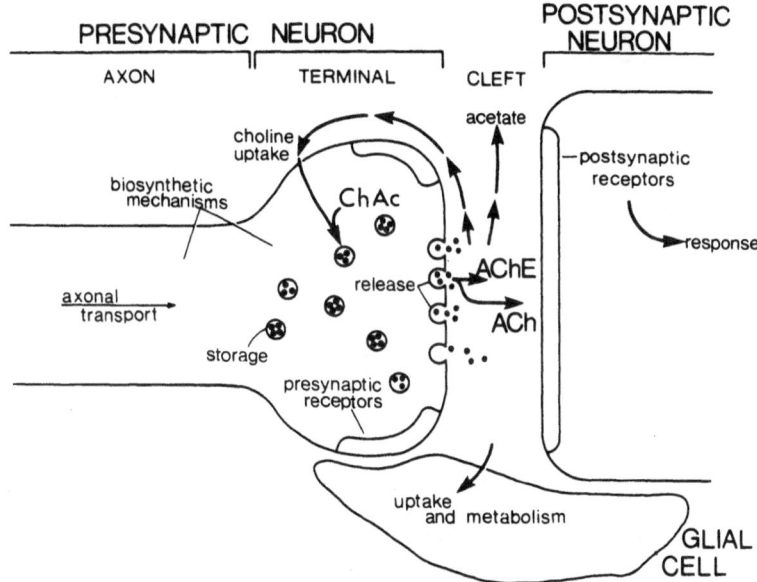

Fig. 6. Schematic representation of the location of the major components of a cholinergic synapse. ChAc, choline acetyltransferase; ACh, acetylcholine; AChE, acetylcholinesterase.

A schematic representation of the location of the various elements of a cholinergic synapse is shown in Fig. 6. Techniques for recording synaptic activity and the application of acetylcholine and related compounds which have been successfully developed at peripheral synapses are more difficult to apply to central synapses. Problems include the introduction and precise location of recording probes and in particular the problem of applying drugs directly to the synapse. Two main methods are used to apply putative transmitters and drugs to synaptic preparations in the central nervous system (Fig. 7). In the first of these (bath application) the compound is simply applied in the perfusion solution. This has the advantage of delivering a known concentration of the drug but clearly it will not be localized to active receptors. So long as all the receptors are available to the drug partitioning between active and inactive receptors need not be a serious problem - the proportion being fixed for a given preparation. Other disadvantages of this method of application include the possibility of specific desensitization of receptors affecting the recorded response and the possibility of restricted access due to physical and chemical barriers. A second major method of application is iontophoresis. By this means a charged compound is delivered from a micropipette following the passage of a pulse

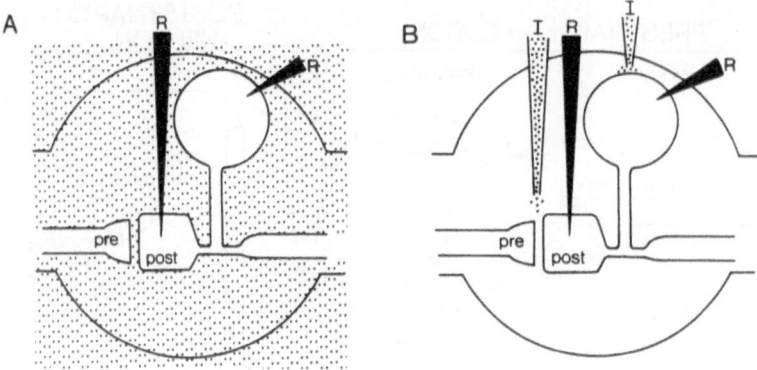

Fig. 7. Schematic illustration of the two main methods used to
apply putative neurotransmitters and related drugs to insect central
neurons. (A) bath application; (B) iontophoresis. R, recording
electrode; I, injection electrode.

of appropriate polarity. The localized application of the putative
transmitter or drug has the advantage that receptor distribution
can be studied. A disadvantage is that the drug concentration
is not accurately known.

Acetylcholine has long been suspected to be an insect
excitatory central neurotransmitter. Numerous studies have now
revealed different components of the cholinergic system in the
central nervous tissues of a variety of insect species. Studies on
the A6 ganglion of Periplaneta americana (see Calhoun, 1963) showed
the presence of acetylcholine (63.0 µg/g tissue) choline acetyltransferase (10.0 mg ACh synthesized/g/hr) and acetylcholinesterase
(314.9 mg ACh hydrolyzed/g/hr). In a recent study of the moth
Manduca sexta the antennal nerves have been shown to be thickly
populated with sensory neurones which contain endogenous acetylcholine and extracts contained choline acetyltransferase and
acetylcholinesterase activity (Sanes & Hildebrand, 1975, 1976a,b;
Sanes, Prescott & Hildebrand, 1977). These sensory fibres make
synapses in the antennal lobes of the brain. Levels of acetylcholine, choline acetyltransferase and acetylcholinesterase are
reduced by amputation of antennae, suggesting a possible role for
acetylcholine as a sensory neurotransmitter (Sanes, Prescott &
Hildebrand, 1977). A similar conclusion derives from the observation that degeneration of sensory axons in leg nerve 5 of the metathoracic ganglion of the locust (Schistocerca) results in a drop
in the level of choline acetyltransferase (Emson, Burrows &
Fonnum, 1974).

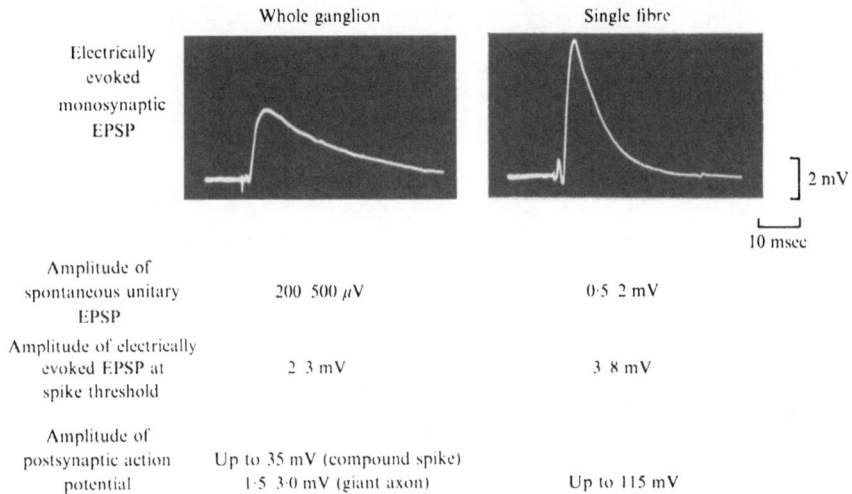

	Whole ganglion	Single fibre
Electrically evoked monosynaptic EPSP		
Amplitude of spontaneous unitary EPSP	200 500 μV	0·5 2 mV
Amplitude of electrically evoked EPSP at spike threshold	2 3 mV	3 8 mV
Amplitude of postsynaptic action potential	Up to 35 mV (compound spike) 1·5 3·0 mV (giant axon)	Up to 115 mV

Fig. 8. A summary of data on the amplitude of excitatory post-synaptic potentials at the cercal nerve, giant fibre synapses, recorded from a whole ganglion and from a single postsynaptic fibre using modified sucrose-gap techniques. (from Callec & Sattelle, 1973).

Study of the acetylcholine sensitivity of insect neurons has involved electrophysiological studies on identified cells and biochemical studies on the binding of acetylcholine and related compounds to various central nervous tissue extracts. Several electrophysiological studies have been performed on the excitatory monosynaptic relay in the terminal abdominal ganglion of Periplaneta americana between sensory axons from the cercal mechanoreceptors and interneurons giving rise to the ascending giant-fibres of the ventral nerve cord. The earlier studies employing hook-electrode recording techniques consistently report a low sensitivity to acetylcholine (Yamasaki & Narahashi, 1960). The use of micro-electrode (Callec, 1974) and sucrose-gap (Callec & Sattelle, 1973; Sattelle, 1977) recording techniques has greatly improved our understanding of this relay (Figs. 8 & 9). Callec (1974) has shown that iontophoretic injection of acetylcholine into the region of the neuropile containing numerous dendrites of the interneuron which gives rise to the medio-ventral giant fibre produces a depolarization (acetylcholine potential) and a diminution of resistance of the postsynaptic membrane. Comparison of the current-voltage curves of the excitatory postsynaptic potential (EPSP) and the acetylcholine potential recorded at this synapse reveals similar reversal potentials (Callec, 1974). In this same study both curare and atropine (5.0 x 10^{-4} g/ml) are shown to block the evoked EPSP and the acetylcholine potential.

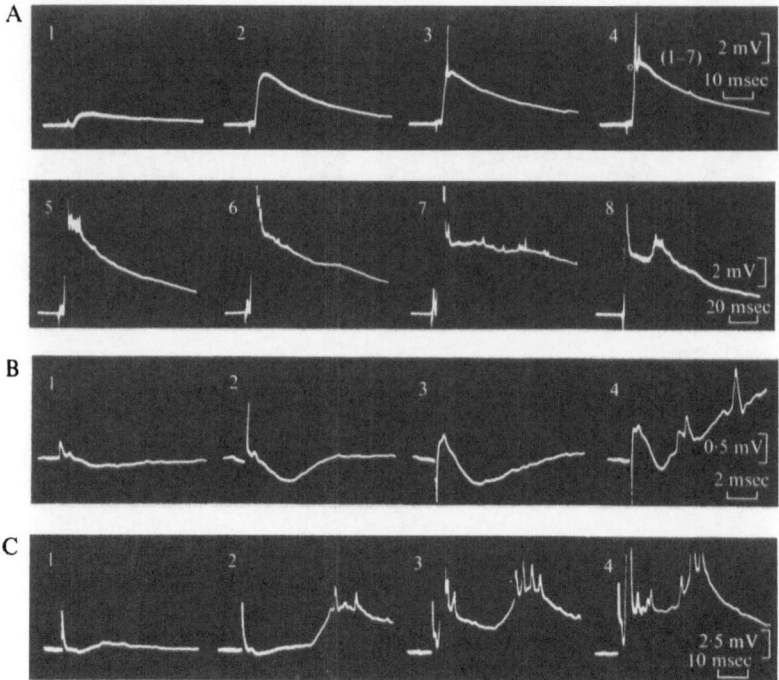

<u>Fig. 9</u>. Postsynaptic events following the electrical stimulation
of cercal nerves Xl, X. A, illustrates the effects of progressively
increasing the stimulation applied to nerve Xl. A_1-A_3, monosynaptic
EPSP. A_4-A_8 evolution of polysynaptic EPSP and compound spike.
B, C, show effects of progressively increasing the stimulation
applied to nerve X. B_1-B_3 shows compound IPSP increasing in
amplitude with higher stimulation. (from Callec & Sattelle, 1973).

Eserine potentiates the effects of acetylcholine and increases
the sensitivity of the cercal nerve, giant fibre synapse to as low
as 10^{-6} - 10^{-7} M acetylcholine (Shankland <u>et al</u>., 1970; Sattelle
<u>et al</u>., 1976; see also Fig. 10). The following agonist spectrum -
nicotine > carbachol > pilocarpine - has been obtained using modified
sucrose-gap recording techniques in conjunction with bath application
of the compounds. Pitman and collaborators (Pitman & Kerkut, 1970;
Kerkut, Pitman & Walker, 1969a,b) applying acetylcholine iontophoretically to nerve cell bodies of <u>Periplaneta americana</u> obtain a
similar agonist spectrum and calculate the threshold amount of
acetylcholine needed for a response to be 1.3 x 10^{-13} moles. These
authors also show that the acetylcholine and EPSP reversal potentials
have similar values. The acetylcholine response is reduced in
sodium-free saline suggesting this cation might be involved in the
acetylcholine response.

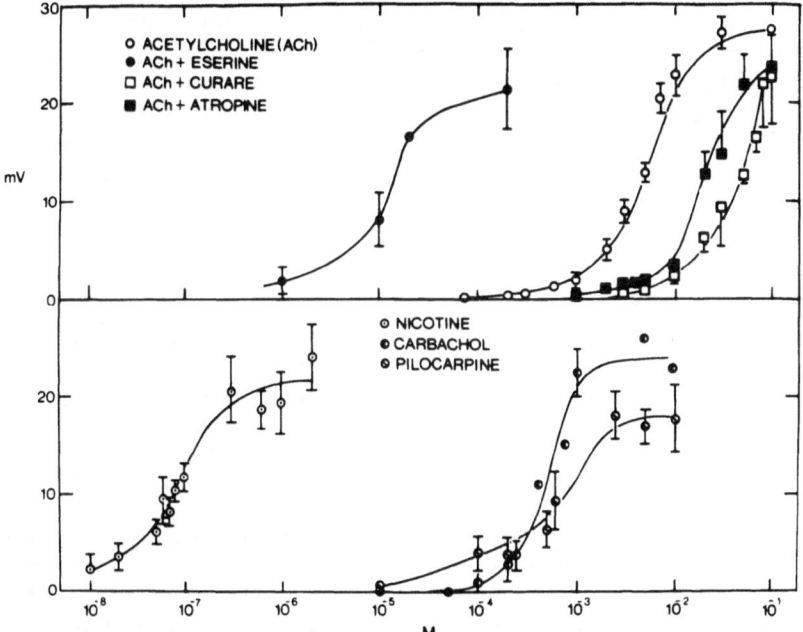

Fig. 10. Actions of acetylcholine and various cholinergic agonists and antagonists on synaptic transmission in the sixth abdominal ganglion of the cockroach. Ganglionic (postsynaptic) depolarization (in mV) is plotted against concentration (M). Vertical bars represent twice the standard error.

Attempts at chemical modification of acetylcholine synthesis in the presynaptic neuron have been less successful. Hemicholinium-3 which acts by inhibiting choline uptake produces progressive but irreversible blockade of synaptic transmission after repeated presynaptic stimulation (Shankland et al., 1971). A study on a group of isothiocyanate compounds which are potent choline acetyltransferase inhibitors (Baillie et al., 1975) resulted in the demonstration of a primarily postsynaptic site of action of these compounds (Sattelle & Callec, 1977) when applied to the cockroach sixth ganglion.

The pharmacology of acetylcholine receptors purified from housefly heads has been investigated (Aziz & Eldefrawi, 1973; Eldefrawi, 1976; Donnellan et al., 1975). These receptors appear to show both muscarinic and nicotinic properties. Not only is their muscarone binding inhibited by nicotine and atropine but also their binding of nicotine is blocked by atropine and vice-versa (Eldefrawi et al., 1971). This has led to the suggestion that insect acetylcholine receptors may be of mixed affinity. Further electrophysiological studies are needed to test this hypothesis.

The snake-venom α-bungarotoxin binds nicotinic acetylcholine receptors in chordates. An ^{125}I α-bungarotoxin binding activity which may
represent acetylcholine receptors has recently been demonstrated in
central nervous extracts from Manduca sexta (Sanes, Prescott &
Hildebrand, 1977) and Drosophila melanogaster (L. Hall, personal
communication).

CONCLUSIONS

This brief report has endeavored to survey those aspects of the
neurobiology of the insect central nervous system which are most relevant to an understanding of the actions of neurotoxic agents including
insecticides. For example, a knowledge of the permeability properties
of the various barriers restricting the exchange of a molecule between
the haemolymph and the neural elements in the central nervous system
is of considerable value in assessing its potency and likely site of
action. It is clear that conduction processes in insect axons closely
resemble those of other invertebrate and vertebrate axons. Evidence
is accumulating for acetylcholine as a likely sensory transmitter in
the insect central nervous system. Further work on acetylcholine
receptors should establish whether or not insect cholinergic receptors differ substantially in their chemosensitivity from other
invertebrate or even vertebrate receptors.

REFERENCES

Ashhurst, D. E.   1968.   The connective tissue of insects.   Ann. Rev.
    Entomol. 13:45.
Ashhurst, D. E. and Costin, N. M.   1971a.   Insect mucosubstances.
    I.   The mucosubstances of developing connective tissue in
    the locust, Locusta migratoria.   Histochem. J. 3:279.
Ashhurst, D. E. and Costin, N. M.   1971b.   Insect mucosubstances.
    II.   The mucosubstances of the central nervous system.
    Histochem. J. 3:297.
Aziz, S. A. and Eldefrawi, M. E.   1973.   Cholingergic receptors of
    the central nervous system of insects.   Pesticide Biochem.
    Physiol. 3:168.
Baillie, A. C., Corbett, J. R., Dowsett, J. R., Sattelle, D. B. and
    Callec, J. J.   1975.   Inhibitors of choline acetyltransferase
    as potential insecticides.   Pestic. Sci. 6: 645.
Berridge, M. J. and Gupta, B. L.   1967.   Fine-structural damage in
    relation to ion and water transport in the rectal papillae
    of the blowfly, Calliphora.   J. Cell Sci. 2:89.
Boulton, P. S. and Rowell, C. H. F.   1968.   Structure and function
    of the extraneural sheath in insects.   Nature 217:379.
Callec, J. J.   1974.   Synaptic transmission in the central nervous
    system of insects.   In Insect Neurobiology (ed. J. E. Treherne),
    pp. 119-186, North Holland, Amsterdam.

Callec, J.J. and Sattelle, D.B. 1973. A simple technique for
    monitoring the synaptic actions of pharmacological agents.
    J. Exp. Biol. 69:725.
Colhoun, E.H. 1963. The physiological significance of acetylcholine
    in insects and observations upon other pharmacologically
    active substances. In Advances in Insect Physiology Vol.1 (eds.
    J.W.L. Beament, J.E. Treherne & V.B. Wigglesworth), pp.1-45,
    Academic Press, London & New York.
Donnellan, J.F., Jewess, P.J. and Cattell, K.J. 1975. Subcellular
    localization and properties of a cholinergic receptor isolated
    from housefly heads. J. Neurochem. 25:623.
Diamond, J.M. and Wright, E.M. 1969. Biological membranes: the
    physical basis of ion and non-electrolyte selectivity.
    Ann. Rev. Physiol. 31:581.
Eldefrawi, A.T. 1976. The acetylcholine receptor and its inter-
    actions with insecticides. In Insecticide Biochemistry and
    Physiology (ed. C.F. Wilkinson), Plenum, New York.
Eldefrawi, M.E., Eldefrawi, A.T. and O'Brien, R.D. 1971. Binding
    of five cholinergic ligands to housefly brain and Torpedo
    electroplax. Mol. Pharmacol. 7:104.
Eldefrawi, M.E. and O'Brien, R.D. 1967. Permeability of the
    abdominal nerve cord of the cockroach Periplaneta americana L.
    to quaternary ammonium salts. J. Exp. Biol. 41:1.
Eldefrawi, M.E., Toppozada, A., Salpeter, M.M. and O'Brien, R.D.
    1968. The location of penetration barriers in the ganglia
    of the american cockroach Periplaneta americana. J. Exp. Biol.
    48:325.
Emson, P.C., Burrows, M. and Fonnum, F. 1974. Levels of glutamate
    decarboxylase, choline acetyltransferase and acetylcholin-
    esterase in identified motoneurons of the locust. J. Neurobiol.
    5:33.
Gerschenfeld, H.M. 1973. Chemical transmission in invertebrate
    central nervous systems and neuromuscular junctions. Physiol.
    Rev. 53:1.
Hall, Z.W., Hildebrand, J.G. and Kravitz, E.A. 1974. Chemistry of
    Synaptic Transmission: Essays and Sources. Chiron Press,
    Newton, Mass.
Hodgkin, A.L. 1951. The ionic basis of electrical activity in
    nerve and muscle. Biol. Rev. 26:339.
Huddart, H. 1972. Fine structure of the neural fat body sheath
    in the stick insect and its physiological significance.
    J. Exp. Zool. 179:145.
Kerkut, G.A., Pitman, R.M. and Walker, R.J. 1969a. Sensitivity
    of neurones of the insect central nervous system to ionto-
    phoretically applied acetylcholine or GABA. Nature 222:1075.
Kerkut, G.A., Pitman, R.M. and Walker, R.J. 1969b. Iontophoretic
    application of acetylcholine and GABA onto insect central
    neurones. Comp. Biochem. Physiol. 31:611.

Lane, N.J. 1972. Fine structure of a lepidopteran nervous system and its accessibility to peroxidase and lanthanum. Z. Zellforsch. 131:205.

Lane, N.J. 1974. The organization of insect nervous systems. In Insect Neurobiology (ed. J.E. Treherne), pp.1-72. North Holland, Amsterdan & Oxford.

Lane, N.J. and Treherne, J.E. 1971. The distribution of the neural fat-body sheath and the accessibility of the extraneural space in the stick insect Carausius morosus. Tissue & Cell 3:589.

Lane, N.J. and Treherne, J.E. 1972. Studies on perineurial junctional complexes and the sites of uptake of microperoxidase and lanthanum in the cockroach central nervous system. Tissue & Cell 4:427.

Locke, M. and Huie, P. 1972. The fiber components of insect connective tissue. Tissue & Cell 4:601.

Maddrell, S.H.P. and Treherne, J.E. 1966. A neural fat-body sheath in a phytophagous insect (Carausius morosus). Nature 211:215.

Moore, J.H., Blaustein, M.P., Anderson, N.C. and Narahashi, T. 1967. Basis of tetrodotoxin's slectivity in blockage of squid axons. J. Gen. Physiol. 50:1401.

Narahashi, T. 1965. The physiology of insect axons. In The Physiology of the Insect Central Nervous System (eds. J.E. Treherne & J.W.L. Beament), pp.1-20, Academic Press, New York.

O'Brien, R.D. 1967. Insecticides, Action and Metabolism. Academic Press, New York & London.

Pichon, Y. 1969. Aspects electriques et ioniques du functionnement nerveaux chez les Insectes. Cas particulier de la chaine nerveuse abdominale d'une Blatte, Periplaneta americana L. These d'Etat, Paris, 247pp.

Pichon, Y. 1974. Axonal conduction in insects. In Insect Neurobiology (ed. J.E. Treherne), pp.73-118. North Holland, Amsterdam & Oxford.

Pichon, Y., Moreton, R.B. and Treherne, J.E. 1971. A quantitative study of the ionic basis of extraneuronal potential changes in the central nervous system of the cockroach (Periplaneta americana L.). J. exp. Biol. 54:757.

Pichon, Y., Sattelle, D.B. and Lane, N.J. 1972. Conduction processes in the nerve cord of the moth Manduca sexta in relation to its ultrastructure and haemolymph ionic composition. J. Exp. Biol. 56:717.

Pichon, Y. and Treherne, J.E. 1970. Extraneuronal potentials and potassium depolarization in cockroach giant axons. J. Exp. Biol. 53:485.

Pitman, R.M. and Kerkut, G.A. 1970. Comparison of the actions of iontophoretically applied acetylcholine and GABA with the EPSP and IPSP in cockroach central neurons. Comp. Gen. Pharmacol. 1:221.

Pitman, R.M. 1971. Transmitter substances in insects: a review. Comp. Gen. Pharmacol. 2:347.

Sanes, J.R. and Hildebrand, J.G. 1975. Nerves in the antennae of pupal Manduca sexta Johanssen (Lepidoptera:Sphingidae). Willhelm Roux Arch. Entwickl. - Mech. Org. 178:71.

Sanes, J.R. and Hildebrand, J.G. 1976a. Structure and development of antennae in the moth Manduca sexta. Devel. Biol. 51:282.

Sanes, J.R. and Hildebrand, J.G. 1976b. Acetylcholine and its metabolic enzymes in developing antennae of the moth Manduca sexta. Devel. Biol. 52:105.

Sanes, J.R., Prescott, D.J. and Hildebrand, J.G. 1977. Cholinergic neurochemical development of normal and deafferented antennal lobes during metamorphosis of the moth Manduca sexta. Brain Res. 119:389.

Sattelle, D.B. 1973. Potassium movements in a central nervous ganglion of Limnaea stagnalis (L.) (Gastropoda:Pulmonata). J. Exp. Biol. 58:15.

Sattelle, D.B. 1974. Electrophysiology of the giant nerve cell bodies of Limnaea stagnalis (L.) (Gastropoda:Pulmonata). J. Exp. Biol. 60:653.

Sattelle, D.B. 1977. A simple assay for the actions of toxic agents on synaptic transmission in the insect central nervous system. In Crop Protection Agents: their Biological Evaulation (ed. N.R. McFarlane), pp.411-426. Academic Press, London, New York.

Sattelle, D.B. and Callec, J.J. 1977. Actions of isothiocyanates on the insect central nervous system. Pestic. Sci. (in press).

Sattelle, D.B. and Howes, E.A. 1975. The permeability to ions of the neural lamella and extracellular spaces in the C.N.S. of Anodonta cygnea. J. Exp. Biol. 63:421.

Sattelle, D.B., McClay, A.S., Dowson,R.J. and Callec, J.J. 1976. The pharmacology of an insect ganglion: actions of carbamylcholine and acetylcholine. J. Exp. Biol. 64:13.

Shankland, D.L., Rose, J.A. and Donninger, C. 1971. The cholinergic nature of the cercal nerve-giant fibre synapse in the sixth abdominal ganglion of the cockroach Periplaneta americana (L.). J. Neurobiol. 2:247.

Smith, D.S. and Treherne, J.E. 1963. Functional aspects of the organisation of the insect central nervous system. In: Advances in Insect Physiology Vol. 1 (eds. J.W.L. Beament, J.E. Treherne & V.B. Wigglesworth), pp.401-484, Academic Press, London & New York.

Smith, D.S. and Treherne, J.E. 1965. Electron microscopical localization of acetylcholinesterase activity in the central nervous system of an insect (Periplaneta americana). J. Cell Biol. 26:445.

Thomas, M.V. 1976a. Insect blood-brain barrier: an electrophysiological investigation of its permeability to the aliphatic alcohols. J. Exp. Biol. 64:101.

Thomas, M.V. 1976b. Insect blood-brain barrier: a radioisotope study of the kinetics of exchange of a liposoluble molecule (n-butanol). J. Exp. Biol. 64:119.

Treherne, J.E. 1965. Some preliminary observations on the effects
    of cations on conduction processes in the abdominal nerve cord
    of the stick insect Carausius morosus. J. Exp. Biol. 42:1.
Treherne, J.E. 1966. The Neurochemistry of Arthropods. Cambridge
    University Press.
Treherne, J.E. 1972. A study of the function of the neural fat
    body sheath in the stick insect (Carausius morosus). J. Exp.
    Biol. 56:129.
Treherne, J.E., Lane, N.J., Moreton, R.B. and Pichon, Y. 1970. A
    quantitative study of potassium movements in the central
    nervous system of Periplaneta americana. J. Exp. Biol. 53:109.
Treherne, J.E. and Maddrell, S.H.P. 1967a. Membrane potentials in
    the central nervous system of a phytophagous insect (Caruasius
    morosus). J. Exp. Biol. 46:413.
Treherne, J.E. and Maddrell, S.H.P. 1967b. Axonal function and
    ionic regulation in the central nervous system of a phyto-
    phagous insect (Carausius morosus). J. Exp. Biol. 47:235.
Treherne, J.E. and Smith, D.S. 1965. The penetration of acetyl-
    choline into the central nervous tissues of an insect (Peri-
    planeta americana). J. Exp. Biol. 43:13.
Tucker, L.E. and Pichon, Y. 1972a. Electrical and radioisotope
    study of an insect 'blood-brain barrier'. Nature New Biol.
    236:126.
Tucker, L.E. and Pichon, Y. 1972b. Sodium efflux from the central
    nervous connectives of the cockroach. J. Exp. Biol. 56:441.
Weidler, D.J. and Diecke, F.P.J. 1969. The role of cations in
    conduction in the central nervous system of the herbivorous
    insect Carausius morosus. Z. Vergl. Physiol. 64:372.
Weidler, D.J. and Diecke, F.P.J. 1970. The regulation of sodium
    ions in the central nervous system of the herbivorous insect
    Carausius morosus. Z. Vergl. Physiol. 67:160.
Werman, R. 1966. Criteria for identification of a central nervous
    system transmitter. Comp. Biochem. Physiol. 18:745.
Wigglesworth, V.B. 1959. The histology of the nervous system of
    an insect Rhodnius prolixus (Hemiptera). II. The central
    ganglia. Quart. J. Micr. Sci. 100:299.
Wigglesworth, V.B. 1960. The nutrition of the central nervous
    system of the cockroach Periplaneta americana. The mobili-
    zation of reserves. J. Exp. Biol. 37:500.
Yamasaki, T. and Narahashi, T. 1958. The effects of potassium and
    sodium ions on the resting and action potentials of the giant
    axon of the cockroach. Nature 182:805.
Yamasaki, T. and Narahashi, T. 1959. The effects of potassium and
    sodium ions on the resting and action potentials of the
    cockroach giant axon. J. Insect Physiol. 3:146.
Yamasaki, T. and Narahashi, T. 1960. Synaptic transmission in
    the last abdominal ganglion of the cockroach. J. Insect
    Physiol. 4:1.

ACETYLCHOLINE RECEPTORS: PURIFICATION, STRUCTURE AND INTERACTION WITH INSECTICIDES[*]

A. T. Eldefrawi, M. E. Eldefrawi, and N. A. Mansour

Department of Pharmacology and Experimental Therapeutics

Univ. of Maryland School of Medicine, Baltimore, Md. 21201

INTRODUCTION

The acetylcholine (ACh) receptor is a regulatory protein in the postsynaptic membrane, which upon binding of the transmitter ACh, changes its conformation and induces increased ion flux across the membrane through opening of gates or channels, leading to changes in membrane potential. Cholinergic transmission in insects plays a vital role. Its importance is underscored by the fact that the majority of insecticides in use today are anticholinesterases. These cause accumulation of ACh, resulting in excessive stimulation of the ACh-receptor followed by blockade of transmission and death of the animal. Other insecticides, such as nicotine, act directly on the ACh-receptor, but they are poor anti-ACh-esterases (Fujita et al., 1970).

For fifty years, pharmacological and physiological studies pointed to the presence of the ACh-receptor (Nachmansohn, 1955), but only in the last four years has the molecule been isolated in pure form and its properties studied.

PURIFICATION AND PROPERTIES OF ELECTRIC ORGAN ACH-RECEPTORS

The ACh-receptor is the first and only neurotransmitter receptor that has been purified, a feat that was feasible for three major reasons. One was the discovery of a tissue that is very rich

[*]The research presented in this report was financed by National Institutes of Health research grants AI 13640 and NS 13231, and National Science Foundation grant BMS 75-06760.

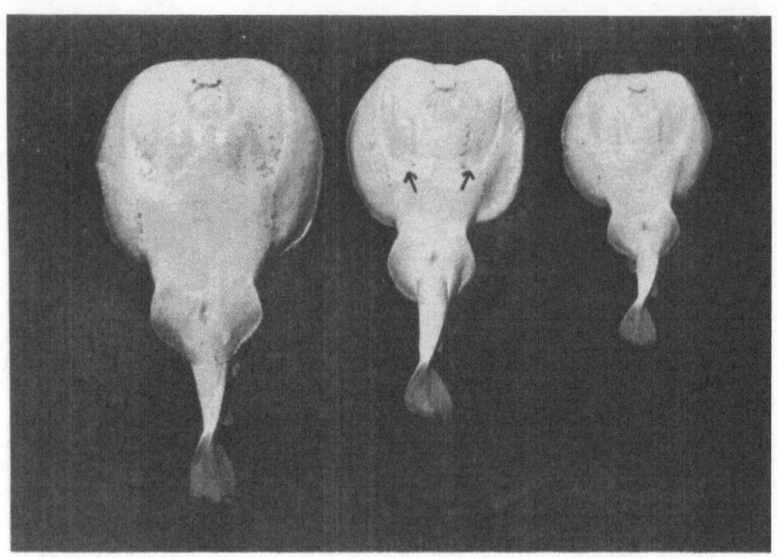

Fig. 1. Ventral view of three electric rays, *Torpedo ocellata*, showing the location of the electric organs, one on each side of the body, pointed to by an arrow. The electric organ extends from the dorsal to the ventral skin and can produce up to 200 volts. The current output can reach 50 A with a potential difference between the two skins of 20-60 V. The weight of fish whose electric organs are used ranges from 1 to 3 lbs, and the organ represents about 20% of the total weight.

in ACh-receptors (Nachmansohn, 1959), namely the electric organ of the electric eel, *Electrophorus electricus*, or the electric ray, *Torpedo* sp. (Fig. 1). These organs derive embryonically from skeletal muscles (Keynes and Martins-Ferreira, 1953); and accordingly their receptors have the same pharmacology as that of muscle ACh-receptors. The second reason was the finding of polypeptide neurotoxins of snake venoms that bind specifically and almost irreversibly to nicotinic ACh-receptors (Lee, 1973; Changeux, 1975; Miledi et al., 1971). The most widely used are α-bungarotoxin (α-BGT) from the venom of the krait *Bungarus multicinctus* and cobra neurotoxins from several cobra *Naja naja* subspecies, which are polypeptides of molecular weight 6000-8000, and are extremely useful in detecting minute amounts of nicotinic ACh-receptors. The third reason was the advent of affinity chromatography or affinity adsorption, introduced by Cuatrecasas (1970), a method where a gel (e.g. Sepharose beads) is used to which a specific ligand (e.g. cobrotoxin) is covalently bound. It now takes us only 24 hours

to purify totally the ACh-receptor of electric organs; starting
with homogenization followed by membrane preparation, its solubilization with the detergent Triton X-100, incubation with the affinity gel to adsorb the ACh-receptor, wash of nonspecific proteins
by series of incubations with buffers followed by filtration,
desorption of the ACh-receptor with a high concentration of a
cholinergic drug (e.g. carbamylcholine) and its collection in the
filtrate, then finally dialysis to remove the drug (Eldefrawi and
Eldefrawi, 1973; Eldefrawi et al., 1975a).

The ACh-receptor is detected in solution by means of its
binding of ACh and specific drugs. One of the methods used to
measure binding is equilibrium dialysis, where a semipermeable
cellophane bag, tied at both ends, is suspended in buffer and specific
radioactive drug is placed in the bath and the flask shaken. The
drug passes through the membrane, and at equilibrium the drug
concentration is equal inside the bag as in the bath. When the
receptor protein is present inside the bag, it binds the radioactive
drug so that at equilibrium, the concentration of the drug is
higher inside the bag than outside. This excess in radioactivity
per unit volume represents the amount bound and is converted to
moles bound per g tissue or mg protein. When a competing nonradioactive drug (an activator or an inhibitor of the ACh-receptor) is
present with the radioactive drug in the bath, binding of the latter
to the receptor is reduced (Eldefrawi, 1976).

During the past three years, a great deal of information has
been gathered on the molecular properties of the ACh-receptor of
electric organs. The following are the highlights: It is an
acidic glycoprotein, with an isoelectric point of 4.5-4.8 (Klett
et al., 1973; Eldefrawi and Eldefrawi, 1973; Meunier et al., 1974;
Raftery et al., 1973; Eldefrawi et al., 1975a). Negatively stained,
it appears as rosette shaped (8-9 nm in diameter) with an electron
dense core (Fig. 2). It is an intrinsic membrane protein, with a
large hydrophobic area, that transverses the membrane, possibly
extruding beyond it at one or both sides and carrying binding sites
for ligands extracellularly.

When the ACh-receptor is excited at 290 nm, it fluoresces with
a maximum at 336 nm; an intrinsic fluorescence that is due to the
2.4 mole percent L-tryptophan in the molecule (Eldefrawi et al.,
1975a). Binding of receptor activators was found to quench this
fluorescence and cobrotoxin to abolish the quenching (Barrantes,
1976; Bonner et al., 1976). The ACh-receptor of electric organs
has a drug specificity that is typical of skeletal muscle nicotinic
ACh-receptor, where the activating effect of ACh is imitated by
nicotine and is inhibited by curare and the specific snake venom
neurotoxins. The other major kind of ACh-receptor present in
brain, smooth muscles and glands of vertebrates is muscarinic in

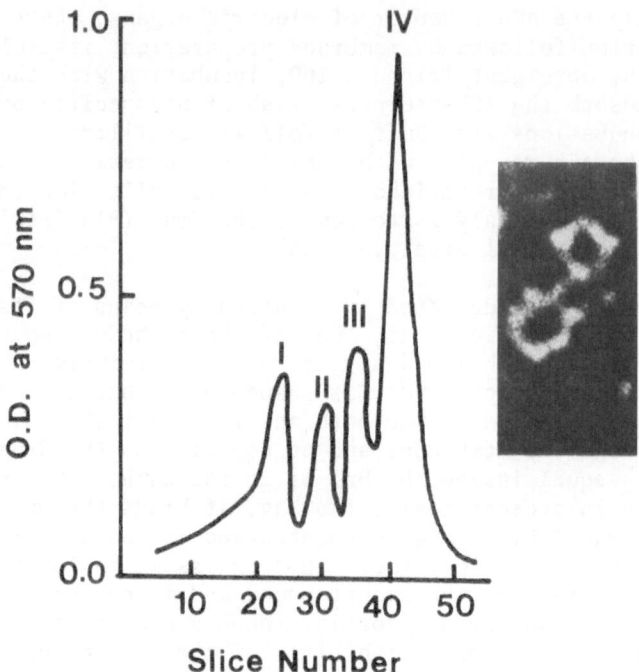

Fig. 2. SDS disc gel electrophoresis of the ACh-receptor purified from *T. ocellata*. Molecular weights of the subunits are I - 81,000; II - 61,000; III - 50,000; IV - 40,000. Inset is electron micrograph of the purified ACh-receptor molecule negatively stained with 2% phosphotungstate (1,093,000x magnification).

its pharmacology, being activated by muscarine and pilocarpine and inhibited by atropine.

The ACh-receptor has a very high affinity for Ca^{2+} such that, when purified in Ringer buffer, 4.7% of its weight is due to bound Ca^{2+} detected by atomic absorption (Eldefrawi et al., 1974). Even when purified in Ca^{2+}-free solution, about 0.5% of the weight of the receptor is due to bound Ca^{2+}. Some of this Ca^{2+}, the receptor releases upon binding of activators as evidenced from studies using the binding of the fluorescent lanthanide terbium, Tb^{3+} (Rübsamen et al., 1976a) or a Ca^{2+} specific dye (Chang and Neumann, 1976).

It has sometimes been assumed that the ACh-receptor molecule may be directly responsible for binding of ACh as well as for cation flux across the membrane. Consequently, attempts were made to reconstitute the purified ACh-receptor molecules in synthetic lipid membranes (Michaelson and Raftery, 1974; Shamoo and Eldefrawi, 1975; McNamee et al., 1976; Eldefrawi et al., 1975b). However, in no case were selective cation fluxes or conductances obtained that were similar, in specificity, magnitude and kinetics, to the physiologic events. Recently, perhydrohistrionicotoxin, the reduced analog of the arrow poison from the skin of a Colombian frog, which was shown in electrophysiological experiments to bind to the ion conductance modulator (ICM) of the ACh-receptor (Albuquerque et al., 1973), was radiolabeled and its specific binding utilized to label the ICM of the ACh-receptor of *Torpedo* electric organ (Eldefrawi et al., in press b). The data suggested that the ICM was closely associated with the ACh-receptor in the membrane, possibly through noncovalent bonding, but the two molecules separate after solubilization with Triton X-100 by selective adsorption or immunoprecipitation. This ICM has recently been partially purified.

By sedimentation equilibrium, the molecular weight of the receptor is 330,000 in the presence of 0.1% Triton X-100 (Edelstein et al., 1975). Values ranging from 260,000 to 360,000 have been obtained for the solubilized receptor by use of other methods (Biesecker, 1973; Meunier et al., 1972; Hucho and Changeux, 1973; Martinez-Carrion et al., 1975). However, using radiation inactivation on the receptor in its membrane, a molecular weight value of 610,000 is obtained (Wunderlich and Eldefrawi, in press). It is suggested that this is the molecular weight of not only the ACh-receptor, but also its ion conductance modulator, which is bound to it noncovalently in the membrane, and each molecule is affected by the other one's binding of ligands (Eldefrawi et al., in press b). After mercaptoethanol and sodium dodecyl sulfate (SDS) treatment followed by electrophoresis, four subunits of the ACh-receptor are isolated, the major one having molecular weight of 40,000 (Fig. 2). That major subunit carries the binding site for activators as well as a separate binding site for inhibitors, such as α-BGT (Biesecker, 1973; Meunier et al., 1974; Weill et al., 1974; Rübsamen et al., 1976a,b; Hucho et al., 1976).

DRUG INTERACTIONS WITH ACH-RECEPTORS

In 1970 it was discovered that the housefly brain was 3-10x richer in cholinergic binding molecules than even the electric organ of *Torpedo* (Eldefrawi and O'Brien, 1970). The housefly head extract bound activators and inhibitors with K_D in the µM range similar to that of the *Torpedo* receptor as shown in Table I. However, their pharmacologies differ. Binding of ACh or muscarone to the *Torpedo* ACh-receptor is blocked by nicotinic drugs (the top six in Table I), but none or little by the muscarinic ones (the following four). On the other hand, binding of [^{3}H]decamethonium to the housefly putative ACh-receptors is inhibited with muscarinic

TABLE I. Blockade of Binding of the Lubrol Solubilized *Torpedo* ACh-receptor (as Detected by [^{3}H]ACh Binding at 0.1 µM) and the Housefly Head Putative ACh-receptors (as Detected by [^{3}H]Decamethonium Binding at 0.1 µM) by Various Drugs and Toxins.

Drug or toxin (10 µM)	% Blockade of binding	
	Torpedo[a]	Housefly[b]
Carbamylcholine	74 ± 16	35.5 ± 6.0
Succinylcholine	75 ± 19	54.0 ± 8.2
Benzoylcholine	12 ± 3	75.2 ± 7.1
Nicotine	41 ± 7	50.0 ± 3.3
Anabasine	19 ± 3	25[c]
d-tubocurarine	60 ± 6	40.4 ± 7.2
Pilocarpine	12 ± 1	83.5 ± 0.9
Arecoline	0[d]	52.9 ± 3.1
Atropine	10 ± 1	80.3 ± 10.4
Scopolamine	0[d]	74.8 ± 5.9
α-Bungarotoxin	100[d,e]	0[d]
Eserine (100 µM)	0[d,g]	78[f]
Neostigmine (100 µM)	35 ± 3[g]	
Pyridostigmine (100 µM)	0[d,g]	
Edrophonium (100 µM)	77 ± 15[g]	
DFP (100 µM)	19[h]	0[d,h]
Tetram (100 µM)	0[d,h]	58[h]
Guthoxon (100 µM)	0[d,h]	24[h]

[a]Data from Eldefrawi et al. (1972).
[b]Data from Mansour et al. (unpublished).
[c]Anabasine blockade was of [^{3}H]muscarone binding to the housefly putative ACh-receptors (Eldefrawi et al., 1970).
[d]Values of 0 and 100 indicate nonsignificant (p > 0.05) and total blockade, respectively.
[e]α-Bungarotoxin was present at 1 µM, and blockade was of [^{3}H]ACh binding to the purified ACh-receptor (Eldefrawi and Eldefrawi, 1973).
[f]Value is for blockade by eserine of [^{3}H]muscarone binding (at 1 µM) to the housefly receptors (Eldefrawi and O'Brien, 1970).
[g]At the higher concentration of 1 mM eserine, neostigmine, pyridostigmine and edrophonium blocked 30, 82, 20 and 100% of [^{3}H]ACh binding to the solubilized *Torpedo* receptor.
[h]Data from Eldefrawi et al. (1971b). In the case of *Torpedo*, values are for blockade of the binding of [^{3}H]nicotine (at 0.1 µM).

TABLE II. Effects of Organic Mercury Fungicides on Binding of
[^{3}H]ACh (at 1 μM) to ACh-receptors and on ACh-esterase Activity
in Electric Organ Membranes of *Torpedo ocellata*.[a]

Drug (100 μM)		% Inhibition	
Chemical Name	EPA[*]Code	ACh-receptor Mean ± SD	ACh-esterase Mean ± SD
Methylmercury chloride	4560	102.2 ± 8.3	4.8 ± 2.4
Ethylmercury chloride	3400	61.8 ± 6.2	0.8 ± 2.8
MEMMI[b]	4440	99.7 ± 6.3	17.5 ± 0.7
Cyano (methylmercury) guanidine	1560	92.2 ± 3.7	11.9 ± 2.4
Phenylmercury acetate	5680	55.5 ± 2.2	11.9 ± 2.4
Phenylmercury chloride	5480	50.3 ± 3.7	6.3 ± 7.6
Diphenylmercury	2640	1.5 ± 2.4	16.3 ± 1.8
Phenylmercury borate[c]	5460	4.5 ± 4.2	12.7 ± 3.4
Phenylmercury hydroxide[c]	5485	1.3 ± 3.1	3.2 ± 2.4
d-Tubocurarine[b]		58.6 ± 1.5	4.8 ± 2.1
DFP[b,d]		0.5 ± 2.0	99.7 ± 0.2
Tetram[b]		1.8 ± 1.5	99.5 ± 0.1

[a]Data from Eldefrawi et al. (in press a).
[b]MEMMI is N-methylmercuri-1,2,3,6-tetrahydro-3,6-endomethano-3,4,
  5,6,7,7-hexachlorophthalimide; DFP is diisopropyl fluorophosphate;
  Tetram is 0,0-diethyl S(β-diethylamino)ethyl phosphorothiolate.
[c]The borate and hydroxide salts of phenylmercury were used at
  10 μM, while all other drugs were used at 100 μM.
[d]DFP is added to the ACh-receptor preparation at 100 μM, and to the
  dialysis bath at 10 μM when binding of [^{3}H]ACh is determined, so
  as to inhibit the ACh-esterase present. The value of 99.7 ± 0.2%
  inhibition of the enzyme by DFP is after 1 h incubation. Higher
  inhibition is obtained with longer incubation.
[*]EPA is the Environmental Protection Agency.

drugs as well as the nicotinic ones. Also, its nicotine binding is
inhibited with toxic nicotinoids but not nontoxic ones (Eldefrawi
et al., 1970) and with atropine, while its atropine binding is
inhibited with nicotine (Eldefrawi et al., 1971a). Thus, these
housefly putative receptors exhibit mixed nicotinic muscarinic

pharmacology. Similar observations were made by Donnellan et al.
(1975) who did ligand binding studies and by Sattelle (this book)
who did electrophysiologic studies.

Organophosphates and carbamates, which are known mainly for
their anticholinesterase activity with K_i in the μM or lower concentrations also bind to the *Torpedo* electric organ ACh-receptor
and block its binding of ACh (Table I), but only at high
concentrations of above 0.1 mM. These anticholinesterases also
bind to the housefly putative ACh-receptors. Nicotine, whose
target appears to be the ACh-receptor, and its K_i for ACh-esterase
is in the 10 mM range, far higher than its toxic concentration,
inhibits binding of muscarone to the housefly receptor, and so does
anabasine (Table I) and toxic nicotinoids, while the nontoxic ones
do not (Eldefrawi et al., 1970). Thus, the insect central nervous
system ACh-receptor may be the target for these drugs. Very recently, muscarinic activators were shown to have acaricidal action
(Bigg and Purvis, 1976).

Another group of drugs that bind to the ACh-receptor of the
electric organ is the organic mercury compounds known mostly for
their fungicidal activity. At 100 μM methylmercury inhibits all the
[^{3}H]ACh binding to the purified *Torpedo* ACh-receptor (Table II).
On the other hand, mercuric chloride does not inhibit any (Shamoo
et al., 1976). When various organic mercurials are compared as to
their effectiveness in inhibiting binding of ACh to the electric
organ receptor and ACh-esterase activity, several are more potent
than d-tubocurarine (a classic nicotinic receptor inhibitor), and
none is as effective an anti-ACh-esterase as DFP or Tetram.

PURIFICATION AND PROPERTIES OF HOUSEFLY ACH-RECEPTORS

For purification of the housefly brain putative ACh-receptors
the supernatant of 100,000 x g, 1 hr is chromatographed on Sephadex
G-200. As shown in Fig. 3, the peak which binds decamethonium,
atropine, ACh and other cholinergic drugs, separates from the ACh-
esterase peaks and from various other proteins. This step purifies
the receptor 10x. The cholinergic binding peak also binds ACh with
K_D of 10 μM (Mansour et al., unpublished); a value similar to that
reported by Sattelle (this book) as causing 50% depolarization of
the cockroach sixth abdominal ganglion.

Affinity chromatography was applied to purify the putative
housefly receptors, binding of ACh and nicotine to the housefly
receptors was not inhibited with the α-BGT or cobra venom. Therefore, the affinity gel with cobra toxin attached, the gel that suc-
ceeded in purifying the *Torpedo* receptor, was ineffective in
adsorbing the housefly putative ACh-receptors. Another affinity

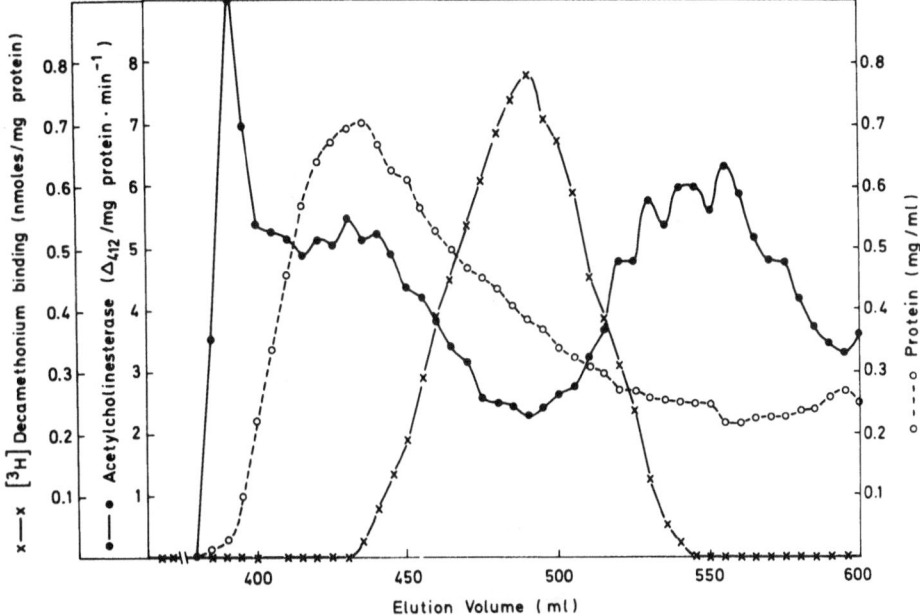

Fig. 3. Gel filtration of the supernatant of 100,000 xg of house-fly brain on Sephadex G-200. Void volume is 400 ml (from Mansour et al., unpublished).

gel with phenyltrimethylammonium as the specific drug, partially purified the housefly receptor but resulted in some loss of binding.

The two protein bands that are suspected of being the putative ACh-receptors are obtained in pure form by semi-preparative disc gel electrophoresis (Fig. 4). It may be that both proteins are ACh-receptors; one may be a byproduct of the other, or only one is the ACh-receptor. It cannot be that one is the muscarinic receptor and the other is the nicotinic receptor, since binding of nicotine is inhibited with atropine, and binding of atropine is inhibited with nicotine (Eldefrawi et al., 1971a) indicating that the same protein binds nicotine and atropine. It may be that in the house-fly brain there are two ACh-receptors, which are both nicotinic and muscarinic. Separation of the two proteins, currently in progress, should resolve that point. The two proteins are labile and most of their binding of drugs is easily lost during purification. However, immunologically they are quite stable.

A rabbit that was inoculated with the two pure housefly proteins had no visible clinical symptoms, and produced a high titre of

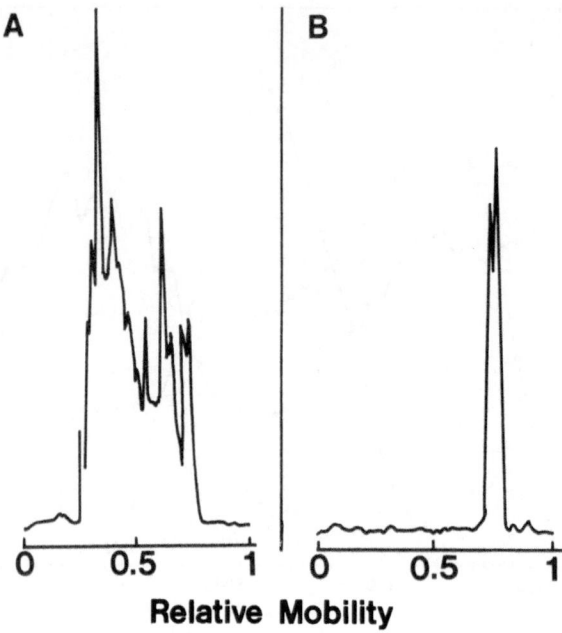

Fig. 4. Disc gel electrophoresis of putative housefly brain ACh-
receptors. A. the peak of [3H]decamethonium binding in Fig. 4
and B. the purified ACh-receptors.

Fig. 5. Double diffusion assay of: *left*. Rabbit antisera for the
two housefly proteins (bottom well) against the two isolated housefly proteins (top left well) and the [3H]decamethonium binding fraction in Fig. 3 (top right well), and *right*. Rabbit antisera for the
two isolated housefly proteins mixed with rabbit antisera for the
purified *Torpedo* ACh-receptor (bottom well) against the purified
Torpedo ACh-receptor (top left well) and the two isolated housefly
proteins (top right well) (from Mansour et al., unpublished).

antibodies. When these antibodies were incubated with the crude housefly extract, its binding of atropine was inhibited by 75%. This proves that the two isolated proteins, though they lost most of their cholinergic binding capacity, are antigenically similar to the cholinergic binding proteins in the housefly head extract; suggesting that the two proteins are the same. In double diffusion tests, a sharp strong line appears between the pure housefly proteins and the antisera against them mixed with the antisera against the pure *Torpedo* ACh-receptor (Fig. 5). A line also appears between this well and the pure *Torpedo* receptor, but the two lines do not connect smoothly, suggesting different antigenic determinants on the two receptors (the *Torpedo* nicotinic receptor and the housefly brain ACh-receptors). In addition, the antisera against the housefly receptors did not inhibit binding of ACh to the pure *Torpedo* ACh-receptor, and the antisera against the *Torpedo* ACh-receptor did not inhibit binding of decamethonium or atropine to the housefly receptor. Therefore, the ACh-receptor of the electric organ appears to be different from the putative housefly ACh-receptors, not only in drug specificity, but also in antigenic determinants. Incubation of rabbit antisera against the purified housefly proteins with synaptosomal membranes of cow brain corpus striatum, then binding of [^{3}H]3-quinuclidinyl benzilate (at 4 nM), that is blocked with 0.01 μM atropine, is inhibited by 69%. Such binding is specific for the muscarinic ACh-receptor (Yamamura and Snyder, 1974). Thus, it appears that the housefly brain putative ACh-receptors and the cow brain muscarinic receptors have similar antigenic determinants. The former receptors have not yet been compared with mammalian brain nicotinic receptors.

A major characteristic of the housefly brain putative ACh-receptors, which differentiates it from ACh-receptors of electric organ or mammalian brain, is the ease of solubilizing it simply by homogenization in low ionic strength solution, though not in Ringer (Aziz and Eldefrawi, 1973). This has been largely responsible for considerable reluctance on our part to accept it as the receptor protein. However, its antigenic similarity to mammalian brain muscarinic ACh-receptors and its high affinity binding of cholinergic drugs supports its identity as ACh-receptor. It may be that there are endogenous detergent-like molecules in fly head tissues, which solubilize intrinsic proteins. In fact, aggregation appears after fractionation of the housefly extract by gel filtration. Also, even the intrinsic membrane bound ACh-receptor of the electric eel has been solubilized by extended dialysis against low ionic strength buffer followed by tryptic digestion (Aharonov et al., 1975). In addition, another putative ACh-receptor from an invertebrate, the squid, *Loligo opalescens*, has been solubilized in salt solution free of detergent, but unlike the housefly putative ACh-receptor, it bound α-BGT significantly (Kato and Tattrie, 1974).

CONCLUSION

We have isolated the housefly brain putative ACh-receptor possibly in a pure form, without any contamination from ACh-esterase,
and its properties are now under extensive studies. Because of the
very low concentration of muscarinic ACh-receptors in mammalian
brain and their instability during purification, it may be some
time before they are isolated in pure form. In the meantime, ACh-
receptors from housefly brain may serve as a model for studying
mammalian brain muscarinic ACh-receptors. This insect brain may
play a role similar to that played by ACh-receptors of electric
organs in the elucidation of structure and function of skeletal
muscle ACh-receptors.

The recent discovery of the ion conductance modulator, as an
entity separate from the receptor, adds another protein to the
growing list of candidates that may be targets for insecticides.
We are at an exciting age where various important molecules of the
nervous system are being isolated and their structure and function
studied. These new developments are generating many relevant
questions. Examples of questions that may be answered in the near
future are:

1. Is it possible to radiolabel or fluorescent tag antibodies
against the housefly ACh-receptors and use them to map ACh-receptors
in mammalian as well as insect brains?

2. Can we utilize differences between insect and mammalian
ACh-receptors to develop new insecticides that act selectively on
the insect ACh-receptor as their target, for example, from amongst
organic mercury compounds?

3. Is it possible that an organophosphate or carbamate resistant insect strain contains modified ACh-receptors, with lower
affinity for ACh, such that the accumulation of ACh resulting from
ACh-esterase inhibition could be better tolerated by the insect?

4. Is anticholinesterase activity sufficient to describe the
mode of action of all organophosphate and carbamate insecticides,
or do some of these insecticides also affect receptor and possibly
ICM function?

REFERENCES

Aharonov, A., Tarrab-Hazdai, R., Abramsky, O., and Fuchs, S., 1975, Immunological relationship between acetylcholine receptor and thymus: A possible significance in myasthenia gravis, *Proc. Nat. Acad. Sci. USA* 72:1456.

Albuquerque, E. X., Barnard, E. A., Chiu, T. H., Lapa, A. J., Dolly, J. O., Jansson, S. E., Daly, J., and Witkop, B., 1973, Acetylcholine receptor and ion conductance modulator sites at the murine neuromuscular junction: Evidence from specific toxin reaction, *Proc. Nat. Acad. Sci. USA* 70:949.

Aziz, S., and Eldefrawi, M. E., 1973, Cholinergic receptors of the central nervous system of insects, *Pestic. Biochem. Physiol.* 3:168.

Barrantes, F. J., 1976, Intrinsic fluorescence of the membrane-bound acetylcholine receptor: Its quenching by suberyldicholine, *Biochem. Biophys. Res. Comm.* 72:479.

Biesecker, G., 1973, Molecular properties of the cholinergic receptor purified from *Electrophorus electricus*, *Biochemistry* 12:4403.

Bigg, D. C. H., and Purvis, S. R., 1976, Muscarinic agonists provide a new class of acaricides, *Nature* 262:220.

Bonner, R., Barrantes, F. J., and Jovin, T. M., 1976, Kinetics of agonist-induced intrinsic fluorescence changes in membrane-bound acetylcholine receptor, *Nature* 263:429.

Chang, H. W., and Neumann, E., 1976, Dynamic properties of isolated acetylcholine receptor proteins: Release of calcium ions by acetylcholine binding, *Proc. Nat. Acad. Sci. USA* 73:3364.

Changeux, J.-P., 1975, The cholinergic receptor protein from fish electric organ, in: *Handbook of Psychopharmacology* (L. L. Iverson, S. D. Iverson, and S. H. Snyder, eds.) 6, pp. 235-301, Plenum Press, New York.

Cuatrecasas, P., 1970, Protein purification by affinity chromatography, *J. Biol. Chem.* 245:3059.

Donnellan, J. F., Jewess, P. J., and Cattell, K. J., 1975, Subcellular localization and properties of a cholinergic receptor isolated from housefly heads, *J. Neurochem.* 25:623.

Edelstein, S. J., Beyer, W. B., Eldefrawi, A. T., and Eldefrawi, M. E., 1975, Molecular weight of the acetylcholine receptors of electric organs and the effect of Triton X-100, *J. Biol. Chem.* 250:6101.

Eldefrawi, A. T., 1976, The acetylcholine receptor and its interactions with insecticides, in: *Insecticide Biochemistry and Physiology* (C. F. Wilkinson, ed.), pp. 297-326, Academic Press, New York.

Eldefrawi, A. T., and O'Brien, R. D., 1970, Binding of muscarone by extracts of housefly brain: Relationship to receptor for acetylcholine, *J. Neurochem.* 17:1287.

Eldefrawi, M. E., and Eldefrawi, A. T., 1973, Purification and molecular properties of the acetylcholine receptor from *Torpedo* electroplax, *Arch. Biochem. Biophys.* 159:362.

Eldefrawi, M. E., Eldefrawi, A. T., and O'Brien, R. D., 1970, Mode of action of nicotine in the housefly, *J. Agr. Food Chem.* 18: 1113.

Eldefrawi, M. E., Eldefrawi, A. T., and O'Brien, R. D., 1971a, Binding of five cholinergic ligands to housefly brain and *Torpedo* electroplax, *Mol. Pharmacol.* 7:104.

Eldefrawi, M. E., Britten, A. G., and O'Brien, R. D., 1971b, Action of organophosphates on binding of cholinergic ligands, *Pestic. Biochem. Physiol.* 1:101.

Eldefrawi, M. E., Eldefrawi, A. T., and Wilson, D. B., 1975a, Tryptophan and cysteine residues of the acetylcholine receptors of *Torpedo* species. Relationship to binding of cholinergic ligands, *Biochemistry* 14:4304.

Eldefrawi, M. E., Eldefrawi, A. T., and Shamoo, A. E., 1975b, Molecular and functional properties of the acetylcholine receptor, *Ann. N. Y. Acad. Sci.* 264:183.

Eldefrawi, M. E., Eldefrawi, A. T., Seifert, S., and O'Brien, R. D., 1972, Properties of Lubrol-solubilized acetylcholine receptor from *Torpedo* electroplax, *Arch. Biochem. Biophys.* 150:210.

Eldefrawi, M. E., Eldefrawi, A. T., Penfield, L. A., O'Brien, R. D., and van Campen, D., 1974, Binding of calcium and zinc to the acetylcholine receptor purified from *Torpedo californica*, *Life Sci.* 16:925.

Eldefrawi, M. E., Mansour, N. A., and Eldefrawi, A. T. Interactions of acetylcholine receptors with organic mercury compounds, in: *Membrane Toxicity* (A. Shamoo,ed.) Plenum Press,N.Y. (in press a).

Eldefrawi, A. T., Eldefrawi, M. E., Albuquerque, E. X., Oliviera, A., Mansour, N. A., Adler, M., Daly, J., Burgermeister, W., and Witkop, B., Binding of [^{3}H]perhydrohistrionicotoxin to the cholinergic ion conductance modulator, *Proc. Nat. Acad. Sci. USA* (in press b).

Fujita, T., Yamamoto, I., and Nakajima, M., 1970, Analysis of the structure-activity relationship of nicotine-like insecticides using substituent constants, in: *Biochemical Toxicology of Insecticides* (R. D. O'Brien and I. Yamamoto, eds.), pp. 21-32, Academic Press, New York.

Hucho, F., and Changeux, J.-P., 1973, Molecular weight and quaternary structure of the cholinergic receptor protein extracted by detergents from *Electrophorus electricus* electric tissue, *FEBS Letters* 38:11.

Hucho, F., Layer, P., Kiefer, H. R., and Bandini, G., 1976, Photo-affinity labeling and quaternary structure of the acetylcholine receptor from *Torpedo californica* 73:2624.

Kato, G., and Tattrie, B., 1974, Solubilization of the acetylcholine receptor protein from *Loligo opalescens* without detergents, *FEBS Letters* 48:26.

Keynes, R. D., and Martins-Ferreira, H., 1953, Membrane potentials in the electroplates of the electric eel, *J. Physiol.* 119:315.

Klett, R. P., Fulpius, B. W., Cooper, D., Smith, M., Reich, E., and Possani, L. D., 1973, The acetylcholine receptor. I. Purification and characterization of a macromolecule isolated from *Electrophorus electricus*, *J. Biol. Chem.* 248:6841.

Lee, C. Y., 1972, Chemistry and pharmacology of polypeptide toxins in snake venoms, *Ann. Rev. Pharmacol.* 12:265.

Martinez-Carrion, M., Sator, V., and Raftery, M. A., 1975, The molecular weight of an acetylcholine receptor isolated from *Torpedo californica*, *Biochem. Biophys. Res. Comm.* 65:129.

McNamee, M. G., Weill, C. L., and Karlin, A., 1975, Purification of acetylcholine receptor from *Torpedo californica* and its incorporation into phospholipid vesicles, *Ann. N. Y. Acad. Sci.* 264:175.

Meunier, J.-C., Olsen, R. W., and Changeux, J.-P., 1972, Studies on the cholinergic receptor protein from *Electrophorus electricus* III. Effect of detergents on some hydrodynamic properties of the receptor protein in solution, *FEBS Letters* 24:63.

Meunier, J.-C., Sealock, R., Olsen, R., and Changeux, J.-P., 1974, Purification and properties of the cholinergic receptor protein from *Electrophorus electricus* electric tissue, *Eur. J. Biochem.* 45:371.

Michaelson, D. M., and Raftery, M. A., 1974, Purified acetylcholine receptor: Its reconstitution to a chemically excitable membrane, *Proc. Nat. Acad. Sci.* 71:4768.

Miledi, R., Molinoff, P., and Potter, L. T., 1971, Isolation of the cholinergic receptor protein of *Torpedo* electric tissue, *Nature* 229:554.

Nachmansohn, D., 1955, Metabolism and function of the nerve cell, *Harvey Lect. (1953/1954)* 49:57.

Nachmansohn, D., 1959, *Chemical and Molecular Basis of Nerve Activity*, Academic Press, New York.

Raftery, M. A., Schmidt, J., Martinez-Carrion, M., Moody, T., Vandlen, R., and Duguid, J., 1973, Biochemical studies on *Torpedo californica* acetylcholine receptors, *J. Supramol. Struct.* 1:360.

Rübsamen, H., Hess, G. P., Eldefrawi, A. T., and Eldefrawi, M. E., 1976a, Interaction between calcium and ligand-binding sites of the purified acetylcholine receptor studied by use of a fluorescent lanthanide, *Biochem. Biophys. Res. Comm.* 68:56.

Rübsamen, H., Montgomery, M., and Hess, G. P., 1976b, Identification of a calcium-binding subunit of the acetylcholine receptor, *Biochem. Biophys. Res. Comm.* 70:1020.

Shamoo, A. E., and Eldefrawi, M. E., 1975, Carbamylcholine and acetylcholine-sensitive, cation-selective ionophore, as part of the purified acetylcholine receptor, *J. Membr. Biol.* 25:47.

Shamoo, A. E., McLennan, D. H., and Eldefrawi, M. E., 1976, Differential effects of mercurial compounds on excitable tissues, *Chem.-Biol. Interactions* 12:41.

Weill, C. L., McNamee, M. G., and Karlin, A., 1974, Affinity-labeling of purified acetylcholine receptor from *Torpedo californica*, *Biochem. Biophys. Res. Comm.* 61:997.

Wunderlich, K., and Eldefrawi, M., Molecular weight of the acetylcholine receptor in *Torpedo* electric organ membranes, *Membrane Biochem.* (in press).

Yamamura, H. I., and Snyder, S. H., 1974, Muscarinic cholinergic receptor binding in the longitudinal muscle of the guinea pig ileum with [^{3}H]quinuclidinyl benzilate, *Mol. Pharmacol.* 10:861.

ISOZYMIC FORMS OF ACETYLCHOLINESTERASE

Ram K. Tripathi

Section of Neurobiology and Behavior
Cornell University
Ithaca, New York 14853

1. INTRODUCTION

Acetylcholinesterase (AChE, EC 3.1.1.7) is widely distributed throughout the animal kingdom and is a vital enzyme in nervous transmission (Nachmansohn, 1970). It catalyzes the reaction of acetylcholine into choline and acetate as follows:

$$(CH_3)_3\overset{+}{N}-CH_2-CH_2-O-\underset{\underset{CH_3}{|}}{C}=O+H_2O \rightleftharpoons (CH_3)_3\overset{+}{N}-CH_2-CH_2OH+CH_3COO^-+\overset{+}{H}$$

| Acetylcholine | Choline | Acetate |

It is a target enzyme for organophosphates and carbamates which are in common use today as insecticides against the insect pests of agriculture and public health (O'Brien, 1967).

Neurotoxic effects of organophosphates and carbamates to vertebrates and insects are due to inhibition of their AChE, although such effects are determined by several factors; including for example, chemical structure, rate of penetration into vital centers, degradation, affinity to AChE, duration of AChE inhibition and other nonspecific reactions. Unlike in vertebrates, AChE inhibition in insects does not result in death by asphyxiation. The ultimate cause of death in insects is not known although the majority of the findings support the view that AChE inhibition is highly correlated with the poisoning process (O'Brien, 1976). Strong evidence comes from the fact that changes in sensitivity to inhibition of AChE by these

43

chemicals can confer high levels of resistance to insects (Iwata
and Hama, 1972; Tripathi and O'Brien, 1973b; Tripathi, 1976; Ayed
and Georghiou, 1975, Plapp and Tripathi, 1977).

AChE from most vertebrates and insects (except house fly) are
highly specific for acetylcholine (ACh) and have little activity
against butyrylcholine (BuCh) as a substrate (Lee et al., 1974;
Guilbault et al., 1970). House fly brain AChE hydrolyzes BuCh at
an almost equal rate to that of ACh (Dauterman et al., 1962;
Metcalf et al., 1955). Butyrylcholine hydrolysis from the crude
homogenates may have been due to the contamination by butyryl-
cholinesterase, but it appears that highly purified AChE showed
the same behavior as described above (unpublished results).
Butyrylcholine hydrolysis by house fly AChE may be due to some
special characteristic of this enzyme.

In addition to difference in butyrylcholine hydrolysis by house
fly AChE, vertebrate and insect AChE show a considerable variation in
their rate of inhibition by organophosphates and carbamates
(Hollingworth et al., 1967; Hellenbrand, 1967; Yu et al., 1972;
O'Brien et al., 1975; Wustner and Fukuto, 1974; Tripathi et al., 1973).

In this chapter I shall use the term "isozyme" to mean multiple molecular forms of an enzyme and shall discuss primarily the
soluble isozymes of house fly brain, which is the richest source.
Markert (1975) stated that once the accepted criteria for defining
a collection of molecules as an enzyme have been successfully
applied, and if these molecules by any means (electrophoretic, iso-
electrofocussing, chromatographic, centrifugation, ultrafiltration,
solubility, immunochemical, etc.) can be separated into distinguishable molecular forms, then these types represent isozymic forms of
the enzyme. In a review, Shaw (1969) classified isozymes into two
major categories: (a) those that are distinctly different molecules
and are presumably produced from different genetic sites; and (b)
those which result from secondary alterations in the structure of
a single polypeptide species, and may, in many cases, be in vitro
artifacts.

2.   OCCURRENCE OF ACETYLCHOLINESTERASE ISOZYMES

It is now well documented that AChE from vertebrate and invertebrate sources occurs as isozymes either in aqueous extracts
(Bernsohn et al., 1962; Maynard, 1966; Christoff et al., 1966;
Krysan and Kruckeburg, 1970; Hollunger and Niklasson, 1973;
Tripathi and O'Brien, 1975; Bajgar, 1975; Steele and Smallman,
1976a) or in saline extracts (Massoulie et al., 1975, Varela, 1975)
or after partial solubilization of the tissue by detergents (Davis
and Agranoff, 1968; Skangiel-Kramska and Niemierko, 1971; Shafai
and Cortner, 1971; Coats and Simpson, 1972; Hall, 1973; Booth

et al., 1975) or in powder remaining after extraction of the
tissues with organic solvents (Jackson and Aprison, 1966; Baldwin
and Hochachka, 1970) or in highly-purified preparations (Dudai et
al., 1973; Chan et al., 1972; Wenthold et al., 1974; Ott et al.,
1975; Bon et al., 1976; Tripathi and O'Brien, 1977).

3. IN VITRO AND IN VIVO STUDIES ON ISOZYMES

Earlier studies on acetylcholinesterase from the house flies
have shown that there are four AChE isozymes in the head and three
quite different ones in the thorax (Tripathi and O'Brien, 1973a).
All the isozymes were found to be AChE as judged by their inhibition with carbamate eserine and organophosphates guthoxon and malaoxon; and their insensitivity to iso-OMPA (Eldefrawi et al., 1970).
Using the kinetic procedure on gel of Chiu et al. (1972), it was
shown that the isozymes varied over a 5-fold range in their reactivity towards acetylthiocholine (Table 1) and over a 2.3-fold range
towards malaoxon (Table II) (Tripathi et al., 1973).

Table I. Michaelis Constants (K_m) and Maximum Velocity (V_{max}) of
ATCh (Acetylthiocholine) for AChE Isozymes of House fly
at 25°C, pH 6.0.

Isozyme	10^4 K_m (M)	V_{max} (arbitrary units)	Fractional[a] Activity	R_m[b]
		Head		
I	1.83 (± 0.31)	1.89 (± 0.07)	0.33	0.22
II	6.87 (± 1.42)	1.97 (± 0.17)	0.22	0.42
III	4.35 (± 0.16)	2.66 (± 0.03)	0.38	0.49
IV	7.70 (± 0.84)	0.56 (± 0.03)	0.07	0.63
		Thorax		
V	1.58 (± 0.23)	0.57 (± 0.003)	0.25	0.29
VI	6.57 (± 0.99)	1.69 (± 0.14)	0.40	0.65
VII	3.86 (± 1.03)	1.32 (± 0.17)	0.35	0.69

Standard errors are shown in parentheses.

[a] Calculated on the basis of relative absorbancy from the stained
zymogram with 1 x 10^{-3} M ATCh.

[b] R_m is expressed as relative mobility of each isozyme, calculated
by the ratio of isozyme to the tracking dye migration.

Table II.   Biomolecular Rate Constants (k_i) of AChE Isozymes of House
            Fly Head with Malaoxon, Tetram, and Eserine at 25°C,
            pH 6.0.

Isozyme	Malaoxon	Tetram	Eserine
	$10^{-5} \times k_i$ (M^{-1} min^{-1})		
I	7.85 ($\pm$ 0.37)	8.80 ($\pm$ 0.63)	25.46 ($\pm$ 1.22)
II	5.34 ($\pm$ 0.23)	8.50 ($\pm$ 0.17)	22.24 ($\pm$ 1.59)
III	4.86 ($\pm$ 0.22)	7.60 ($\pm$ 0.29)	15.99 ($\pm$ 0.77)
IV	3.42 ($\pm$ 0.45)	5.90 ($\pm$ 0.21)	29.71 ($\pm$ 2.10)

Standard errors are shown in parentheses.

Isozymes were found to differ a great deal in their inhibition
patterns when the insect was poisoned with various organophosphate
insecticides. Fig. 1 shows that during poisoning by an LD_{50} dose
of paraoxon applied to the tip of the abdomen, none of the head isozymes were severely inhibited and the three thoracic isozymes differed profoundly in their inhibition behavior. Table III shows the
results with four different organophosphates. By comparing the
sensitivities of isozymes to these different organophosphates, it
was concluded that inhibition of thoracic isozyme V was the most
significant in poisoning. Zettler and Brady (1975) from their

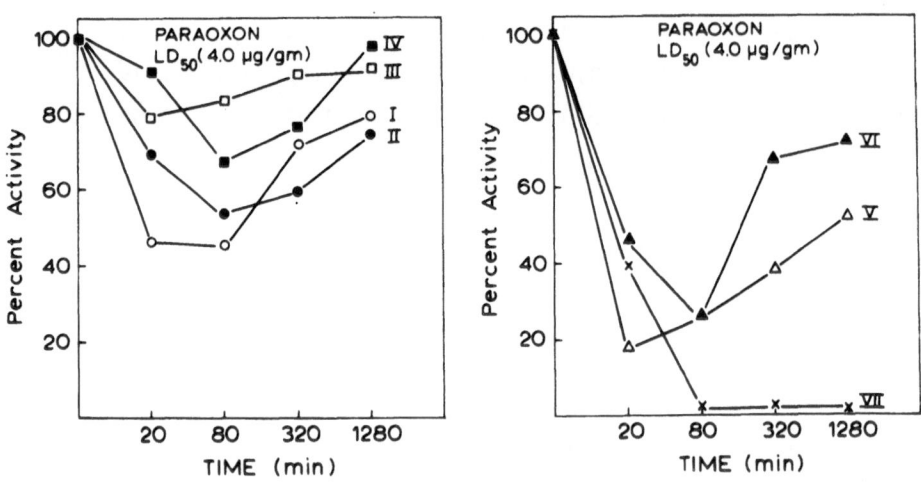

Fig. 1.   The effects of paraoxon on the isozymes of head (left) and
          thorax (right).

Table III.   The Minimal Percent Activity of AChE After Poisoning
             With an LD_{50} Dose.

Isozyme	Malaoxon	Paraoxon	Diazinon	Dichlorvos	Range [a]
			Head		
I	18	45	54	39	36
II	42	53	28	72	44
III	51	78	32	57	46
IV	28	67	67	70	42
Total[b]	36	61	41	55	25
			Thorax		
V	15	18	22	21	7
VI	5	38	1	16	37
VII	1	1	1	1	0
Total[b]	6	20	7	12	14

[a] Range of minimal activities shown in table.

[b] Equals Σfm, where f is the fractional activity of each isozyme
(from Table I) and m is the percentage minimal activity (from
this table).

studies in vivo on thoracic isozymes also concluded that the isozymes
differed in their inhibition behavior by two different organophosphates.

4.   MOLECULAR CHARACTERIZATION OF ISOZYMES

4.1 Ferguson Plot

The relative mobilities (RM) of the four crude AChE isozymes
with respect to a dye marker were determined on 5-10% gels and the
data were arranged as described by Ferguson (1964). A plot of log
RM against the gel concentration is shown in Fig. 2. In this plot
the slope of the line (denoted by a retardation coefficient K_r) is
directly related to the molecular weight (MW) of the protein (Hedrick and Smith, 1968; Rodbard and Chrambach, 1971). Size isomeric
proteins will show nonparallel Ferguson lines extrapolating to a

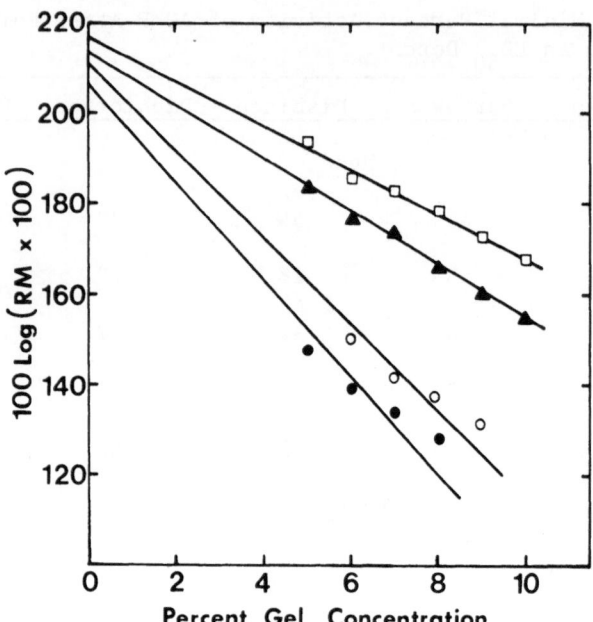

Fig. 2.   Ferguson plots of various AChE forms. Best straight lines
          were determined by unweighted least-square linear regres-
          sion of the data.

common point in the vicinity of 0% gel concentration. Charge isomeric proteins will show parallel lines. Proteins differing in both
charge and size will show nonparallel lines intersecting at gel concentrations other than 0%. Over the gel concentration range of
5-10% the Ferguson plots of the isozymes showed straight nonparallel
lines intersecting at gel concentration other than 0%. This suggested that AChE isozymes belong to size and charge isomer family.
From the MW versus K_r relationship established for the experimental
system by the use of marker proteins, the MW of isozyme I, II, III
and IV was calculated as 375,000, 255,000, 160,000 and 110,000
respectively (Table IV).

4.2 Gel Filtration on Sepharose 6B

Sepharose 6B separates proteins on the basis of effective size,
i.e. on the Stokes radius, which is the radius of a sphere having
hydrodynamic properties identical with the protein. Fractionation of
crude AChE on Sepharose 6B showed 3 peaks of activity (Fig. 3) which
are termed A, B and C in order of decreasing Stokes radius. The

Table IV. Physico-chemical Properties of House Fly Brain AChE.

ISOZYMES	MOLECULAR WEIGHTS			SEDIMEN-TATION COEFFICIENT	STOKES RADIUS nm
	Ferguson Plot	Sedimen-tation	Gel Filtration		
I	375000	307000	491000	11.5	9.36
II	255000	-	-	-	-
III	160000	152000	181000	7.2	5.65
IV	110000	87000	-	5.0	-

Subunit in SDS 82000

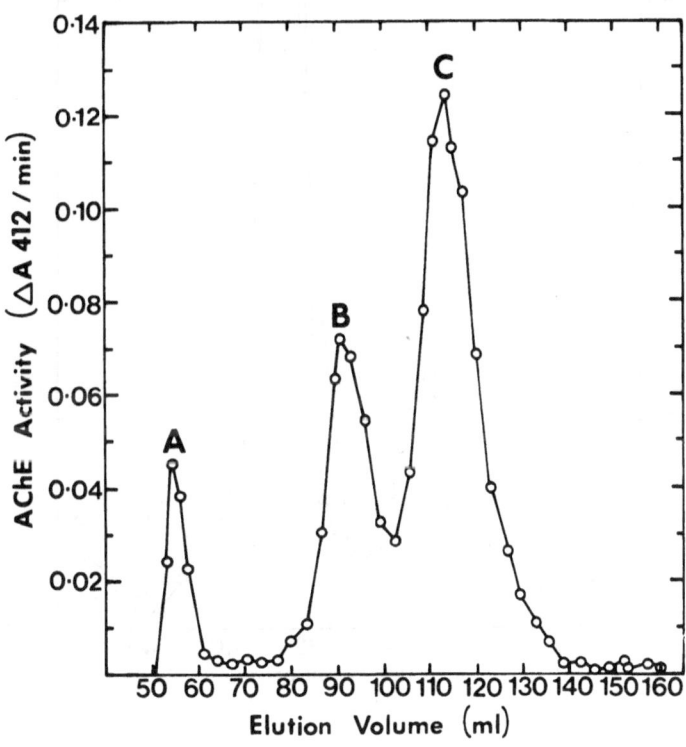

Fig. 3. Elution profiles of crude AChE on Sepharose 6B.

first eluted peak of activity coincided with the void volume of the
column. When all the peaks were analyzed by 7% polyacrylamide gel
electrophoresis, Peak A did not enter the gel; Peak B corresponded
to isozyme I and Peak C corresponded to isozyme III. The molecular
weights (Table IV) estimated according to the method of Siegel and
Monty were found to be 491,000 for Peak B and 181,000 for Peak C.
The Stokes radius, determined by the standard curve were found to be
9.36 nm for Peak C (Table IV).

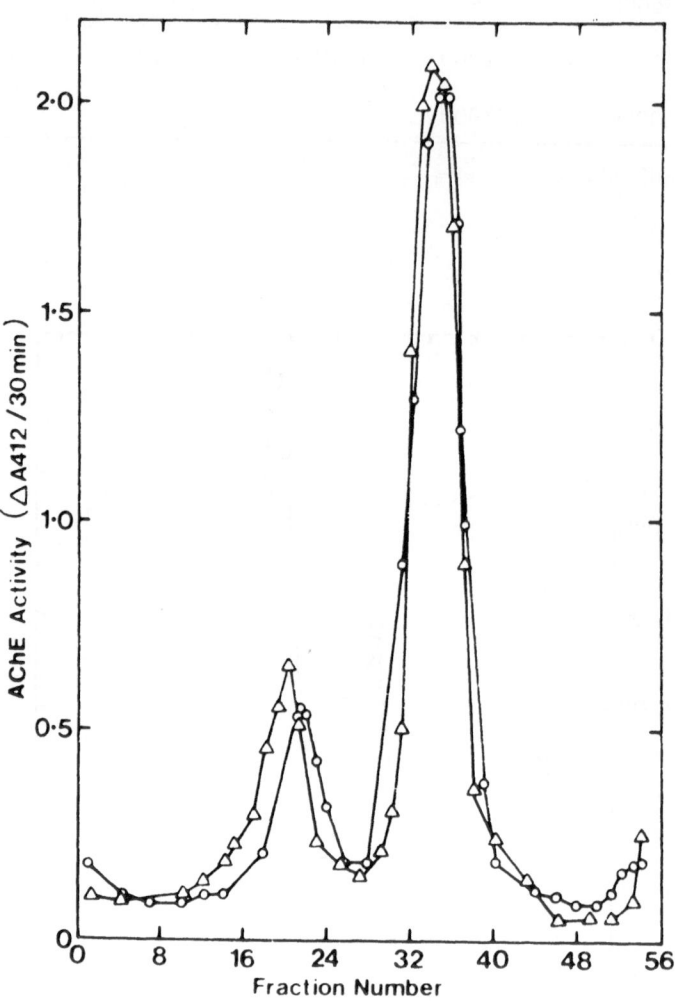

Fig. 4.   Sucrose density gradient pattern of AChE (a) Crude(o-o)
          (b) purified (Δ-Δ)。

4.3 Sucrose Density Gradient Centrifugation

Sucrose density gradient fractionation separates proteins on the basis of their sedimentation velocities, which are a function of molecular size, shape and density. Crude AChE, on 5–20% linear sucrose density gradient showed two peaks (Fig. 4a) of activity when assayed according to the method of Ellman et al., (1961), which agreed with Krysan and Chadwick (1966). On the other hand, when sucrose density gradients were run with 7% acrylamide and (after polymerization) stained with the histochemical method of Karnovsky and Roots (1964) using acetylthiocholine, three species with sedimentation coefficient (Table IV) of 5.0, 7.2 and 11.5 were observed (Fig. 5). The mol wts, calculated by the simple ratio of Martin and Ames (1961) were 87,000, 152,000 and 307,000 using aldolase as standard (Table IV). The calculation assumes that the standard and the acetylcholinesterases were all globular and had the same density.

4.4 Isoelectric Focussing

Isoelectric focussing separates molecules on the basis of differences in isoelectric point. Crude AChE was separated by

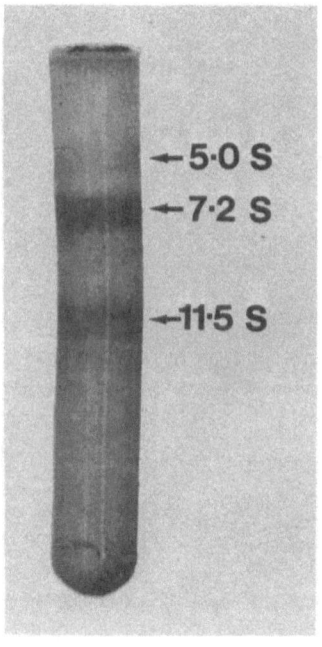

Fig. 5.   Sucrose density gradient profile of crude AChE, containing 7% acrylamide.

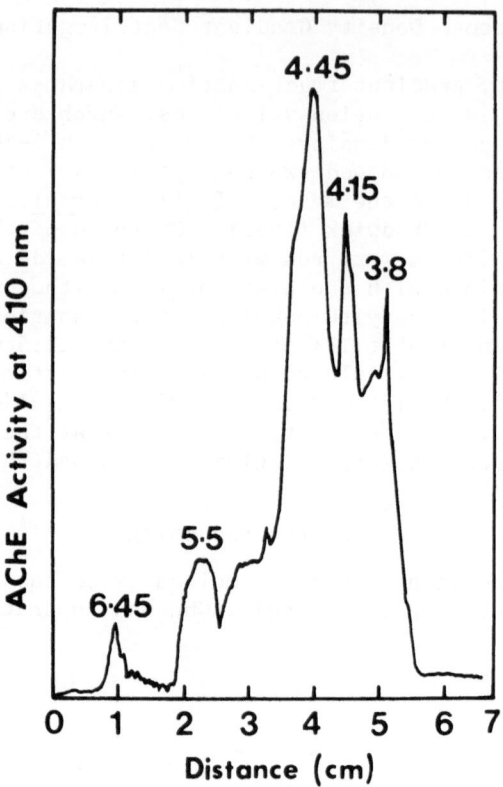

Fig. 6.   Densitometric scan of AChE fractionated on isoelectric
          focussing gel.

isoelectric focussing in polyacrylamide gels containing ampholytes
of pH 3.5-10 range.   AChE activity bands were visualized by the
method of Karnovsky and Roots (1964).   Five activity peaks with
isoelectric point (PI) of 3.8, 4.15, 4.45, 5.5, and 6.45 were observed (Fig. 6).

5.   PURIFICATION OF ACETYLCHOLINESTERASE

AChE from the heads of house fly (Musca domestica, tetrachlor-
vinphos resistant strain) was purified by affinity chromatography
(Tripathi and O'Brien, 1977).   The enzyme from the crude extract of
100,000 g, 1 hr supernatant was adsorbed on an affinity column containing trimethyl (p-aminophenyl) ammonium chloride hydrochloride,

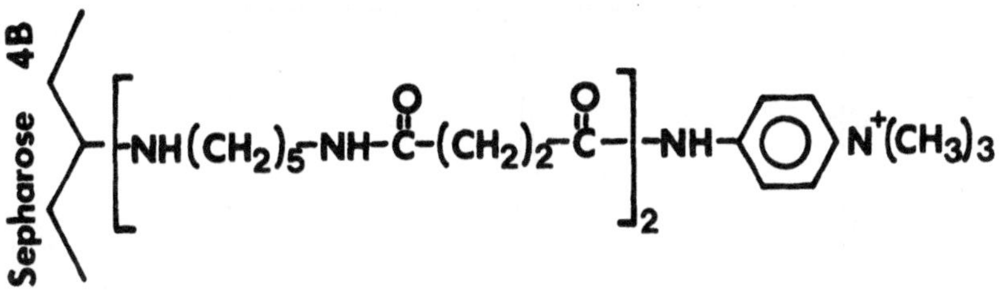

Fig. 7. Affinity chromatography resin linked to the inhibitor.

covalently linked to Sepharose 4B (Fig. 7). After extensive washing, the AChE was eluted with a solution of a selective reversible
inhibitor BW 284C51. The AChE was freed from the inhibitor by passing through Sephadex G-50 and then concentrated in a collodion membrane bag.

A typical purification is shown in Table V. The enzyme has been
purified 1223-fold in one step with a recovery of 34%. The specific
activity was 752 units/mg protein, which is similar to the values
reported for house fly brain AChE previously (Huang and Dauterman,
1973; Steele and Smallman, 1976b).

On analytical polyacrylamide gel electrophoresis, purified
AChE revealed five protein bands, four corresponding to the enzyme
activity bands and one devoid of enzyme activity (Fig. 8). Periodic
acid-Schiff stain indicated that the isozyme I was glycoprotein
(Tripathi and O'Brien, 1977). On storage at 0°C, it was observed
that the activity of isozyme I and II deteriorated much more than
that of isozymes III and IV; the activity of I and II was lost in
less than two weeks.

Table V. Purification of House Fly Brain AChE.

Purification Stage	Total Activity (Units)	Specific Activity (Units/mg)	Yield %	Purification Factor
Crude Extract	99.22	0.614	100	1
Purified AChE	33.10	752.0	34	1223

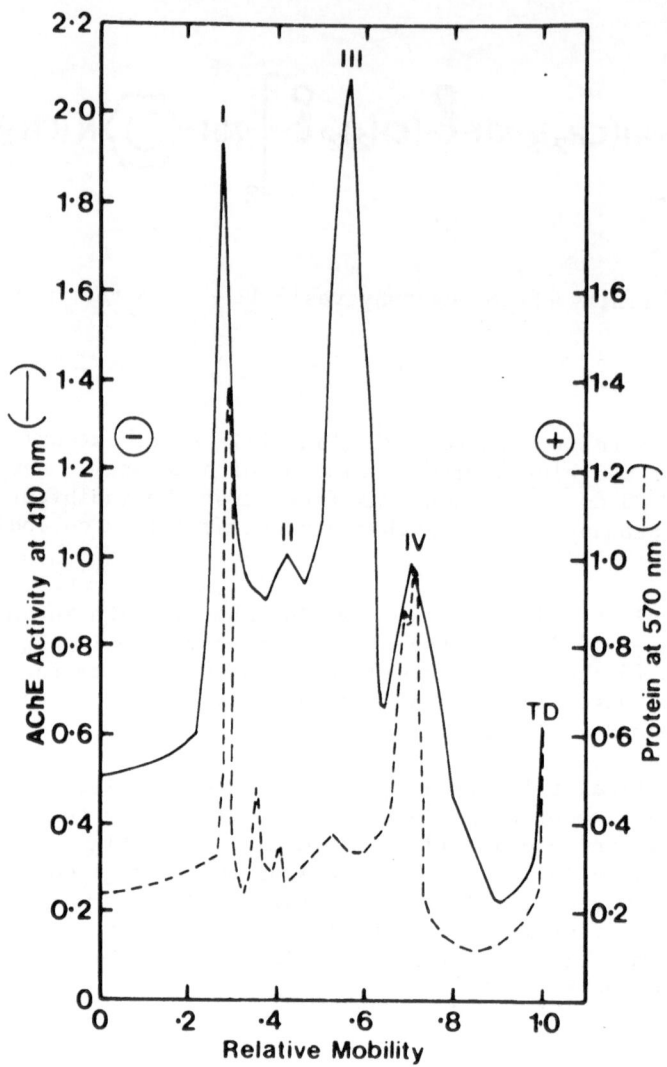

Fig. 8.   Electrophoretograms of purified housefly AChE. Scan of gel
stained for protein with coomassie blue (------); scan of
gel stained for AChE (————). TD denotes the portion of
tracking dye. AChE isozymes are numbered I through IV in
order of increasing anodic mobility in the separating gel.

Purified AChE on sucrose density gradient centrifugation showed
two major species exactly like the crude preparation (Fig. 4b).
Polyacrylamide disc gel electrophoresis showed that the heavy peak
corresponded to the slowest moving isozyme I, and the light to the

fast moving isozyme III (Fig. 8). The molecular weights and sedimentation coefficients of these two major species were 306,000 (±11,150) for heavy (S_{20w} = 11.50 ± 0.28S) form and 143,000 (± 4,700) for light (S_{20w} = 6.9 ± 0.5S) form (Tripathi and O'Brien, 1977); the calculations assume, as before, globular proteins with the same density as the standard.

The partial specific volume ($\bar{v}$) (i.e. the reciprocal of the density) of the purified AChE was determined according to the method of O'Brien et al. (1977) and was found to be 0.75 ml/g (unpublished results).

The subunit structure of purified AChE was determined on polyacrylamide gel electrophoresis in the presence of sodium dodecyl sulphate (SDS) and β-mercaptoethanol according to the method of Weber and Osborn (1969). A subunit weight of 82,000 was found in fresh preparations; however, two to three additional bands were observed in older preparations (unpublished results).

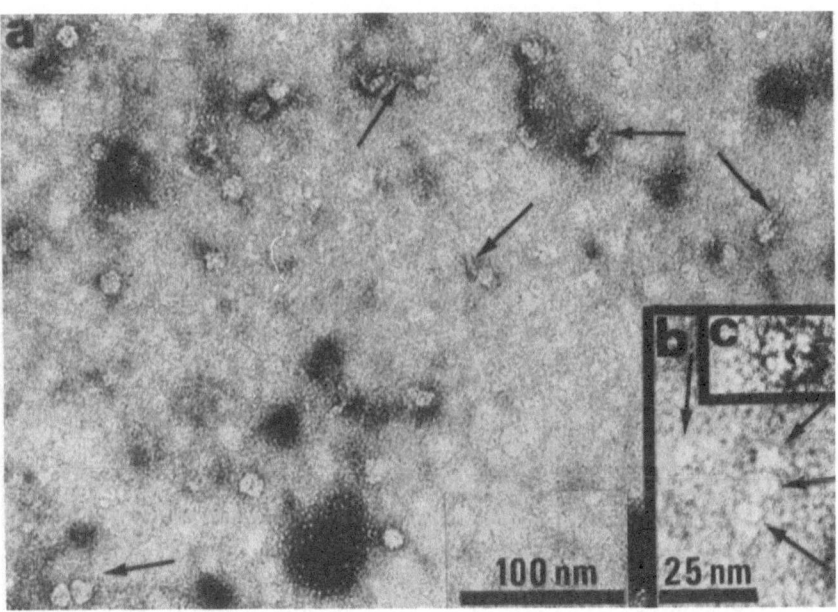

Fig. 9.   Electron micrograph of AChE. (a) A field view illustrating the components making up the sample. Arrows indicate particles showing a tail-like structure. (b) A higher magnified view of several single subunits (arrows) each having an overall diameter of 5-7 nm. Each subunit is separated into two smaller parts by an electron dense line. (c) AChE showing 4 subunits in a separated array (tetramer).

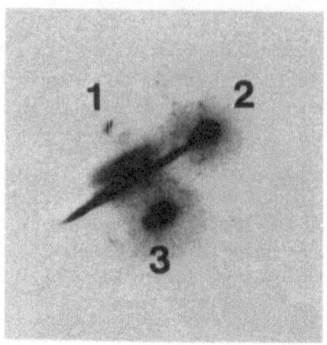

Fig. 10.   Immunodiffusion analysis (Ouchterlony) of purified AChE.
           1. purified AChE   2. control rabbit serum   3. rabbit
           antiserum

Purified AChE after negative staining with 0.5% uranyl formate
under the electron microscope revealed two components (Fig. 9).   The
major component (approx. 90%) appears to be a tetramer of about
12-15 nm across.   In a few cases an attached "tail" is observed which
is 45 nm long and 2 nm thick.   The minor component (approx. 10%) is
made up of a single unit 5-7 nm across (Telford et al., 1977).

Antiserum was prepared by immunizing rabbit with purified AChE.
The Ouchterlony double-diffusion technique showed a sharp precipi-
tine line (Fig. 10).

6.   CONCLUSION

It is apparent that AChE from house flies is a mixture of isozymes, and their difference appears to be due to size and charge
properties.   The exact cause of multiplicity of AChE is not known,
although in some vertebrates it has been attributed to aggregation
of subunits (Adamson, 1977; Adamson et al., 1975; Gordon et al.,
1976).   Data presented in Table IV indicate the similar possibility
for house fly isozymes as they appear to be the multiples of a subunit
weight of 82,000.   However, they may not be simple aggregates as they
differ in their tissue distribution and physiological behavior
(Tripathi and O'Brien, 1973a; Bajgar, 1975).   It is possible that
different forms reported here may arise due to different amounts of
carbohydrates as reported for isozyme I (Tripathi and O'Brien,
1977) or lipids attached to them.   Such a possibility is being
explored further.

7. ACKNOWLEDGEMENTS

I am most grateful to Dr. R. D. O'Brien for his critical review of the manuscript. Experimental work reported herein from this laboratory was supported by NIH Grant ES 00901.

8. REFERENCES

Adamson, E. D., 1977, Acetylcholinesterase in mouse brain, erythrocytes and muscle, J. Neurochem. 28:605.

Adamson, E. D., Ayers, S., Deussen, Z. A. and Graham, C. F., 1975, Analysis of the forms of acetylcholinesterase from the adult mouse brain, Biochem. J. 147:205.

Ayed, H., and Georghiou, G. P., 1975, Resistance to organophosphates and carbamates in Anopheles albimanus based on reduced sensitivity of acetylcholinesterase, J. Econ. Entomol. 68:295.

Bajgar, J., 1975, Characterization and properties of multiple molecular forms of acetylcholinesterase. Possible evaluation in histochemistry, Acta histochemica, supplement XV, S. 123.

Baldwin, J., and Hochachka, P. W., 1970, Functional significance of isoenzymes in thermal acclimatization. Acetylcholinesterase from trout brain, Biochem. J. 116:883.

Bernsohn, J., Barron, K. D., and Hess, A. R., 1962, Multiple nature of acetylcholinesterase in nerve tissue, Nature 195:285.

Bon, S., Huet, M., Lemonnier, M., Rieger, F., and Massoulié, J., 1976, Molecular forms of electrophorus acetylcholinesterase. Molecular weight and composition, Eur. J. Biochem. 68:523.

Booth, G. M., Stratton, C. L., and Larsen, J. R., 1975, Localization and substrate-inhibitor specificity of insect esterase isozymes, in:Isozymes Developmental Biology, Academic Press, New York, p. 721.

Chan, S. L., Shirachi, D. Y. Bhargava, H. N., Gardner, E. and Trever, A. J., 1972, Purification and properties of multiple forms of brain acetylcholinesterase, J. Neurochem. 19:2747.

Chiu, Y. C., Tripathi, R. K., and O'Brien, R. D., 1972, A gel scanning method for kinetic studies on an acetylcholinesterase isozyme, Anal. Biochem. 45:480.

Christoff, N., Anderson, P. J., Slotwiner, P., and Song, S. K., 1966, Electrophoretic and histochemical evaluation of anticholinesterase drugs, Ann. N. Y. Acad. Sci. 135:150.

Coats, P. M., and Simpson, N. E., 1972, Genetic variation in human erythrocyte acetylcholinesterase, Science 175:1466.

Dauterman, W. C., Talens, A., Van Asparen, K., 1962, Partial purification and properties of house fly head cholinesterase, J. Insect Physiol., 8:1.

Davis, G. A., and Agranoff, B. W., 1968, Metabolic behavior of isoenzymes of acetylcholinesterase, Nature, (London) 220:277.

Dudai, Y., Herzberg, M., and Silman, I., 1973, Molecular structure of acetylcholinesterase from electric organ tissue of the electric eel, Proc. Natl. Acad. Sci. 70:2473.

Eldefrawi, M. E., Tripathi, R. K., and O'Brien, R. D., 1970, Acetylcholinesterase isoenzymes from house fly brain, Biochim. Biophys. Acta 212:308.

Ellman, G. L., Courtney, K. D., Andres, Jr., V., and Featherstone, R. M., 1961, A new and rapid colorimetric determination of acetylcholinesterase activity, Biochem. Pharmacol. 7:88.

Ferguson, K. A., 1964, Starch gel electrophoresis application to the classification of pituitary proteins and polypeptides, Metabolism 13:985.

Gordon, M. A., Chan, S. L., and Trevor, A. J., 1976, Active site determination on forms of mammalian brain and eel acetylcholinesterase, Biochem. J. 157:69.

Guilbault, G. G., Kuan, S. S., and Sadar, M. H., 1970, Purification and properties of cholinesterase from honey bee, Apis millifera, L., and boll weevils, Anthonomus grandis, B., J. Agric. Food Chem. 18:692.

Hall, Z. W., 1973, Multiple forms of acetylcholinesterase and their distribution in endplate and non-endplate regions of rat diaphragm muscle, J. Neurobiol. 4:343.

Hedrick, J. L., and Smith, J. L., 1968, Size and charge isomer separation and estimation of molecular weights of proteins by disc gel electrophoresis, Arch. Biochem. Biophys. 126:155.

Hellenbrand, K., 1967, Inhibition of house fly acetylcholinesterase by carbamates, J. Agric. Food Chem. 15:825.

Hollingworth, R. M., Fukuto, T. R., and Metcalf, R. L., 1967, Selectivity of sumithion compared with methyl parathion: influence of structure on anticholinesterase activity, J. Agric. Food. Chem. 15:235.

Hollunger, E. G., and Niklasson, B. H., 1973, The release and molecular state of mammalian brain acetylcholinesterase, J. Neurochem. 20:821.

Huang, C. T., and Dauterman, W. C., 1973, Purification of fly head cholinesterase, Insect Biochem. 3:325.

Iwata, I., and Hama, H., 1972, Insensitivity of cholinesterase in Nephotettix cincticeps resistant to carbamate and organophosphorus insecticides, J. Econ. Entomol. 65:643.

Jackson, R. L., and Aprison, M. H., 1966, Mammalian brain acetylcholinesterase. Purification and properties, J. Neurochem. 13:1351.

Karnovsky, M. J., and Roots, L., 1964, A direct coloring" thiocholine method for cholinesterases, J. Histochem. Cytochem. 12:219.

Krysan, J. L., and Chadwick, L. E., 1966, The molecular weight of cholinesterase from the house fly Musca domestica, J. Insect Physiol. 12:781.

Krysan, J. L., and Kruckeburg, W. C., 1970, The sedimentation properties of cholinesterases from a mayfly, Hexagenia bilineata (Say); Ephemeroptera, and the honey bee Apis millifera L., Int. J. Biochem. 1:241.

Lee, A. H., Metcalf, R. L., and Kearns, C. W., 1974, Purification and some properties of house cricket, Acheta domesticus, acetylcholinesterase, Insect Biochem. 4:267.

Markert, C. L., 1975, Biology of isozymes in:Isozymes Molecular Structure, Markert, C. L. (Ed), Academic Press, New York.

Martin, R. G., and Ames, B. N., 1961, A method for determining the sedimentation behavior of enzymes: application to protein mixtures, J. Biol. Chem. 236:1372.

Massoulié, J., Bon, S., Rieger, F., and Vigny, M., 1975, Molecular forms of acetylcholinesterase, Croatica Chem. Acta 47:163.

Maynard, E. A., 1966, Electrophoretic studies of cholinesterases in brain and muscle of the developing chicken, J. Exp. Zool. 161:319.

Metcalf, R. L., March, R. B., and Maxon, M. G., 1955, Substrate preferences of insect cholinesterases, Ann. Ent. Soc. Amer. 48:222.

Nachmansohn, D., 1970, Proteins in excitable membranes, Science 168:1059.

O'Brien, R. D., 1967, Insecticide Action and Metabolism, Academic Press, New York.

O'Brien, R. D., 1976, Acetylcholinesterase and its inhibition in:
    Insecticide Biochemistry and Physiology, Wilkinson, C. F. (Ed),
    Plenum Press, New York.

O'Brien, R. D., Timpone, C. A., and Gibson, R. E., 1977, The
    measurement of partial specific volumes and sedimentation co-
    efficients by sucrose density centrifugation, J. Biol. Chem.,
    submitted.

O'Brien, R. D., Hetnarski, B., Tripathi, R. K., and Hart, G. J.,
    1975, Recent studies on acetylcholinesterase inhibition in:
    Mechanism of Pesticide Action, Vol. 2, American Chemical Society,
    Washington, D. C., p. 1.

Ott, P., Jenny, B., and Brodbeck, W., 1975, Multiple forms of puri-
    fied human erythrocyte acetylcholinesterase, Eur. J. Biochem.
    57:469.

Plapp, F. W., Jr., and Tripathi, R. K., Genetic and biochemical
    studies on an insecticide-resistant house fly strain with an
    altered acetylcholinesterase, Biochem. Genetics, in press.

Rodbard, D., and Chrambach, A., 1971, Estimation of molecular radius
    free mobility, and valence using polyacrylamide gel electrophore-
    sis, Analyt. Biochem. 40:95.

Shafai, T., and Cortner, J. A., 1971, Human erythrocyte acetylchol-
    inesterase. I. Resolution of activity into two components, Bio-
    chem. Biophys. Acta 236:612.

Shaw, C. R., 1969, Isozymes: classification, frequency, and signifi-
    cance, Int. Rev. Cytol. 25:297.

Siegel, L. M., and Monty, K. J., 1966, Determination of molecular
    weights and frictional ratios of proteins in impure systems by use
    of gel filtration and density gradient centrifugation, applica-
    tion to crude preparations of sulphite and hydroxylamine reduct-
    ases, Biochim. Biophys. Acta 112:346.

Skangiel-Kramska, J., and Niemierko, S., 1971, Isozymes of acetyl-
    cholinesterase in the sciatic nerve of rabbit and their molecular
    weight, Bull. Acad. Pol. Sci. 19:389.

Steele, R. W., and Smallman, B. N., 1976a, Acetylcholinesterase from
    house fly head, molecular properties of soluble forms, Biochim.
    Biophys. Acta 445:131.

Steele, R. W., and Smallman, B. N., 1976b, Acetylcholinesterase of
    the house fly head, affinity purification and subunit composition
    Biochim. Biophys. Acta 445:147.

Telford, J. F., Tripathi, R. K., and O'Brien, R. D., 1977, Electron microscopy of acetylcholinesterase from house fly brain, J. Mol. Biol., submitted.

Tripathi, R. K., 1976, Relation of acetylcholinesterase sensitivity to cross-resistance of a resistant house fly strain to organophosphates and carbamates, Pestic. Biochem. Physiol. 6:30.

Tripathi, R. K., and O'Brien, R. D., 1973a, Effects of organophosphates in vivo upon acetylcholinesterase isozymes from house fly head and thorax, Pestic. Biochem. Physiol 2:418.

Tripathi, R. K., and O'Brien, R. D., 1973b, Insensitivity of acetylcholinesterase as a factor in resistance of house flies to the organophosphate Rabon, Pestic. Biochem. Physiol. 3:495.

Tripathi, R. K., and O'Brien, R. D., 1975, The significance of multiple molecular forms of acetylcholinesterase in the sensitivity of house flies to organophosphorus poisoning in: Isozymes Physiology and Function, Markert, C.L. (Ed.), Academic Press, New York, p. 395.

Tripathi, R. K., and O'Brien, R. D., 1977, Purification of acetylcholinesterase from house fly brain by affinity chromatography, Biochim. Biophys. Acta 480:382.

Tripathi, R. K., Chiu, Y. C., and O'Brien, R. D., 1973, Reactivity in vitro, towards substrate and inhibitors of acetylcholinesterase isozymes from electric eel electroplax and house fly brain, Pestic. Biochem. Physiol. 3:55.

Varela, J. M., 1975, Potentials in exploring the physiological role of acetylcholinesterase isozymes in: Isozymes Physiological Function, Markert, C. L. (Ed.), Academic Press, New York, p. 315.

Weber, K., and Osborn, M., 1969, The reliability of molecular weight determinations by dodecyl-sulphate polyacrylamide gel electrophoresis, J. Biol. Chem. 244:4406

Wenthold, R. J., Mahler, H. R., and Moore, W. J., 1974, Properties of acetylcholinesterase from rat brain, J. Neurochem. 22:945.

Wustner, D. A., and Fukuto, T. R., 1974, Affinity and phosphorylation constants for the inhibition of cholinesterases by the optical isomers of O-2-butyl S-2 (dimethylammonium)ethyl ethyl phosphonothioate hydrogen oxalate, Pestic. Biochem. Physiol. 4:365.

Yu, C., Metcalf, R. L., and Booth, G. M., 1972, Inhibition of acetylcholinesterase from mammals and insects by carbofuran and its related compounds and their toxicities towards these animals, J. Agric. Food Chem. 20:923.

Zettler, J. L., and Brady, U. E., 1975, Acetylcholinesterase iso-
    zymes of the house fly thorax: in vivo inhibition by organophos-
    phate insecticides, Pestic. Biochem. Physiol. 5:471.

NOVEL INHIBITORS OF INSECT CHOLINE ACETYLTRANSFERASE AND THEIR EFFECTS ON SYNAPTIC TRANSMISSION AT AN INSECT CHOLINERGIC SYNAPSE

M. E. Schroeder, A. C. Boyer, R. F. Flattum, and
K. G. R. Sundelin

Shell Development Company, Biological Sciences
Research Center, Modesto, California 95352

INTRODUCTION

Synaptic transmission in the insect central nervous system is at least partly mediated by acetylcholine (Gerschenfeld, 1973). The significance of this transmitter in impulse propagation is reflected in the fact that many of our most effective insecticides act in some way to disrupt transmission at the insect cholinergic synapse.

Choline acetyltransferase (E.C. 2.3.1.6) catalyzes the synthesis of acetylcholine and its potential as a target for new insecticides has been suggested (O'Brien, 1967; Yu and Booth, 1971; Baillie et al.,1975). Since very little is known about the active center of insect choline acetyltransferase, previous studies have concentrated on analogs of choline in their attempts to identify new inhibitors of the enzyme. Baillie et al.(1975) have reported a choline analog with a K_i value of 0.06 µM against house fly choline acetyltransferase. Although this is apparently the most powerful inhibitor yet identified for this enzyme, neurophysiological studies indicate that the primary site of action of the inhibitor is on the acetylcholine receptor of the insect rather than on choline acetyltransferase.

Since cholinergic neurons occur to a greater or lesser extent in representatives of practically every phylum in the animal kingdom, it would seem from the standpoint of specificity that attempts to inhibit such an ubiquitous enzyme as choline acetyltransferase represents an unfeasible strategy of insect control. However, the insect enzyme appears different in several aspects

63

from that of other species. Some differences are the notably
lower temperature optima, the apparent absence of reactive sulf-
hydryl groups and a lack of association of mitochondria in choline
acetyltransferase derived from insect sources (Chadwick, 1963;
Boccacci et al., 1960). Furthermore, the insect enzyme shows
differences with respect to substrate specificity (Mehrotra and
Dauterman, 1963) and affinity (Mehrotra, 1961) as well as in its
response to certain nonsulfhydryl reactive inhibitors (Yu and
Booth, 1971). These differences are potentially useful in the
design of selective inhibitors of insect choline acetyltransferase.
If it can be demonstrated that inhibition of this enzyme can
constitute a lethal lesion or sufficiently debilitate the insect
so that it cannot function normally, a selective control agent
may result. This paper is a summary of an investigation into the
inhibitory activity of about 500 compounds on insect choline
acetyltransferase and the neurophysiological effects of selected
inhibitors on synaptic transmission at an insect cholinergic
synapse.

METHODS

Enzyme Purification

Three grams of house fly (Musca domestica L.) heads were homogenized in 10 ml of 0.001 M Tris pH 7.0 buffer using a Potter
Elvehjem homogenizer. The crude homogenate was partially purified
in order to reduce the activity of acetylcoenzyme A hydrolase.
This enzyme hydrolyzes acetylcoenzyme A to coenzyme A and acetate
ion at a rate which is six times faster than the utilization of
acetylcoenzyme A by the transferase. The purification was
accomplished by filtering the crude homogenate through cheesecloth
to remove debris and then centrifuging at 30,000 g for 30 minutes.
The entire supernatant was then applied to a Cellex-D (Bio-Rad
Laboratory with a capacity of 0.9 meq/g dry weight) column (30 cm
x 1.2 cm) in the sodium form equilibrated at pH 7.0 in 0.001 M
Tris buffer, pH 7.0. The column was washed with 60 ml of 0.1 M
Tris buffer, pH 7.0. Choline acetyltransferase was eluted with
1.0 M Tris buffer, pH 7.0. Eight-milliliter fractions were
collected using an unrestricted gravity flow rate. Ammonium
sulfate was added to the tubes with maximum amount of choline
acetyltransferase until the solution had reached 60% saturation
with respect to the ammonium sulfate. This mixture was then
centrifuged for 30 minutes at 30,000 x g. The precipitate was
suspended in 1.0 ml of a mixture containing Tris buffer (0.01 M,
pH 7.0), ammonium sulfate (60% saturated with respect to ammonium
sulfate). This preparation was diluted 1:20 in 0.1 M sodium
phosphate buffer, pH 7.0, prior to use. All operations were
carried out at $2^{\circ}C$.

Enzyme Assay

The enzyme (0.08 ml) was preincubated with 9.1×10^{-3} μmoles dichlorvos (phosphoric acid, 2,2-dichlorovinyl dimethyl ester) or eserine and 3 μmoles potassium phosphate buffer, pH 7.0, in a total volume of 0.12 ml for 20 minutes at 36°C. A 0.12 ml aliquot of this mixture was mixed with 0.04 ml of a solution containing 0.21 μmoles acetylcoenzyme A, 0.43 μmoles choline chloride, 7.26×10^{-4} μmoles 1-^{14}C-acetylcoenzyme A (0.047 μCi). After five minutes at 36°C, 0.08 ml of 0.1 M acetylcholine iodide was added and the tube was heated in a boiling water bath for 1.5 minutes. The tube was rapidly cooled and centrifuged for five minutes at 2,000 rpm to sediment the denatured protein. One-hundred microliters of the supernatant was then applied to a Micro BioRex-70 column (Bio-Rad Laboratory with a capacity of 10.2 meq/g dry weight and a mesh size of 100-200) in the sodium form equilibrated at pH 7.0 in water. Micro columns were prepared by placing resin in Pasteur pipettes with glass wool plugs. Teflon spaghetti tubing was used to keep the liquid in the column. The pipette was filled to the indentation mark. This was equivalent to approximately 0.5 g of resin in the sodium form. The column was then washed with 9.0 ml of 1×10^{-3} M sodium acetate. The acetyl-1-^{14}C choline was eluted with 9.0 ml of 1.0 $\underline{N}$ HCl into a scintillator vial. Thirteen milliliters of Triton X-100 scintillation fluid (mixture of 46% Triton X-100 and 54% Toluene liquid scintillation fluid consisting of one part Packard Instrument Company Permafluor to 24 parts toluene) was added with mixing and the sample was counted in a Packard TriCarb scintillation spectrometer.

Enzyme Inhibition

To determine the inhibitory activity of the candidate compounds the assay procedure was modified in terms of the concentration of reagents used. The concentration of acetylcoenzyme A was changed to its K_m value of 0.064 μmoles and choline chloride to its value of 0.055 μmoles. The candidate inhibitor (0.016 μmoles) was also added to the mixture prior to the five-minute incubation period. An amount of solvent equivalent to that used in the test assay was added to the control assay. In this study I_{50} is defined as the concentration of compound required to inhibit 50% of the enzymatic activity within the five-minute incubation period and in the presence of K_m amounts of both substrates.

Neurophysiological Studies

Inhibitors selected on the basis of their activity in the
in vitro enzyme assay were tested for their ability to disrupt
synaptic transmission at an insect cholinergic synapse. The
tissue chosen for this study was the sixth abdominal ganglion
preparation of the American cockroach, Periplaneta americana (L.).
This ganglion is the site of cholinergic synapses between afferent
sensory neurons of the cerci and the giant interneurons of the
ventral nerve cord (Shankland et al., 1971; Flattum and Shankland,
1971).

Shankland et al. (1971) have shown that repetitive stimulation
of the cercal afferents leads to a blockade of synaptic transmission in ganglia which have been treated with hemicholinium-3.
This drug indirectly inhibits acetylcholine synthesis by preventing
the resorption of choline into the presynaptic terminal (MacIntosh,
1961). The blockade is presumably due to depletion of endogenous
stores of transmitter.

For similar reasons, inhibition of choline acetyltransferase
would be expected to produce a synaptic blockade in preparations
subjected to repetitive presynaptic stimulation. To test this
hypothesis a portion of the cockroach ventral nerve cord consisting
of both cercal nerves 8 (Guthrie and Tindall, 1968), the sixth,
fifth, and fourth abdominal ganglia, and the interganglionic
connectives was removed from the body cavity and transferred to a
lucite bathing chamber. Stimulating and recording electrodes were
of the suction-electrode type (Florey and Kriebel, 1966). The
sixth abdominal ganglion was desheathed with a pair of finely
sharpened forceps and the entire preparation was irrigated with
saline (Yamasaki and Narahashi, 1959) for 20 minutes at a flow
rate of 1.5 ml/minute. This was followed by irrigation with a
suspension of inhibitor in saline for 30 minutes. The suspensions
were made by squirting 0.5 ml of an acetone stock solution of the
inhibitor into 100 ml of saline. In all experiments the final
concentration of acetone in saline never exceeded 0.5%. Separate
control experiments showed that this concentration of acetone had
no deleterious effect on synaptic transmission during the test
period. The performance of the cercal nerve-giant fiber synapse
was checked periodically during inhibitor irrigation and in all
cases was found to function normally. All solutions were delivered
to the preparation from elevated reservoirs.

At the end of the 30-minute irrigation period, but in the
continued presence of the drug, the preparation was stimulated at
a frequency of 30 Hz (0.1 msec duration) at increasing super-
threshold voltages until 10 volts per stimulus was reached and
synaptic transmission failed. Stimulation at this voltage and

frequency was continued for an additional three minutes after which the stimulus was reduced to 1.0 volt above the original threshold and the frequency was reduced to 1 per five seconds. These conditions produced a synaptic blockade in both inhibitor treated and control preparations. In the latter, however, synaptic transmission always returned within a few minutes after the stimulus voltage and frequency were reduced with a mean recover time of 7.8 ± 0.42 minutes (n = 9). The resumption of normal synaptic transmission following a period of post-tetanic depression is a reflection of the mobilization of transmitter into readily releasable storage sites which had been depleted during the period of tetanic stimulation (Callec, 1974). In this study, therefore, the elapsed time for the reappearance of synaptic transmission was considered to be a neurophysiological expression of the amount of transmitter available for release and, indirectly, an indication of synthesis. Recovery time was measured with time zero starting at the reduced voltage and frequency condition.

The functionality of the postsynaptic acetylcholine receptors of ganglia blocked by an inhibitor was determined by challenge with nicotine (5×10^{-6} M) or acetylcholine (1×10^{-5} M). The latter compound was applied to ganglia which had been pretreated with eserine (10^{-6} M) for 10-15 minutes prior to challenge.

In some experiments the stimulation protocol described above was applied to preparations in which synaptic activity was monitored with the mannitol gap recording technique (Callec and Sattelle, 1974). This technique offers distinct advantages over conventional suction electrode methods. It permits the application of drugs to selected areas of the preparation. It also allows slow DC potential changes in the ganglion to be monitored and permits simultaneous observation of both presynaptic spikes and excitatory postsynaptic potentials (EPSP). These advantages permit a more critical assessment of a possible site of action of a drug in the ganglion.

In Vivo Toxicity

Compounds which were effective at reasonable concentrations in preventing the resumption of synaptic transmission in the isolated sixth abdominal ganglion preparation were tested for their ability to induce similar symptoms in whole insects. Adult male American cockroaches were injected with suspected inhibitors in 1 μl acetone. Control animals were injected with acetone only. After varying intervals of time, nerve cord preparations were removed and subjected to the stimulation regime described above.

In another series of experiments an attempt was made to
induce hyperactivity in cockroaches treated with inhibitors under
the hypothesis that paralysis or prostration should occur sooner
in those insects subjected to conditions promoting depletion of
endogenous stores of transmitter. Two groups of seven roaches
each were injected with 20 µg of inhibitor in 0.5 µl acetone.
Each group was placed in an eight-ounce jar which was then rotated
on a turntable (30 rpm) held at a 45° angle to the vertical. The
jar was fitted with plastic partitions and lightly coated on the
inside with a silicone lubricant. This arrangement provided a
tumbling type of action by preventing the insects from sliding on
the bottom or grasping the sides of the jar as it was rotated on
the turntable. Each group was tumbled twice daily for ten-minute
intervals. Periods of tumbling were separated by at least six
hours of rest. Control groups were injected with 0.5 µl acetone
and tumbled the same as the treated groups. Another set of
controls was injected with 20 µg of the inhibitor in 0.5 µl
acetone but not tumbled. Mortality was recorded before each period
of tumbling. As roaches from each group became prostrate, nerve
cord preparations were removed and tested for their ability to
recover after high frequency stimulation of the cercal nerve-
giant fiber synapse.

RESULTS AND DISCUSSION

Inhibition of House Fly Choline Acetyltransferase

Under the conditions employed in this study, the in vitro
synthesis of acetylcholine was linear with time and enzyme concentration when either the crude or purified enzyme preparation was
used provided the appropriate concentrations of substrates were
present. The Michaelis-Menten constants (K_m) of house fly choline
acetyltransferase for acetylcoenzyme A was 3.8×10^{-4} M and $3.7 \times
10^{-4}$ M for choline. These values agree with those previously
reported for this enzyme (Mehrotra, 1961).

Novel inhibitors of house fly choline acetyltransferase,
comprising three different structural classifications, were found
among over 500 compounds tested.

S-phenyl-α-halothioacetates

Initial screening revealed the significant inhibitory activity
of compounds possessing the

$$-S-\overset{\overset{\displaystyle O}{\|}}{C}-C-$$

moiety. The data in Tables 1 and 2 show that only those compounds
having a single halogen atom alpha to the carbonyl group are good
inhibitors, with bromine being the best, followed by iodine and
chlorine. Similar results were reported by Yu and Booth (1971)
who showed that a bromine atom on the alpha-carbon was necessary
for activity in a series of S-alkyl thioacetate inhibitors of
house fly choline acetyltransferase. These data indicate that
nucleophilic displacement of the alpha substituent may be an
important step in enzyme inhibition. Bulk intolerance by the
enzyme may explain the inactivity of the alpha-trichloro (X) and
the thiocyanate (IV) analogs, although side reactions may also
pertain to the latter.

To test for electronic interactions, analogs with various
aromatic substituents were tested. Data for the para-substituted
compounds, where steric interactions would be minimized, gave no
clear indication whether electron donating or withdrawing substituents are required for biological activity.

Compounds XVII, XVIII, XIX, and XX were prepared to determine
if hydrophobic bonding to the enzyme could be utilized to increase
inhibitory activity. These compounds, however, were inactive.

Table 2 shows that for alpha-chloro compounds, a phenyl ring
attached directly to the sulfur is required for activity. Substitution of the ring by methyl or naphthyl groups, or insertion of
methylene groups between the sulfur and phenyl ring, results in
a loss of activity. These results are in apparent conflict with
those of Yu and Booth (1971) who reported that methyl, ethyl,
n-propyl, and n-butyl bromothioacetates were good inhibitors of
house fly choline acetyltransferase. This conflict may be
resolved, however, by the fact that Yu and Booth used the alpha-
bromo analog, whereas the present study uses the alpha-chloro
derivatives. As Table 1 shows, substitution of bromine for
chlorine in the alpha position increases inhibitory activity by
a factor of 40. In agreement with Yu and Booth, the present study
shows that substitution of the sulfur atom of I with oxygen (XXVII)
or nitrogen (XXIX) results in a loss of activity (Table 2).

Maleimides

Available cyclic compounds containing the

$$R-N-\overset{\overset{\displaystyle O}{\|}}{C}-\overset{\overset{\displaystyle}{|}}{\underset{|}{C}}-Cl$$

fragments were tested as inhibitors of choline acetyltransferase.
Such analogs are represented by the maleimide derivetive, XXX
(Table 3). These compounds were weakly active with I_{50} values

Table 1

$$\text{R}_4 \bigcirc \text{-S-C-C-R}_3 \quad \overset{\overset{\displaystyle O}{\|}}{\underset{\displaystyle R_2}{C}} \overset{R_1}{\underset{R_2}{|}}$$

No.	R_1	R_2	R_3	R_4	I_{50} ChA Inhibition
I	H	H	Cl	—	2.5×10^{-5} M
II	H	H	Br	—	6.3×10^{-7} M
III	H	H	I	—	3.3×10^{-6} M
IV	H	H	SCN	—	$> 10^{-3}$ M
V	H	—	=CH-CH$_3$	—	$> 10^{-3}$ M
VI	H	H	H	—	$> 10^{-3}$ M
VII	H	CH$_3$	Cl	—	$> 10^{-3}$ M
VIII	H	Cl	Cl	—	$> 10^{-3}$ M
IX	Cl	Cl	Cl	—	$> 10^{-3}$ M
X	H	H	Cl	2,3,4-tri Cl	$> 10^{-3}$ M
XI	H	H	Cl	p-CH$_3$	1.3×10^{-4} M
XII	H	H	Cl	p-OCH$_3$	6.3×10^{-5} M
XIII	H	H	Cl	p-NO$_2$	1.0×10^{-4} M
XIV	H	H	Cl	p-Br	$> 10^{-3}$ M
XV	H	H	Cl	p-Cl	2.5×10^{-5} M
XVI	H	H	Cl	p-F	2.5×10^{-5} M
XVII	H	H	Cl	p-n-Butoxy	10^{-3} M
XVIII	H	H	Cl	p-Benzyloxy	$> 10^{-3}$ M
XIX	H	H	Cl	p-Benzyl	$> 10^{-3}$ M
XX	H	H	Cl	p-Phenyl	$> 10^{-3}$ M

Table 2

$$R-\overset{O}{\underset{\|}{C}}-CH_2-Cl$$

No.	R	I_{50} ChA Inhibition
XXI	phenyl$-CH_2-S$	1.6×10^{-3} M
XXII	naphthyl$-S$	1.3×10^{-4} M
XXIII	phenyl$-\overset{CH_3}{\underset{}{CH}}-S$	$> 10^{-3}$ M
XXIV	CH_3-phenyl$-CH_2-S$	$> 10^{-3}$ M
XXV	CH_3-S	$> 10^{-3}$ M
XXVI	phenyl$-CH_2-CH_2-CH_2-S$	$> 10^{-3}$ M
XXVII	phenyl$-O-$	$> 10^{-3}$ M
XXIX	phenyl$-NH-$	$> 10^{-3}$ M

Table 3

No.	R_1	R_2	R_3	I_{50}
XXX	Cl	Cl		5×10^{-4} M
XXXI	H	H		$> 10^{-3}$ M
XXXII	H	Cl		$> 10^{-3}$ M
XXXIII	Cl	Cl	H	$> 10^{-3}$ M
XXXIV	Cl	Cl	$ClCH_2-$	6.3×10^{-4} M
XXXV	Cl	Cl	$BrCH_2-$	2.5×10^{-4} M
XXXVI	Cl	Cl	$(Cl_3)CS-$	6.3×10^{-4} M
XXXVII	H	H	NO_2	$> 10^{-3}$ M
XXXVIII	Cl	Cl		$> 10^{-3}$ M
XXXIX	Cl	Cl	CH_2	$> 10^{-3}$ M
XL	Cl	Cl		1×10^{-4} M

no better than 1×10^{-4} M. Structure activity relationships indicate that chlorines at R_1 and R_2 are essential for activity. Groups which can be substituted on the nitrogen appear to be limited in size as indicated by the inactivity of substituted phenyl or benzyl analogs. However, this does not explain the relatively high activity of compound XL with the 3-chlorotetrahydropyran-2-yl substituent on the nitrogen as compared to its deoxy analog, XXXVIII.

$SCCl_3$-Substituted Hydantoins

Additional screening revealed a class of inhibitors containing the $-S-C-(Cl)_3$ fragment. Table 4 shows the inhibitory activity of a series of hydantoin compounds containing this moiety. These compounds are generally good inhibitors of house fly choline acetyltransferase with I_{50} values for the active compounds in the 10^{-5} to 10^{-6} M range. A comparison of XLI with XLII shows that the $-S-C-(Cl)_3$ group is essential for activity. Furthermore, a comparison of XLIX with L or XLV with XLIII indicates that, although this group may be positioned on either the imide or amide nitrogen, the latter position is preferred.

Neurophysiology

Representative compounds were selected from each class of choline acetyltransferase inhibitors and tested for their ability to prevent recovery of synaptic transmission after repetitive stimulation of the cereal nerve-giant fiber synapse.

The data presented in Table 5 show that, except for the S-phenyl chlorothioacetates (I, X, LI), a correlation can be made between activity in the in vitro enzyme assay and inhibition of synaptic transmission. Those compounds active as enzyme inhibitors (XLIII, XXX) also prevented the recovery of synaptic transmission during the one-hour test period. Likewise, the hydantoin (XLIV) and maleimide (XXXII) analogs, which were inactive on the enzyme, were also ineffective on the ganglion.

In order to more critically evaluate events contributing to synaptic block, inhibitors were applied to nerve preparations under mannitol-gap recording conditions. The advantages of this technique over conventional suction electrode methods were described previously.

Table 4

No.	R_1	R_2	R_3	R_4	I_{50}
XLI	H	H	H	H	$> 10^{-3}$ M
XLII	H	H	H	$(Cl_3)CS-$	1.1×10^{-5} M
XLIII	CH_3	CH_3	H	$(Cl_3)CS-$	2×10^{-5} M
XLIV	CH_3	CH_3	H	H	$> 10^{-3}$ M
XLV	CH_3	CH_3	$(Cl_3)CS-$	H	3.9×10^{-6} M
XLVI	CH_3	C_2H_5	H	$(Cl_3)CS-$	3.9×10^{-6} M
XLVII	CH_3	C_4H_9	H	$(Cl_3)CS-$	1×10^{-5} M
XLVIII	C_2H_5	C_4H_{11}	H	$(Cl_3)CS-$	3.9×10^{-6} M
XLIX	H	⬡	$(Cl_3)CS-$	H	6.3×10^{-6} M
L	H	⬡	H	$(Cl_3)CS-$	1.6×10^{-5} M

Preparations treated with either the active hydantoin (XLIII) or maleimide (XXX) inhibitors showed no significant change in the level of ganglionic polarization during the development of the block. Furthermore, these same ganglia showed no change in their sensitivity to threshold concentrations of cholinergic agonists. Both nicotine (5×10^{-6} M) and acetylcholine (1×10^{-5} M), the latter when applied to eserinized preparations, produced ganglionic depolarizations of 15-20 mV. These responses, which were similar in magnitude to control preparations, indicate that postsynaptic receptor desensitization is probably not a contributing factor to the development of the block.

Application of either XLIII or XXX to a region of the connective between the fifth and sixth abdominal ganglia produced no significant change in the amplitude or rise time in the monophasic action potential recorded under mannitol-gap conditions. Likewise, in the sixth abdominal ganglion, even after the excitatory post-synaptic potential had been depressed by inhibitor treatment, an action potential could still be observed invading the presynaptic terminal. Axonal conduction, therefore, in both pre- and post-synaptic elements was not impaired by either inhibitor.

These neurophysiological experiments suggest a presynaptic site of action for XLIII and XXX in the ganglion. More specifically, an effect on those processes concerned with synthesis and/ or release of transmitter into the synaptic cleft is indicated. Of these two possibilities, an effect on transmitter synthesis is suggested by the fact that the development of the block in ganglia treated with either inhibitor was highly dependent upon the frequency of presynaptic stimulation. Stimulation at 5 Hz for 70 minutes had no effect on synaptic transmission, whereas stimulation at 30 Hz always produced a block in 30-70 minutes. This implies that exhaustive presynaptic stimulation, and the accompanying release of presynaptic stores of transmitter, are necessary prerequisites for the development of synaptic blockade. Shankland et al. (1971) have shown that similar conditions of stimulation are necessary to produce a block in ganglia treated with hemicholinium-3, which indirectly inhibits acetylcholine synthesis by preventing the resorption of choline into the pre-synaptic terminals. On the other hand, conditions which produce a synaptic block by inhibiting transmitter release, such as high Mg^{++}, low Ca^{++} saline, do not show such a dramatic dependence on presynaptic stimulation.

Although neurophysiological evidence is consistent with the hypothesis that inhibition of acetylcholine synthesis is a significant factor in the synaptic blockade induced by the maleimide and hydantoin compounds, the situation with respect to the phenyl thioacetate group of inhibitors appears to be much

Table 5

Structure	I_{50}	Recovery Time (Minutes)	Nicotine Response 10^{-5} M
(I)	2×10^{-5} M	> 60 @ 1×10^{-4} M 14.6 @ 1×10^{-5} M	-*
(X)	$> 10^{-3}$ M	> 60 @ 1×10^{-5} M	-*
(LI)	$> 10^{-3}$ M	8.5 @ 9.6×10^{-5} M	+
(XLIII)	2×10^{-5} M	> 60 @ 1×10^{-5} M	+
(XLIV)	$> 10^{-3}$ M	> 60 @ 10^{-4} M	+

Table 5 (Contd.)

Structure	I_{50}	Recovery Time (Minutes)	Nicotine Response 10^{-5} M
(XXX)	5×10^{-4} M	> 60 @ 2×10^{-6} M	+
(XXXII)	$> 10^{-3}$ M	8.0 @ 5×10^{-6} M	+

* The response to nicotine of ganglia blocked by I and X was negative when the entire nerve cord preparation was bathed in the inhibitor. When inhibitor was applied selectively to the ganglionic region under mannitol-gap recording conditions, the response to nicotine was positive.

more complex. As shown in Table 5, there is no consistent correlation between enzyme inhibitory activity and effects on the ganglion. Compound X, which was inactive on the enzyme, was better than the active analog I in preventing the recovery of synaptic transmission. Furthermore, although both compounds produced synaptic blockade, they also antagonized the response of the ganglion to nicotine. These results suggest that the block may involve an effect on the postsynaptic acetylcholine receptors. However, the situation is complicated by the fact that ganglia blocked by I or X applied selectively to the ganglionic region under mannitol-gap conditions showed a positive response to nicotine (Table 5). It is difficult to reconcile these conflicting results with different methods of drug application, except to postulate multiple sites of action for these compounds, one within the ganglion and another extraganglionic site. This hypothesis is also suggested by the dramatically different times required for a block to develop depending on the site of application of the compound. When the whole nerve preparation was

bathed in I, synaptic blockade occurred between one and four
minutes after stimulation was initiated, whereas it took between
20 and 40 minutes for the block to develop when I was applied only
to the region of the ganglion. In any event, the data do not
support inhibition of choline acetyltransferase as a site of
primary action for the phenyl thio acetate class of compounds.

In Vivo Toxicity

Since XLIII and XXX produced neurophysiological effects in
vitro which indicated that inhibition of acetylcholine synthesis
was a mode of primary action, they were tested for their ability
to induce similar symptoms in whole insects.

Cockroaches injected with 20 µg of XLIII or XXX in 0.5 µl of
acetone appeared normal during a nine-day period of observation.
Each day after injection nerve cord preparations were sampled from
each group and stimulated as described previously. These experiments were conducted in normal physiological saline so that any
effect on transmission was due to compound present in the
preparation at the time of sacrifice. Compound XLIII was effective
in preventing synaptic recovery between three and four days post-
injection (Figure 1). Compound XXX showed a similar, though less
dramatic, trend and in both cases the effect was reversible.

Insects injected with either inhibitor developed no symptoms
indicative of significant neurological impairment. However, nerve
cord preparations sampled from these same insects became blocked
when subjected to repetitive stimulation in vitro (Figure 1). The
implication is that, although sufficient inhibitor was present in
the nervous system to block transmission, the effect could only
develop under conditions of excessive transmitter release induced
by repetitive presynaptic stimulation. Therefore, even if acetylcholine synthesis was inhibited, either totally or partially
in vivo, it is possible that normal synaptic transmission was
sustained in the whole insect by an undepleted residual supply of
transmitter, in addition to any new transmitter that may have been
synthesized by a partially inhibited enzyme. If this hypothesis
is correct, then synaptic blockade and prostration should occur
in vivo if acetylcholine depletion could be significantly augmented
during choline acetyltransferase inhibition. One way to increase
transmitter turnover in vivo is to induce hyperactivity. Figure 2
shows the results of an experiment in which groups of cockroaches
were injected with 20 µg of XLIII and XXX in acetone and then
subjected to mechanical stimulation in a rotating jar. Although
this procedure induced significant mortality in the control group,
the effect occurred earlier and more dramatically in the groups
treated with the inhibitors. Furthermore, nerve cord preparations

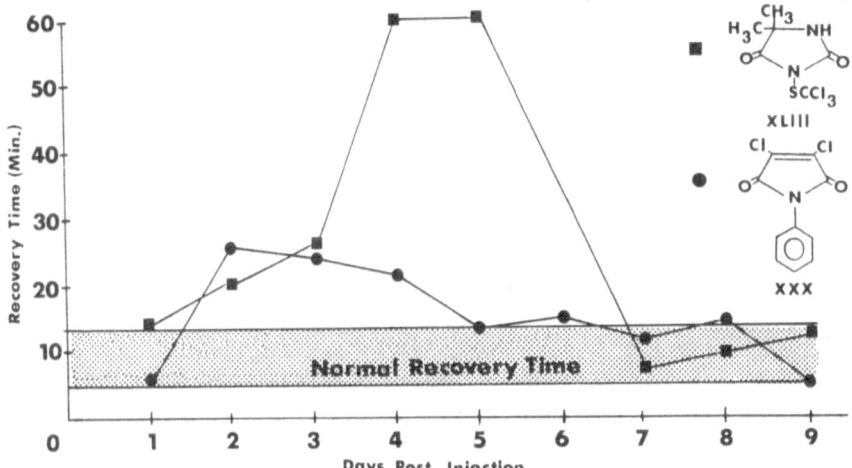

Figure 1. Nerve cord preparations sampled from cockroaches injected with 20 µg of XLIII failed to resume synaptic transmission following a period of induced post-tetanic depression at the cercal nerve-giant fiber synapse. The maximum effect occurred between 3 and 4 days post injection. Compound XXX showed a similar trend, although the effect was not as great. In both cases, the effect was reversible.

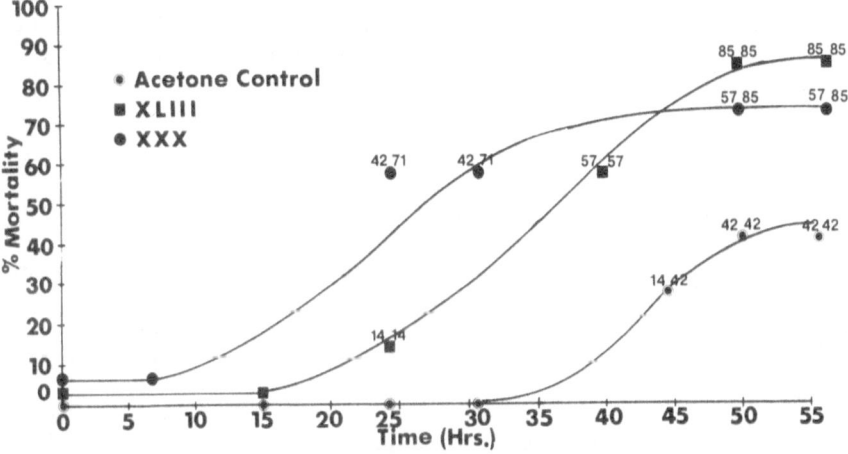

Figure 2. Cockroaches injected with 20 µg of compounds XXX or LVIII followed by periods of induced hyperactivity showed earlier and greater mortality than acetone controls. Each point represents the average of 2 replicates whose individual values are indicated at the corresponding point. Cockroaches injected with inhibitors or acetone only and not stressed showed no mortality.

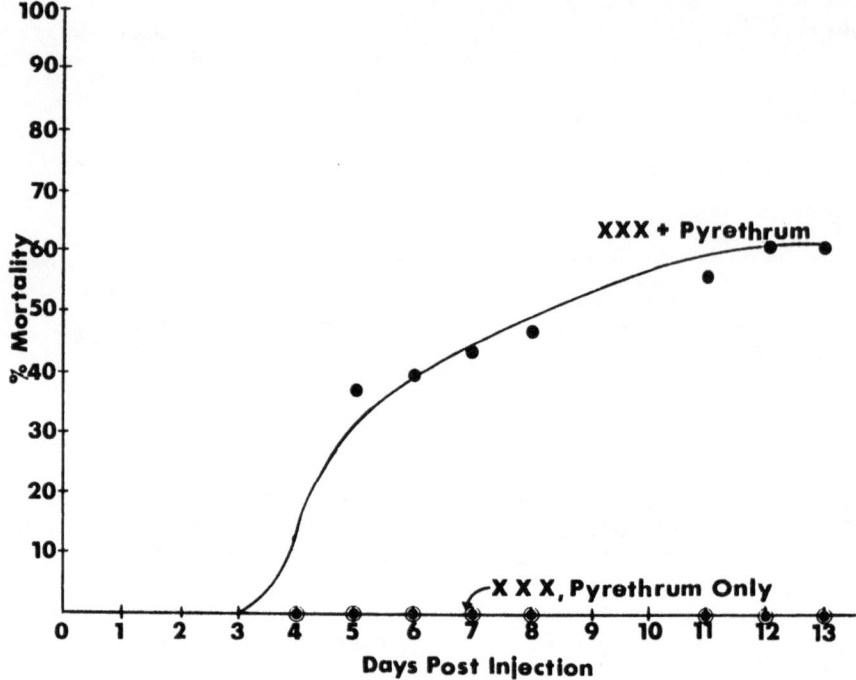

Figure 3.   Cockroaches injected with 20 µg of compound XXX followed
daily by sublethal, topical doses (0.3 µg) of natural pyrethrum
showed an apparent synergistic interaction.   Cockroaches injected
with XXX or treated daily with topical doses of pyrethrum only
showed no mortality.

sampled from prostrate roaches in the treated groups showed
either a complete blockade of the synaptic transmission or a
highly variable response to even low-frequency (1/sec) presynaptic
stimulation, which rapidly culminated in a blockade.   Separate
control groups injected with inhibitors and not subject to
mechanical stimulation showed no mortality or aberrant synaptic
transmission.

This experiment was given more practical significance in a
test in which groups of cockroaches were injected with a sublethal
dose of XXX followed daily by topical, sublethal applications of
natural pyrethrum (20 µg in acetone).   An apparent synergistic
interaction between XXX and pyrethrum is evident in which the
combination treatment induced 61% mortality after 12 days, whereas
XXX or pyrethrum alone was not toxic (Figure 3).

Assuming that choline acetyltransferase was at least partially inhibited by XXX or XLIII, it is evident from these in vivo experiments that the effect does not, by itself, constitute a lethal lesion. When used in combination with agents that induce neural hyperactivity, however, the inhibitor may act to intensify the effects of the hyperactive agent.

CONCLUSIONS

The ultimate purpose of this study was to identify novel inhibitors of insect choline acetyltransferase and assess their potential as practical insect control agents. The first goal has essentially been realized. Three new classes of compounds were found which showed significant inhibitory activity against house fly choline acetyltransferase. Neurophysiological experiments tend to confirm the hypothesis that, at least for two of the groups, enzyme inhibition is a significant factor in their mode of action. The second goal, that of practical utility, remains to be demonstrated. The data presented in this paper indicate that enzyme inhibition is, by itself, insufficient to induce significant mortality. A potential role for inhibitors as synergists, when used in combination with agents that induce neural hyperactivity, such as conventional insecticides, remains to be explored. This study lends credence to that possibility. When viewed in this context, it is conceivable that an active inhibitor with sufficient species specificity and field stability could become an important component in a strategy of integrated pest management by reducing the amount of insecticide used to provide an adequate control program.

REFERENCES

Baillie, A. C., Corbett, J. R., Dowsett, J. R., Sattelle, D. B., and Callec, J. J., 1975, Inhibitors of choline acetyltransferase as potential insecticides, Pestic. Sci. 6:645.

Boccacci, M., Natalizi, G., and Bettini, S., 1960, Research on the mode of action of halogen containing thiol alkylating agents on insects. Effect of iodoacetic acid on choline acetylase, J. Ins. Physiol. 4:20.

Callec, J-J., 1974, Synaptic transmission in the central nervous system of insects, in: Insect Neurobiology (J. E. Treherne, ed.), pp. 119-185, North-Holland Publishing Co., Amsterdam.

Callec, J-J., and Sattelle, D. B., 1973, A simple technique for monitoring the synaptic actions of pharmacological agents, J. Exp. Biol. 59:725.

Chadwick, L. E., 1963, Systematic pharmacology of the anti-cholinesterase agents. Actions on insects and other invertebrates, in: Handbuch der Experimentellen Pharmakologie, (G. B. Koelle, ed.), pp. 741-798, Springer-Verlag, Berlin.

Flattum, R. F., and Shankland, D. L., 1971, Acetylcholine receptors and the diphasic action of nicotine in the American cockroach, Periplaneta americana (L.), Comp. Bioc. Physiol. 2:159.

Florey, E., and Kreibel, M. E., 1966, A new suction electrode system, Comp. Bioc. Physiol. 18:175.

Gerschenfeld, H. M., 1973, Chemical transmission in invertebrate central nervous systems and neuromuscular junctions, Physiol. Rev. 53:1.

Guthrie, D. M., and Tindall, A. R., 1968, The Biology of the Cockroach, St. Martin's Press, New York.

MacIntosh, F. C., 1961, Effect of HC-3 on acetylcholine turnover, Fed. Proc. 20:262.

Mehrotra, K. N., 1961, Properties of choline acetylase from the house fly, Musca domestica (L.), J. Ins. Physiol. 6:215.

Mehrotra, K. N., and Dauterman, W. C., 1963, The N-alkyl group specificity of choline acetylase from the house fly, Musca domestica L., and the two-spotted spider mite, Tetranychus telarius L., J. Ins. Physiol. 9:293.

O'Brien, R. D., 1967, Insecticides, Action and Metabolism, Academic Press, New York.

Shankland, D. L., Rose, J. A., and Donniger, C., 1971, The cholinergic nature of the cercal nerve-giant fiber synapse in the sixth abdominal ganglion of the American cockroach, Periplaneta americana (L.), J. Neurobiol. 2:247.

Yamasaki, T., and Narahashi, T., 1959, The effects of potassium and sodium ions on the resting and action potentials of the cockroach giant axons, J. Ins. Physiol. 3:146.

Yu, C-C, and Booth, G. M., 1971, Inhibition of choline acetylase from the house fly (Musca domestica L.) and mouse, Life Sci. II,110:337.

INSECTICIDE-INDUCED RELEASE OF NEUROSECRETORY HORMONES

Manthri Samaranayaka-Ramasamy

Department of Zoology, University of Cambridge, U.K.

Present Address: College of Medicine, King Faisal
        University, P.O. Box 2114, Dammam, Saudi Arabia

The nervous system is the primary site of action of most
insecticides. However, it is possible that the initial nervous
impairment is insufficient to kill an insect. Damage to the
nervous system is followed by other changes and the latter may
have lethal consequences. Spiller (1955) and Jochum (1956)
studying the way in which insecticides kill insects have implicated a chain of events following the initial attack on the
nervous system.

In insects as in other animals the central nervous system is
closely linked with other organ systems, in particular the neuroendocrine (neurohaemal) organs. For example, in the desert locust
Schistocerca gregaria, the principal neurohaemal organ the corpus
cardiacum is in close association with the central nervous system
(Highnam, 1961). Therefore, it is very likely that when insecticides affect the nervous system, there are changes in the normal
flow of information from the brain to the corpus cardiacum; i.e.
it will disrupt the normal feed-forward and feed-back control
systems that exist in the insect, thereby interfering with the
normal transfer of information. Hormone release will be affected
and this would eventually disturb the normal physiological and
biochemical activities in the insect. In a review on the mode of
action of insecticides, Roan and Hopkins (1961) conclude that
"...many of the symptoms of insecticide poisoning appear to be
very similar to those produced by neuroendocrine material; this
suggests a relationship between the two."

Neurosecretory control systems in insects have been well investigated. Most neurosecretory materials act as hormones and are
important in the life of insects (Goldsworthy and Mordue 1974;

83

Maddrell, 1974). For instance, the hormone implicated in the
control of urine formation in insects (Maddrell, 1966; Mordue, 1969)
are products of neurosecretory cells in the central nervous system.
The intrinsic neurosecretory cells of the glandular lobes of the
corpus cardiacum of locusts produce the peptidergic adipokinetic
hormone (Goldsworthy et al. 1972b) and one of the hyperglycaemic
peptides (Mordue and Goldsworthy, 1969). The hyperglycaemic hormone of Periplaneta americana is also found in the corpus cardiacum
(Steele, 1961). Information from the brain via the nerves connec-
ting the brain to the corpus cardiacum is necessary for the normal
release of adipokinetic and hyperglycaemic hormones (Goldsworthy
et al. 1972a; Gersch, 1974). Hence, the primary effect of insecticides on the central nervous system will have consequences on the
releasing mechanisms of the corpus cardiacum.

Effective insecticide treatment of insects nearly always lead
to the expression of symptoms of poisoning which are manifested as
changes in behavior. It is also known that abnormal physiological
events occur in the insect at the time when behavioral changes are
observed.

The fat body is the primary storage organ in insects. It also
acts as the major metabolic centre and contains large reserves of
glycogen and fats (Tietz, 1967). Changes in storage levels of carbohydrates and fats are associated with neurosecretory hormones.
The hyperglycaemic hormone has a strong glycogenolytic action on
the fat body, this effect being due to its ability to increase the
activity of the enzyme phosphorylase (Steele, 1963; Goldsworthy,
1970). When carbohydrate levels in poisoned Schistocerca were estimated, it was observed that the glycogen content in the fat body
showed an almost ten fold decrease compared to non-poisoned insects
(Table 1). In a rather similar way, the total haemolymph carbohydrate also showed a significant decrease at early prostration as
shown in Table 2. These abnormal levels of fat body glycogen and
blood carbohydrates of poisoned Schistocerca suggest the release of
the hyperglycaemic hormone during poisoning (Samaranayaka, 1974).

Early work on the effects of DDT (Merrill et al. 1946; Ludwig,
1946) showed that the glycogen and glucose content of insects decreased during poisoning. These authors did not correlate these
effects with neurosecretions. More recently, however, Granett and
Leeling (1972) made similar observations on Periplaneta americana
and they suggested that the changes were probably associated with
the release of a hyperglycaemic factor.

Table 1. Changes in fat body glycogen with time on poisoning with 500 $\mu g\ g^{-1}$ 5 μl^{-1} lindane. (Insecticide applied topically).

	2.5 hours (tremors)	5 hours (hyperactivity)	15 hours (late prostration)
Poisoned:	16.53 ± 4.61(8)	24.87± 8.53(6)	1.69 ± 0.53(8)
Controls:	28.53 ± 5.93(8)	17.99± 4.77(6)	10.07 ± 1.84(8)
	N.S.	N.S.	$p < 0.001$

Values are mean micrograms of glycogen per milligram wet weight ± standard error (S.E.) of the mean. The number of determinations is given in parentheses. Significance in this experiment and in all subsequent experiments was determined by the Student's 't' test.

Table 2. Effect of 500 $\mu g\ g^{-1}$ 5 μl^{-1} lindane on total carbohydrate (anthrone positive material) in the haemolymph.

Expt. 1. Hyperactivity

	Control	Test
Before treatment	371.2 ± 33.85	366.0 ± 30.14
After treatment	457.2 ± 28.19 (5) N.S.	439.6 ± 30.17 (5) N.S.

Expt. 2. Early prostration

	Control	Test
Before treatment	382.33 ± 28.84	355.67 ± 36.78
After treatment	338.67 ± 39.24 (5) N.S.	117.33 ± 32.12 (5) $p < 0.001$

Results are mean micrograms of total anthrone positive material in 5 μl of haemolymph ± S.E. The number of determinations is given in parentheses.

Normally, the adipokinetic hormone of Schistocerca is released from the glandular lobes of the corpus cardiacum at the
onset of flight and it elevates the diglyceride content in the
haemolymph (Mayer and Candy, 1969; Goldsworthy et al. 1972a and b).
When Schistocerca was poisoned with insecticides the blood lipid
level was markedly increased (Table 3). Lipid content in poisoned
Schistocerca begins to rise at the early stages of prostration;
the bulk of this lipid was shown to be diglyceride (Samaranayaka,
1974). Therefore, it was inferred that the increase in blood
lipid in poisoned insects was due to the release of the adipokinetic hormone.

Table 3. Changes in haemolymph lipid at early prostration.

Insecticide	Before treatment	After treatment	% Change	Significance of change
1. Diazinon(7)	4.95 ± 0.93:	9.58±1.90:	+89.54± 10.9	$p < 0.05$
2. DDVP(9)	4.41 ± 0.45:	12.4±2.11:	+173.1± 28.8	$p < 0.01$
3. Baythion(8)	4.23 ± 0.47:	12.2±0.82:	+202.8± 26.7	$p < 0.001$
4. NRDC 107(7)	5.91 ± 0.47:	10.8±1.48:	+80.53± 16.7	$p < 0.01$
5. NRDC 119(6)	5.22 ± 0.30:	13.9±1.46:	+168.2± 31.2	$p < 0.001$
6. Zectran(8)	3.97 ± 0.38:	11.8±0.89:	+224.3± 47.2	$p < 0.001$
7. Control(9) (acetone)	5.40 ± 0.37:	5.2 ±0.36:	-3.4 ± 5.64	N.S.

Insecticides 1-3 are organophosphates - and Baythion is an
emulsifiable concentrate containing 500 g l^{-1} phoxim. 4-5 are
pyrethroids and 6 is a carbamate. The figures given are for mg.
lipid/cm^3 haemolymph and are expressed as the mean ± S.E. The
number of determinations is given in parentheses.

Results of Tables 1-3 suggest that the hyperglycaemic and
adipokinetic hormones are released after poisoning. If this is
indeed the case, then decapitation ought to prevent such release
by removing the corpora cardiaca which are the release sites for
these hormones. In a series of experiments Schistocerca were decapitated before treatment with 500 µg g $^{-1}$ 5 µl^{-1} of lindane
(Samaranayaka, 1974). There was a significant difference (p<0.001)

between the fat body glycogen content of decapitated poisoned insects (12.0 ± 2.0 µg mg^{-1} glycogen) and intact poisoned insects
(3.0 ± 1.0 µg mg^{-1} glycogen). Similarly, decapitated poisoned
insects showed only a very slight elevation in blood lipid (44.1 ±
19.1%) compared to intact lindane poisoned insects (223.9 ± 37.3%).
The percentage change in blood lipid in the two groups of insects
is highly significant (p<0.001). There is no evidence of hormone
release in decapitated poisoned insects and this demonstrates that
hyperglycaemic and adipokinetic hormones are released from their
natural release sites (corpus cardiacum) on poisoning.

When normal insects are injected with hormone extract, its
effect lasts for sometime,after which metabolic levels return to
normal values (Goldsworthy, 1970: Goldsworthy et al. 1972b). In
insecticide poisoning however, metabolic levels never return to
normal values. If hormones which are released on poisoning are
inactivated or excreted (as would normally happen), then metabolites should return to original levels. The persistance of abnormal amounts of carbohydrates and lipids could be due to two
reasons. Either hormones are released initially in quantities
much larger than those released under normal physiological conditions, or, hormones are continually released due to the breakdown
of internal control mechanisms.

Multiple neurohormone release during poisoning has been demonstrated in Rhodnius prolixus (Maddrell and Reynolds, 1972). Insecticides induce the release of the diuretic hormone and the plas-
ticizing factor in Rhodnius during the paralytic stage of poisoning, by the same pathways used in the natural release of these substances. In Schistocerca, at least two metabolic hormones - hyperglycaemic and adipokinetic hormones are released in a similar way
and the release of adipokinetic hormone starts at the early stages
of poisoning (Samaranayaka, 1974).

However, these may not be the only hormones released in abnormal quantities. Other hormones could well be released. For
instance, in poisoned Schistocerca there is a massive movement of
fluid into the anterior region of the gut. It is not known if
water flow into the gut is under hormonal control. If such control exists in Schistocerca however, it is very likely that insecticide poisoning would produce the observed effects through
induced hormone release (Samaranayaka, 1977b).

Insecticide-induced hormone release from the corpus cardiacum
of Schistocerca has been studied at the ultrastructural level. The
glandular region of the gland contains electron dense granules.
Two types of granules can be identified, the larger with a diameter
of 1000-1300 A and the smaller granules range from 250-450 A. According to Knowles (1967), the larger granules are peptidergic and

the smaller granules are aminergic. Corpora cardiaca of Schistocerca were stimulated with insecticide and fixed in situ. Under
the electron microscope the larger granules showed characteristic
exocytotic profiles, indicating the release of their contents
(Normann and Samaranayaka - in preparation).

If hormone release is a general feature of insecticide
poisoning, then, is there a correlation between the primary or
principal site/mode of action of insecticides and its subsequent
effect of abnormal hormone release? For this, it is necessary to
know the mode of action of insecticides. The mode of action of
organophosphorus and carbamate insecticides is well documented;
they are anticholinesterases (Aldridge, 1971) and the persistance
of acetylcholine in the synapse prolongs the excitatory post synaptic potential - eventually blocking nervous transmission (Narahashi,
1971). Organophophates induce the release of adipokinetic hormone
(Table 3). In vitro and in vivo studies using acetlycholine, cholinergic antagonists and agonists (Samaranayaka, 1977a) have shown
that the synaptic build up of the cholinergic transmitter (acetylcholine) initiates the events leading to organophosphate-induced
release of adipokinetic hormone. These synapses are present in the
brain-corpus cardiacum complex of Schistocerca.

The corpus cardiacum of Schistocerca also has varicose fibres
containing dopamine and 5-HT alternating with neurosecretory fibres
(Klemm, 1971). Adipokinetic hormone release induced by anticholinesterases is significantly reduced by depleting the content of
monoamines in the nervous system using reserpine (Samaranayaka,
1976). Depletion initially occurs in the fibres (Frontali, 1968).
Therefore, in Schistocerca depletion of monoamines may well com-
mence in the aminergic fibres of the corpus cardiacum, and it is
these fibres that are in close association with neurosecretory
fibres. Pharmacological studies show that monoamines participate
in the pathway of release of adipokinetic hormone. The receptor
for the aminergic transmitter/transmitters is a composite dopamine/
5-HT receptor (Samaranayaka, 1976).

From these studies it is possible to work out the sequence of
events leading to anticholinesterase insecticide-induced release of
adipokinetic hormone. The primary site of action is the cholinergic
synapse in the brain-corpus cardiacum complex where acetylcholine
receptors have nicotinic and muscarinic properties (Samaranayaka,
1977a). Activation of these receptors leads to the stimulation of
aminergic fibres which innervate the corpus cardiacum. The aminergic transmitter brings about the release of adipokinetic hormone
from the corpus cardiacum neurosecretory cells by exocytosis.

Several metabolic pathways for hormones exist in insects.
Their homeostasis depends upon the integrated function and communication within the various components of the pathways. Dysfunctions

and breakdowns result when communication in either direction fails. This may well happen in insecticide-induced hormone release.

Symptoms of insecticide poisoning can be interpreted as disruptions of the nervous system followed by disorders of various other tissues. The immediate symptoms of poisoning are not necessarily the prime cause of death of the insect. Many functions in insects are not centralized, and therefore, it is unlikely that death is caused by the disturbance of just one organ or system; it seems that insecticides have complicated multiple actions which can exert a cumulative effect. Multiple neurohormone release is not the only effect of poisoning. Among others, the amount of water and the ionic composition of the haemolymph is altered (Samaranayaka, 1977b). Many processes so far not investigated could also exhibit abnormalities which can be harmful to the insect. Therefore, we can predict a multicomponent scheme of insecticide action. Figure 1 illustrates a possible mechanism for such a scheme as it operates in Schistocerca. It should be emphasized that which component or different combinations of components predominate in a scheme like this will depend on the nature of the insecticide, the physiology and physiological state of the insect and the environmental stresses imposed upon it at the time of poisoning.

It has been reported by several workers including Sternburg and Kearns (1952), Shankland and Kearns (1959) and Sternburg (1963) that hyperactivity caused by insecticides liberated a toxin or toxins into the haemolymph. Sternburg (1963) states "...excessive stress on insects can lead to the release of pharmacologically active substances. ...active compounds liberated during stress must presumably have a normal function... . However, when released in greater than normal amounts as a result of intensive stress, some of these active substances appear to lead to either abnormal behavioral characteristics or even paralysis and death." Sternburg concludes that"...stress in chemical poisoning presumably originates at the primary target of the insecticide, and the abnormal release of pharmacologically active substances would seem to be secondary, although they may subsequently enter into the sequence of events leading to death. The close resemblance of stress paralysis to insecticidal prostration suggests that the most advanced symptoms of poisoning may be related to abnormal concentrations of physiologically active substances. Hormonal release normally must be precise in quantity and time; abnormal release may cause profound pathological and physiological consequences."

Hormones are vital for the life of insects. Many of these are peptides (Mordue and Goldsworthy, 1969; Mayer and Candy, 1969; Aston and White, 1974) and studies on the structures of hormones are still at an early stage. However, the adipokinetic hormone of the locust has been purified and identified (Stone et al. 1976). When

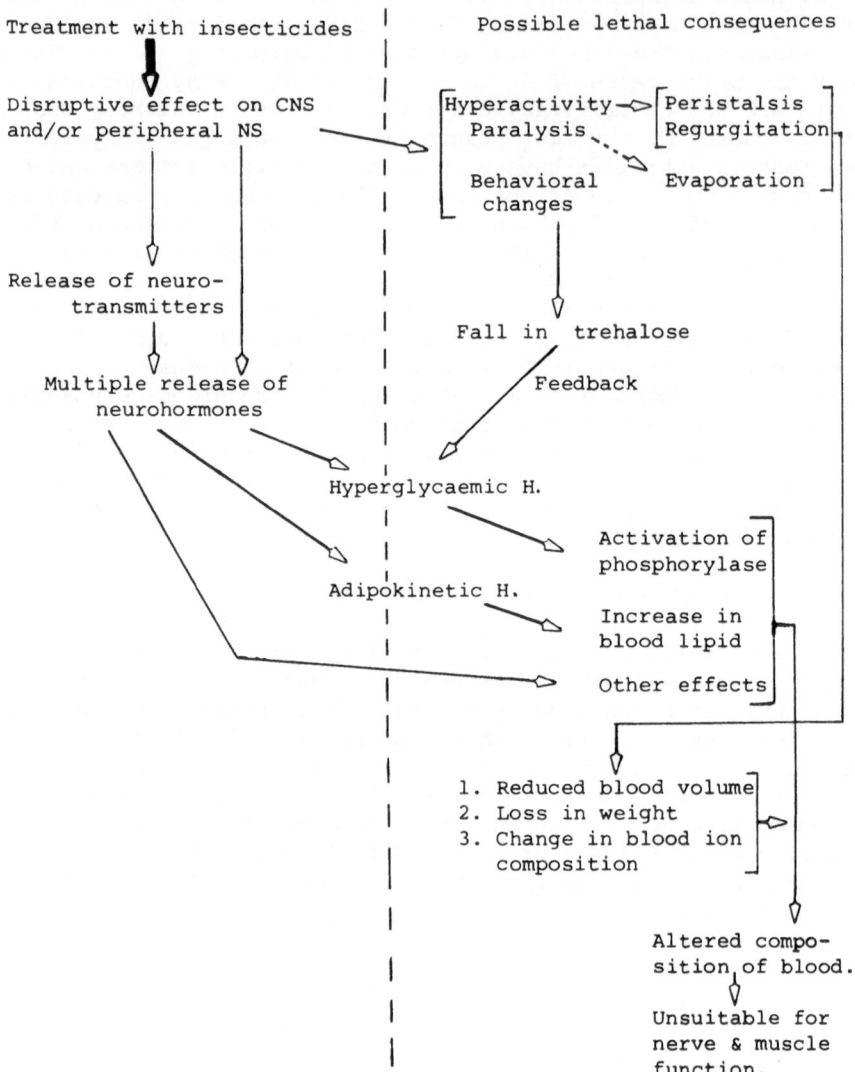

Figure 1.   Probable chain of events following treatment with
            insecticides and their consequences on the insect.

structures of insect hormones are known, the possibility exists that hormones or their synthetic analogues may be used in a manner similar to juvenile hormone analogues.

Detailed investigations on the mechanisms by which hormones are released has implications for the development of new compounds which will be potent in affecting the hormonal balance in insects. Until such time as the nature of insect hormones is known and the neuropharmacology of insects is better understood, the attractive prospect of using many insect hormones and their analogues as insecticides on the same scale as the conventional poisons will remain a theoretical plan. Even then, it remains to be seen whether the idea is economically feasible.

REFERENCES

Aldridge, W.N., 1971, The nature of the reaction of organophosphorus compounds and carbamates with esterases. Alternative Insecticides for Vector Control. Bull. Wld. Hlth. Org. 44:25.

Aston, R.J., and White, A.F., 1974, Isolation and purification of the diuretic hormone from Rhodnius prolixus, J. Insect Physiol. 20:1673.

Frontali, N., 1968, Histochemical localization of catecholamines in the brain of normal and drug treated cockroaches, J. Insect Physiol. 14:881.

Gersch, M., 1974, Selektive Freisetzung des hyperglykamischen Faktors aus den corpora cardiaca von Periplaneta americana in vivo, Experientia 30:767.

Goldsworthy, G.J., 1970, The action of hyperglycaemic factors from the corpus cardiacum of Locusta migratoria on glycogen phosphorylase. Gen Comp. Endocr. 14:78.

Goldsworthy, G.J., Johnson, R.A., and Mordue, W., 1972a, In vivo studies on the release of hormones from the corpora cardiaca of locusts. J. Comp. Physiol. 79:85.

Goldsworthy, G.J., Morude, W., and Guthkelch, J., 1972b, Studies on insect adipokinetic hormones, Gen Comp. Endocr. 18:545.

Goldsworthy, G.J., and Mordue, W., 1974, Neurosecretory hormones in insects, J. Endocr. 60:529.

Granett, J., and Leeling, N.C., 1972, A hyperglycaemic agent in the serum of DDT prostrate American cockroaches, Periplaneta americana, Ann. Entomol. Soc. Amer. 65:299.

Highnam, K.C., 1961, The histology of the neurosecretory system of the adult female desert locust Schistocerca gregaria, Q. J. Microsc. Sci. 102:27.

Jochum, F., 1956, Changes in the reaction chains in the insect organism caused by diethyl-p-nitrophenylthiophosphate, Hofchen-Briefe 9:289.

Klemm, N., 1971, Monoaminhaltige Zellelemente im stomatogastrischen Nervensystem und in corpora cardiaca von Schistocerca gregaria Forsk (Insecta, Orthoptera), Z. Naturforsch. 26b:1085.

Knowles, F.G.W., 1967, Neuronal properties of neurosecretory cells, in: Neurosecretion (F. Stutinsky ed.), pp 8-19, Springer-Verlag, Berlin, Heidelberg, New York.

Ludwig, D., 1946, The effect of DDT on the metabolism of the Japanese beetle, Popillia japonica. Newman, Ann. Entomol. Soc. Amer. 39:496.

Maddrell, S.H.P., 1966, The site of release of the diuretic hormone in Rhodnius - a new neurohaemal system in insects. J. Exp. Biol. 45:499.

Maddrell, S.H.P., 1974, Neurosecretion, in: Insect Neurobiology (J.E. Treherne ed.) pp. 306-357, North Holland, Amsterdam.

Maddrell, S.H.P., and Reynolds, S.E., 1972, Release of hormones in insects after poisoning with insecticides, Nature 236:404.

Mayer, R.J., and Candy, D.J., 1969, Control haemolymph lipid concentration during locust flight-an adipokinetic hormone from the corpus cardiacum, J. Insect Physiol. 15:611.

Merrill, R.S., Savit, J., and Tobias, J.M., 1946, Certain biochemical changes in DDT poisoned cockroach and their prevention by prolonged anesthesia, J. Cell. Comp. Physiol. 28:465.

Mordue, W., 1969, Hormonal control of Malpighian tube and rectal function in the desert locust, Schistocerca gregaria, J. Insect Physiol. 15:273.

Mordue, W., and Goldsworthy, G.J., 1969, The physiological effects of corpus cardiacum extracts in locusts, Gen. Comp. Endocr. 12:360.

Narahashi, T., 1971, Effects of insecticides on excitable tissues, in: Advances in Insect Physiology (J.W.L. Beament, J.E. Treherne and V.B. Wigglesworth eds.)8:1 Academic Press, New York.

Roan, C.C., and Hopkins, T.L., 1961, Mode of action of insecticides, Ann. Rev. Entomol. 6:333.

Samaranayaka, M., 1974, Insecticide-induced release of hyperglycaemic and adipokinetic hormones of Schistocerca gregaria, Gen. Comp. Endocr. 24:424.

Samaranayaka, M., 1976, Possible involvement of monoamines in the release of adipokinetic hormone in the locust Schistocerca gregaria, J. Exp. Biol. 65:415.

Samaranayaka, M., 1977a, Role of acetylcholine in organophosphate-induced release of adipokinetic hormone in the locust Schistocerca gregaria, Pestic. Biochem. Physiol. (in press).

Samaranayaka, M., 1977b, The effect of insecticides on osmotic and ionic balance in the locust Schistocerca gregaria, Pestic. Biochem. Physiol. (in press).

Shankland, D.L., and Kearns, C.W., 1959, Characteristics of blood toxins in DDT-poisoned cockroaches, Ann. Entomol. Soc. Amer. 52:386.

Spiller, D., 1955, Effects of the insecticide DDT on the physiology of an insect, Rhodnius prolixus, Ph.D. Thesis, University of Cambridge.

Steele, J.E., 1961, Occurence of a hyperglycaemic factor in the
    corpus cardiacum of an insect, Nature 192:680.
Steele, J.E., 1963, The site of action of the insect hyperglycaemic
    hormone, Gen. Comp. Endocr. 3:46.
Sternburg, J., 1963, Autointoxication and some stress phenomena,
    Ann. Rev. Entomol. 8:19.
Sternburg, J., and Kearns, C.W., 1952, The presence of toxins other
    than DDT in the blood of DDT-poisoned roaches, Science 116:144.
Stone, J.V., Mordue, W., Batley, K.E., and Howard, R.M., 1976,
    Structure of locust adipokinetic hormone, a neurohormone that
    regulates lipid utilisation during flight, Nature 263:207.
Tietz, A., 1967, Fat transport in the locust: the role of digly-
    cerides, Eur. J. Biochem. 2:236.

THE INSECT NEUROMUSCULAR SYSTEM AS A SITE OF INSECTICIDE ACTION

T. A. Miller

Department of Entomology

University of California, Riverside, CA   92521

INTRODUCTION

It has been known for some time that the insect skeletal
(somatic) neuromuscular junction is different from vertebrate
neuromuscular junction in terms of underlying neurochemistry and
therefore responds to a completely different array of compounds.
Because of its promise as a model site of action, around which it
might be possible to develop selective insecticides, the insect
nerve-muscle synapse has attracted considerable interest over the
past 12 years.

There are a large number of different types of nerve-muscle
synapses in insects. The more familiar synapses are those of the
fast, slow and inhibitory units which have been described for
locust and cockroach skeletal muscles including fibrillar flight
muscles. The remaining types of nerve-muscle synapses are found
mainly in the visceral, cardiac and hyperneural muscle systems and
may be referred to collectively as visceral neuromuscular junctions.

Excitatory Nerve-Muscle Synapses

Of all of the insect nerve-muscle synapses, those which convey
excitation to ambulatory muscles have received the largest amount
of attention in basic physiological and toxicological research.
Several recent reviews give a fairly accurate picture of what has
been learned about the action of agents on the insect skeletal
nerve-muscle synapse (McDonald, 1975; Usherwood and Cull-Candy,
1975; Usherwood, 1974; Smyth *et al.*, 1973; Gerschenfeld, 1973).

From a toxicological standpoint, there have been two major
problems or stumbling blocks to the development of the excitatory
skeletal synapse as a site of action for insecticides. The first
comes with the suggestion that L-glutamate is the neurotransmitter
and the second is the handicap inherent in the lack of a variety
of drugs which act as agonists or antagonists to transmission.

The blood glutamate paradox. Since glutamate was first proposed as an arthropod neuromuscular transmitter, an explanation has
been sought for the apparent paradox of the presence of extremely
large amounts of glutamate in the blood of insects, while the perfusion of similar concentrations of glutamate reportedly causes
tetanic contractions in isolated muscle preparations.

The presence of glutamate in insect blood has been checked and
rechecked by several different groups who admit a difficulty in
separating glutamate and glutamine. However, literature values
reported are 0.7 m$\underline{M}$ (Stevens, 1961), 0.27 m$\underline{M}$ (Evans, 1975) and
about 2.3% or 1 m$\underline{M}$ glutamate in whole blood of *Periplaneta
americana* (Osborne and Neuhoff, 1974). So all of these values for
American cockroach blood list the amount of glutamate at somewhere
around millimolar or slightly less.

Contrast the values of glutamate present in the blood with the
responses reported for perfusion of glutamate over isolated muscle
preparations: Various reports claim a threshold for response to
bath applied glutamate somewhere above $10^{-12}\underline{M}$ (Kerkut and Walker,
1966; Usherwood and Machili, 1968) which causes a slight potentiation of neurally-evoked contractions in locust or cockroach. In
locust retractor unguis muscle this is thought to be a presynaptic
action because the frequency but not amplitude of miniature postsynaptic potentials is increased (Dowson and Usherwood, 1972) and
the effects are reversed by high Mg (30 m$\underline{M}$) and low Ca (0.5 m$\underline{M}$).
Clements and May (1974a), however, reported no potentiation below
$10^{-6}\underline{M}$ glutamate in locust retractor unguis.

No contractile effect is seen in the perfused muscle preparation until concentrations of bath applied glutamate reach the
region of $10^{-6}\underline{M}$ or above (10^{-6} g/ml, Kerkut and Walker, 1966).
Between $10^{-7}\underline{M}$ and $10^{-3}\underline{M}$ concentrations of bath applied glutamate,
excitatory postsynaptic potentials (EPSP) increase amplitudes, then
at the highest concentrations, maximal contraction is attained
along with varying degrees of desensitization. Clements and May
(1974a) reported $4\times10^{-4}\underline{M}$ glutamate generally blocked neuromuscular
transmission completely in the isolated retractor unguis prepara-
tion from locusts.

Murdock and Chapman (1974) analyzed the blood of *Locusta
migratoria* for glutamate by a specific enzymic-fluorometric assay
method. They reported a blood concentration of about $0.7\times10^{-4}\underline{M}$

L-glutamate. They also reported a marked depolarization of the
membrane potential of extensor tibia muscle of *Locusta* when perfused with $1.5 \times 10^{-4}M$ glutamate. Since the threshold concentration
for depressing synaptic transmission by bath applied glutamate was
below the concentration of glutamate found in the blood, some form
of functional barrier was thought to exist.

Clements and May (1974a) reported blood glutamate in *Schisto-*
cerca gregaria adult males averaged $2.2 \times 10^{-4}M$, and complete block
of neuromuscular transmission was obtained for the retractor unguis
preparation upon perfusion of $4 \times 10^{-4}M$ glutamate.

The glutamate paradox, then, simply stated for cockroach or
locust is that while whole blood contains somewhat less than millimolar glutamate, when bath applied to nerve-muscle preparations,
this amount of glutamate causes contraction and desensitization.

Various attempts have been made to explain why live insects
are apparently insensitive to the presence of what to the synapse
is a massive and ever-present dose of a supposed neurotransmitter
molecule in their hemolymphs. Some workers claim various barriers
exist between blood and neuromuscular synapses; others have
suggested the blood glutamate is bound in a form which is unavail-
able for pharmacological responses; still others claim an efficient
uptake mechanism exists which reduces the concentration of glutamate near the actual synapses (cf. Usherwood, 1974; Clements and
May, 1974a; Murdock and Chapman, 1974).

Despite the fact that Clements and May (1974a) did find a significant difference in the response to glutamate of blood-bathed
muscles compared to saline-bathed locust muscles, the barrier
explanations for a lack of action of blood glutamate on excitatory
nerve-muscle synapses are unsatisfactory, especially for cockroach
or maggot muscle. To cite two examples: the hyperneural muscle of
American cockroach enters a sustained tetany in the presence of
bath applied $10^{-4}M$ glutamate, even though glutamate does not appear
to be acting as a neurotransmitter in this case (Miller and James,
1976). For another instance, the intersegmental muscle of maggot
is very sensitive to the presence of glutamate such that injection
of *Calliphora erythrocephala* or *Lucilia sericata* with glutamate
causes immediate paralysis (Irving *et al.*, 1976). The hyperneural
muscle is thin to the point of transparency and offers no anatomical structure which could function as a barrier. The maggot
muscle is reported to have a single enveloping sheath of sarco-
lemma without invagination, and all synaptic junctions are located
externally adjacent to the hemolymph and without glial covering.
Thus in these 2 cases, it is difficult to postulate a physiological
barrier which prevents glutamate from coming in contact with
synaptic membranes.

A novel explanation for the glutamate paradox is the report by Irving *et al.* (1976) that glutamate is virtually absent from the hemolymph of arthropods. These authors found that fresh hemolymph was without effect on muscles of *Lucilia sericata*, but aged *Lucilia* blood gained pharmacological activity in agreement with similar experiments performed on *Schistocerca gregaria* (Miller *et al.*, 1973). Amino acid analysis showed the presence of large amounts of glutamine in freshly drawn hemolymph samples of *Periplaneta americana* and the presence of glutamate in hemocytes; however, a gradual appearance of a glutamate peak in the hemoplasm component occurred only upon allowing the hemolymph sample to clot or age somehwat.

This result clearly contradicts a large number of published and unpublished studies which report substantial amounts of glutamate present. The explanation given by Irving *et al.* (1976) for the disparity in results cited the conversion of glutamine to glutamate brought about by handling, such as use of extremes of pH or extraction at room temperature, and improper correction for glutamate in hemocytes.

There appears to be some basis for the presence of mechanisms in insects for conversion of glutamate to glutamine. Murdock and Koidl (1972a,b) found a restriction to the passage of glutamate into the hemolymph when injected into the gut. They found a rapid conversion of glutamate to glutamine with appearance of glutamine in the hemocoel. They found a similar rapid formation of glutamine when glutamate was injected into the hemocoel of locusts, *Locusta migratoria*.

Holden (1974, personal communication, and Fig. 1) reported a half-life of 17 min for glutamate when injected into the hemocoel of *Periplaneta americana* and a half-life of 16 min for aspartate. Both aspartate and glutamate were removed rather rapidly compared to the other amino acids - alanine and proline (Fig. 1).

Uptake studies of quite a different sort, using autoradiography, have shown a preferential uptake of L-glutamate at the vicinity of the synaptic terminals. Salpeter and Faeder (1971) showed an accumulation of radiolabeled glutamate in the sheath cell area of neuromuscular junctions. Roger Botham (1976, personal communication) showed uptake of labeled glutamate near excitatory nerve-muscle synapses on the locust extensor tibia muscle. He also showed a lack of similar uptake patterns from applications of radiolabeled leucine.

The effect caused by injection of glutamate into insects varies depending on who you are talking to and which insect was used. Some say massive doses injected into cockroaches, *Periplaneta americana* or *Blattella germanica*, produce very little

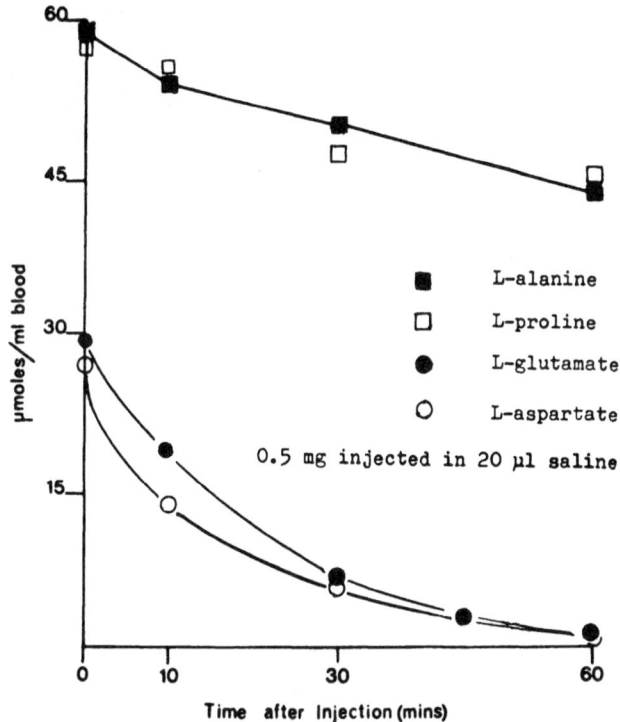

Fig. 1. Clearance of amino acids from the blood of the cockroach, *Periplaneta americana*. Reproduced with permission from Holden, 1974.

effect and no toxicity; others say blowfly larvae are paralyzed immediately by low doses, but recover eventually and blowfly adults are unaffected by low doses. Still others claim that locusts are paralyzed by injections of glutamate and others claim no effect (Clements and May, 1974a).

Neal (1975a,b) offers a possible explanation for differential effects caused by injection of glutamate. He examined the gluta-mate responses of three muscles from the fleshfly, *Sarcophaga bullata*. The metathoracic retractor unguis muscle was most suscep-tible to glutamate with the EPSP abolished after 2 min perfusion by 10^{-4} w/v. For the mesothoracic trochanteral depressor muscle, 10^{-4} w/v glutamate abolished neurally-evoked contractions in 4 min. 10^{-4} w/v glutamate perfused for 15 min onto the dorsolongitudinal flight muscles caused only a 10% reduction in the EPSP amplitude.

Thus, of the 3 muscles examined, the unguis had the most accessible synaptic sites and was most responsive to glutamate, while the fibrillar flight muscle with less accessible synaptic terminals was least susceptible to perfused glutamate.

When injected into tethered and flying *Lucilia sericata*, various putative neurotransmitters produced characteristic effects on the pattern of nerve impulses in the dorsolongitudinal flight motor units (for a discussion of the technique see Miller and Kennedy, 1972). Normal flight motor potentials recorded differentially from two muscles show an alternating pattern which is thought to be determined by central coordination (Fig. 2A).

A disruption in the central nervous system was caused by injection of 11 mM/kg of acetylcholine (Fig. 2B) or by 30 mM/kg of aminobutyric acid (GABA) (Fig. 2C). The effect was seen as a

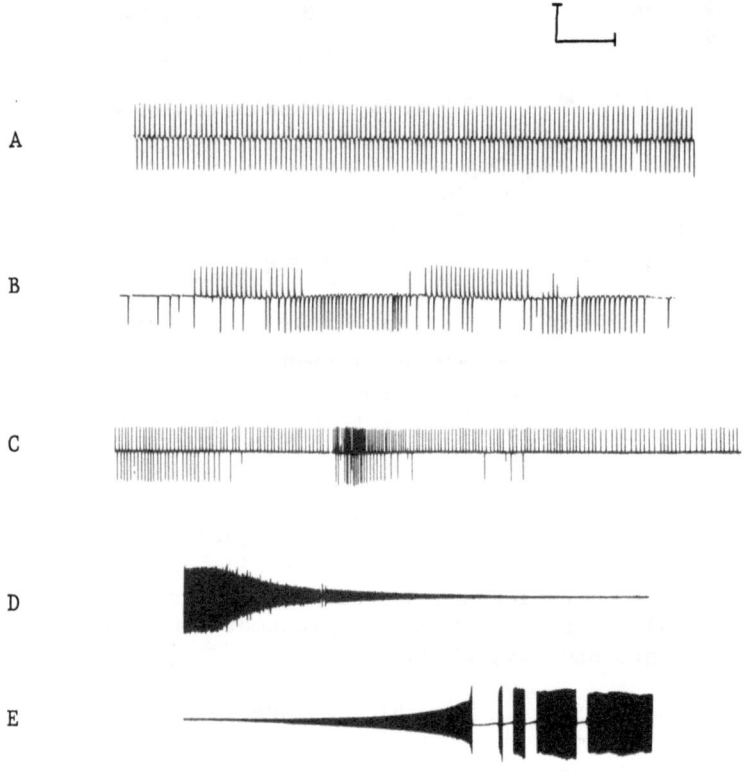

Fig. 2. Dorsolongitudinal flight muscle (DLM) potentials from adult male *Lucilia sericata* recorded during flight upon injection of putative neurotransmitters. A, control trace of activity from dorsal-most pair of DLM recorded differentially; right DLM downward deflection, left DLM upward potentials. B, following injection of 60 μg acetylcholine; C, 51 μg γ-aminobutyric acid; D and E, 12 μg glutamate. Calibration vertical: 50 mv, horizontal: A and C, 5 sec; B, 1 sec; D and E, 1 min. Reproduced with permission from R. J. Hart, Wellcome Research Laboratories, Berkhamsted, Herts., England.

reversible loss of coordination between the 2 flight motor potentials, termed uncoupling (Miller and Kennedy, 1972). Both acetylcholine and GABA are thought to act on the central nervous system
causing excitation, but to be relatively inert, requiring moderately high concentrations to produce convulsions.

Injection of between 0.4 and 6 mM/kg of L-glutamate into
Lucilia sericata caused a completely different response (Fig. 2D
and E). Instead of a loss in coordination, the muscle potentials
were reversibly decreased in amplitude starting about 1 min after
injection. The effect lasted from 4 to 200 min. It was accompanied by complete paralysis and was followed by gradual recovery
and recommencement of flight. The traces appear as a solid black
line because they were recorded at slow speed (Fig. 2D and E).
Injections of more than 6 mM/kg glutamate were lethal. Thus,
injections of compounds into flying *Lucilia* caused responses
similar to those reported by Neal for *Sarcophaga* in terms of EPSP
amplitude depression.

Since *Lucilia* weigh between 24 and 38 mg, a dose of glutamate
of 0.4 mg/g means injection of 12 μg on the average. With perfect
mixing, this would mean a concentration of about 1 g/1 or 6.8 mM
assuming a blood volume of 12 μl. Naturally, the site of injection
would receive the highest concentration. Injection of more than
180 μg was lethal.

Clements and May (1974a) reported the effects of injection of
glutamate into adult locusts. They found no discernable effect in
walking or flight on injection of 20 μl of 0.1 M sodium glutamate,
even though this should have raised blood glutamate levels to at
least 3 mM assuming a blood volume of 680 μl.

When 2-3 ml of locust saline was passed into a tethered adult
locust over 30 min, then 0.1 M glutamate was injected, it required
at least 40 μl before walking or flight behavior was seriously
impaired. Again assuming perfect mixing, this is still a glutamate
concentration on the order of 4-10 mM or roughly the same order of
magnitude to begin to produce effects in *Lucilia*.

From a toxicological standpoint, this rapid metabolism of
glutamate and glutamine might be of interest. However, while disruption of glutamate metabolism by blocking aminotransferases, for
example (Chen and Oechslin, 1976), might be harmful to insects,
the ubiquitous occurrence of this biochemical pathway in nature
means selectivity would be obtained only by handling methods or
some form of lethal synthesis strategy.

It was originally thought that phenylhydrazine caused potentiation of neurally-evoked contractions in insect skeletal muscles
by inhibiting glutamate decarboxylase, thereby freeing more gluta-

mate at the synapse. This was based on a close analogy with the
known effect of cholinesterase inhibitors on the cholinergic
synapse, and it was assumed that glutamate decarboxylase might
perform a similar role in glutaminergic synapses. However, this
toxicological strategy was shown to be a false promise when Ted
McDonald reported that phenylhydrazine had to form a free radical
intermediate before it was active on insect neuromuscular transmission (McDonald, 1972, 1975). When McDonald perfused phenylhydrazine with ascorbic acid and EDTA, which prevent phenylhydrazine oxidation, no effect was found on neuromuscular transmission
by $10^{-3}\underline{M}$ phenylhydrazine. More recently, Clements and May (1974b)
have shown that neither amino-oxyacetic acid nor other inhibitors
of glutamate decarboxylase affect neuromuscular transmission.
This work has rather reemphasized the role of uptake of glutamate
by nerve-muscle tissues which in the absence of any alternative
pathways remains one of the sole mechanisms for removal of glutamate. One other possible mechanism is the apparent existence of
an equilibrium between glutamate and glutamine which heavily favors
the formation of glutamine in the insect blood.

The unpleasant part of writing this review is the enormous
number of loose ends which are left unanswered. Even the most
casual perusal of work in this area will show the large number of
inconsistent results. The question of the amount of glutamate in
the blood is only the most obvious discrepancy, but other observations are equally perplexing. In fact, very few observations stand
without being contradicted elsewhere in the literature.

Whatever the ultimate conclusion concerning glutamate, the
whole area of insect neuromuscular transmission suffers from a
lack of those drugs which would serve to modify the actions of
bath perfused glutamate (Dowson *et al.*, 1975). The review by
Usherwood and Cull-Candy (1975) listed page after page of analogs
and drugs which had been tested for agonistic or antagonistic
actions with glutamate. Despite enormous efforts by the chemical
industry and university groups, the insect equivalent to the
vertebrate curare or atropine or eserine simply has not been
found, and most compounds have activity at excessively high concentrations.

A few compounds of great value have derived from natural
product chemistry and the actions of these are somewhat surprising.

Glutamate agonists. At one time L-glutamate was virtually
alone in stimulating the insect or crustacean muscle to contract
and this alone could argue in favor of its being a neurotransmitter
practically by default.

Those of us who used this argument that no other compound
mimicked neuromuscular transmission of insect muscle at concentra-

tions anywhere near as low as glutamate received somewhat of a shock when quisqualic acid was isolated in Japan and assayed on arthropod muscle. Quisqualic acid is a heterocyclic amino acid (II) first extracted from the seed of *Quisqualis indica* which, when assayed on crayfish, was found to be 500 to 1000 times more potent in depolarizing muscle cells on bath application than glutamic acid itself (I) (Shinozaki and Shibuya, 1974).

When synaptic transmission was blocked in zero Ca, which is thought to prevent release of presynaptic neurotransmitter, quisqualic acid depolarized the muscle by the same amount as under conditions of normal calcium. Those doses of L-glutamate desensitizing the muscle also prevented the action of quisqualic acid and vice versa. Thus quisqualic acid did indeed appear to be mimicking glutamate action.

In insects, while conductance of single membrane channels was virtually identical for quisqualic acid or glutamate, quisqualic acid evidently produced channels of a half-life 1.8 times longer than glutamate-produced channels (Anderson *et al.*, 1976).

Studies on the action of ibotenic acid (III) on locust coxal adductor muscles led to the conclusion that glutamate and ibotenate were competing for extra-synaptic glutamate sensitive sites and that ibotenate had no action at synaptic sites (Lea and Usherwood, 1973). Further investigation showed that extra-synaptic glutamate receptors could be classified into a D receptor which caused depolarization to glutamate, but was insensitive to DL-ibotenate, and an H receptor which hyperpolarized in the presence of either glutamate or ibotenate (Cull-Candy, 1975).

I   II

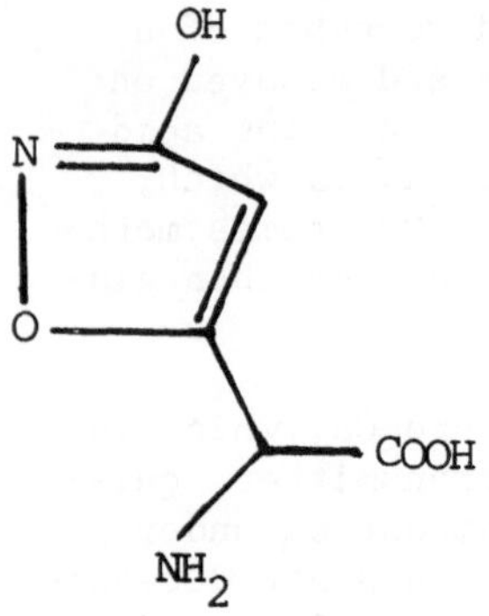

OH

N

O ─── COOH

NH$_2$

III

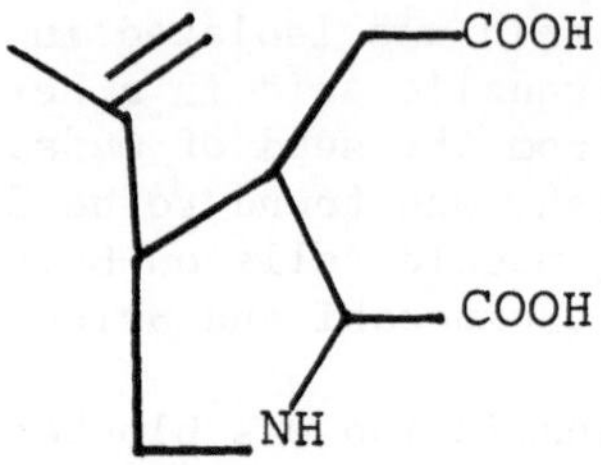

COOH

COOH

NH

IV

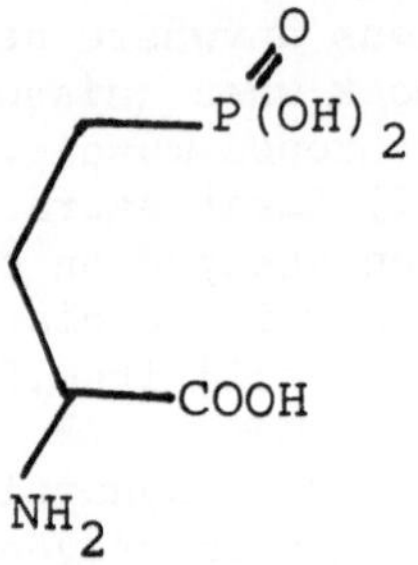

$\overset{O}{P}(OH)_2$

COOH

NH$_2$

V

Kainic acid is another natural product derived from plants, in this case seaweed, and it also has some resemblance to glutamate (IV). Kainic acid was reported to potentiate the action of glutamate at extra-synaptic receptors in crayfish muscle and to be inactive at the neuromuscular junction itself (Takeuchi and Onodera, 1975).

When examined on locust extensor tibiae nerve-muscle preparations, kainic acid potentiated glutamate potentials and EPSP amplitudes with a threshold at $5 \times 10^{-5}\underline{M}$. Since miniature EPSP frequency was increased, but not amplitude, kainic acid was thought to have both pre- and post-synaptic actions on locust muscle (Daoud and Usherwood, 1975). A concentration of kainic acid of $10^{-3}\underline{M}$ was required to depress EPSPs by about 70%, but kainic acid had no effect on effective membrane resistance of either retractor unguis or extensor tibiae muscles of the locusts. Therefore, kainic acid served as a poor glutamate agonist.

Taken together these observations imply that the conformation of the quisqualate molecule fits the insect neuromuscular receptor site far better than the kainic acid molecule, and ibotenate is not recognized at all by the receptor.

A recent report provided evidence that 2-amino-4-phosphono-butyric acid (APB) (V) acts as a glutamate antagonist at the insect neuromuscular junction (Cull-Candy et al., 1976). APB inhibited binding of glutamate to receptor-like proteolipid extracts from locust muscle, and iontophoretic pulses of APB caused no effect, but rapidly reduced depolarizations from coincident pulses of glutamate in double-barrelled pipettes. The unfortunate drawback to APB is its lack of antagonism to ionto-phoresed glutamate when APB was applied in the bathing saline at $5 \times 10^{-4}\underline{M}$. To explain the lack of action, one is forced again to

use the barrier argument and these experiments are forced into
the realm of microelectrodes rather than the more applicable bioassay of bath-applied drugs.

Inhibitory Nerve-muscle Synapses

If one were to consider figure 2 at length, two things may be
learned concerning the injection of putative neurotransmitters
into insects. The first thing is that glutamate falls into one
category by producing an action on EPSP amplitude and both
acetylcholine and GABA (γ-aminobutyric acid) fall into a separate
category in that they both produced disruptions in the activity
of the central nervous system.

The toxicological implications of the action of acetylcholine are obvious since the vast majority of modern insecticides, being organophosphorus and carbamate chemicals, are
cholinergic poisons. However, the lesion implied by the GABA
effect has never been exploited by toxicologists. The putative
neurotransmitter role of GABA at the arthropod nerve-muscle
synapse has been far less controversial than the role hypothe-
sized for glutamate, and the GABA synapse system has received
far less attention both by toxicologists and physiologists.

Those interested in GABA have had from the outset the advantage of a good antagonist in picrotoxin. Picrotoxin is sold as a
plant extract mixture of equimolar amounts of picrotin and picro-
toxinin, the active form. Even after several years of unrefriger-
ated shelf life, picrotoxin may be dissolved sparingly in saline
to 10^{-6}M concentration and bath applied to the insect inhibitory
nerve-muscle preparation where it produces a remarkably specific
reversible blockage of inhibitory transmission.

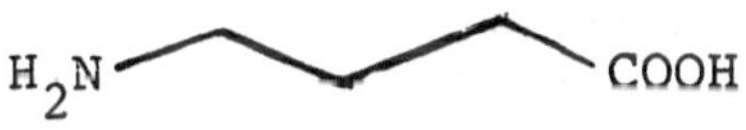

VI

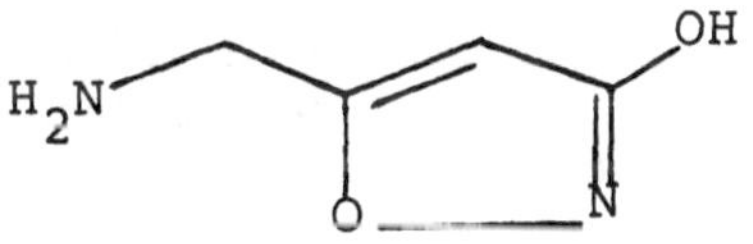

VII

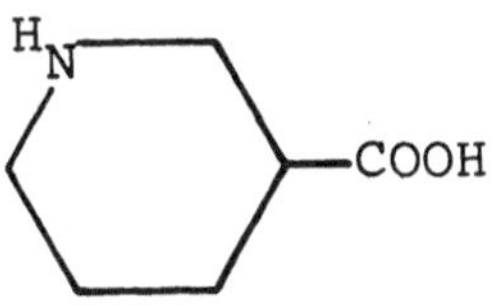

VIII

The central nervous activity of glutamate decarboxylase in
cockroaches produces 60 μMoles of GABA/g wet weight/hr from L-
glutamate. This is considerably higher than crustacean, amphibian,
avian or mammal, but is similar to rates in other insects (Baxter
and Torralba, 1975).

The GABA (VI) agonist muscimol (VII) is 5-10 times more
potent than GABA on suspected GABA receptor fractions, and is 1000
times more active on suspected GABA receptor than on suspected
GABA transport sites from crayfish and rat brain (R. W. Olsen,
1977, personal communication; Johnston, 1976). Although both sites
bind GABA, suspected GABA synaptic receptor sites are distinguished
from extract fractions showing transport in that the latter are
sodium-dependent. Muscimol also blocks IPSPs in cockroach coxal
muscle (Miller, 1976, unpublished).

On·the other hand, nipecotic acid (VIII) appears to be a
potent GABA blocker in having a higher affinity for protein fractions suspected of serving a function in GABA transport (Johnston,
1976; Johnston *et al.*, 1976). Nipecotic acid does not block IPSPs
of cockroach coxal muscle when perfused at 10^{-4}M (Miller, 1976,
unpublished). The work on GABA agonists and antagonists has come
mostly from mammalian neuropharmacology and has not yet been
examined in detail on insects except for a few measurements.

Picrotoxin provides more practical toxicological information.
House flies are not affected by massive topical doses of picrotoxin. A 50 μg topical treatment in acetone is not toxic, so the
native LD_{50} is somewhere above 2500 μg/g . However, when topically
applied with synergist piperonyl butoxide, the LD_{50} is about 75
μg/g, a value which is not impressive to the toxicologist. Compare
this for instance to DDT whose topical LD_{50} is 14 μg/g (5.5 with
synergist) on house fly or carbofuran with an LD_{50} of 6.7 μg/g on
house fly (2.5 with synergist).

When treated on the isolated thoracic ganglion of house flies,
carbamate insecticides produce convulsions in 5-20 min at nominal
concentrations around 10^{-5}M. Phosphate insecticides take longer
as a rule (Miller, 1976). When comparing the action of picrotoxin
with insecticides on the desheathed thoracic ganglion of house
fly, picrotoxin appears to be far more potent in producing disruption in the coordination of the flight motor system.

These observations suggest that the house fly is able to with-
stand enormous amounts of topically applied picrotoxin. The large
synergistic ratio on house fly suggests that picrotoxin may be
metabolized fairly rapidly, but the exact extent of protection
against picrotoxin has not been examined.

Picrotoxin action on the inhibitory nerve-muscle synapse is

completely reversible upon washing. Completely reversible inhibitors of acetylcholinesterase are not toxic as a rule (Chiu *et al.*,
1973), and therefore a toxicological strategist would not expect
picrotoxin or its analogs to be insecticidal as a reasonable
guess. However, disruption of an inhibitory synapse in the
central nervous system is a good toxicological strategy.

We suspect that many motor programs in insects are held off
by inhibitory influences. Probably the best known example of this
inhibition is the depression of the flight motor by tarsal contact
and release of the flight motor pattern triggered by loss of tarsal
contact. It is now widely accepted that coordinated behavior
patterns are inherent characteristics of the central nervous
systems in insects (P. L. Miller, 1974).

Preliminary recordings from central interneurons indicate
motor neurons are not inherently rhythmically active, that rather
they are driven by a very few interneurons which control whole
behavior patterns by an alternating excitation and inhibition
input (Burrows, 1974, 1975).

Lateral inhibition is thought to control the coordination of
firing of flight motor neurons during asynchronous flight in
Diptera (Mulloney, 1976), and lateral inhibition appears to play a
role in visual perception (Fraser Rowell and O'Shea, 1976). Thus
inhibition plays a key role in many central processes. The neurochemistry underlying central inhibition does not necessarily always
involve GABA; other neurotransmitters may be employed at inhibitory
synapses. At least, a model poison like picrotoxin does have
fairly impressive toxic actions on certain parts of the insect
central nervous system.

Visceral Nerve-muscle Synapses

A large number of synapses in the central and peripheral
nervous systems of insects are known to be insensitive to glutamate, GABA or acetylcholine. Dopamine, adrenalin and octopamine
have been found to mimic the role of neurotransmitter at many of
these "neurosecretomotor" synapses in insects (cf. Miller, 1975;
Robertson and Juorio, 1976; Hoyle, 1975; House *et al.*, 1973; Oertel
and Case, 1976). Brian Brown, after a monumental 8 year effort,
isolated and identified proctolin, a pentapeptide (Brown, 1975;
Starratt and Brown, 1975). Brown and his colleagues have proposed
that proctolin is the neurotransmitter at rectal longitudinal
muscle of *Periplaneta americana* where it causes contractions at
extremely low concentrations (ca. $10^{-9}\underline{M}$).

After some preliminary work, it is now evident that proctolin
has effects on cockroach heart (Miller, 1976, unpublished observa-

tions) and hyperneural muscle also at low concentrations (typically $10^{-9}\underline{M}$), and proctolin has actions on certain skeletal muscles of locusts (C. W. Kearns, 1976, personal communication) also at extremely low concentrations.

The toxicological strategies which might be developed around neurosecretomotor synapses or peptide neurotransmitters are not yet clear, but there is an enormous excitement connected with this subject. It cannot be emphasized too strongly how little is known about the neurochemistry involved in neuroendocrine control processes and the possible consequences of their untimely activation at a critical point in insect development. We already suspect that at certain stages the hormonal production of some organs such as the corpora allata are inhibited by a nervous influence from the brain (Granger and Sehnal, 1974; Sehnal and Granger, 1975). Thus, removal of inhibition in the neuroendocrine system is also a legitimate strategy for the toxicologist to consider.

REFERENCES

Anderson, C. R., Cull-Candy, S. G., and Miledi, R., 1976, Glutamate and quisqualate noise in voltage-clamped locust muscle fibres, *Nature* 261:151-153.

Baxter, C. F., and Torralba, C. F., 1975, γ-aminobutyric acid and glutamate decarboxylase (L-glutamate 1-carboxylase E. C. 4.1.1.1.5) in the nervous system of the cockroach, *Periplaneta americana*. I. Regional distribution and properties of the enzyme, *Brain Res.* 84:383-397.

Brown, B. E., 1975, Proctolin: a peptide transmitter candidate in insects, *Life Sci.* 17:1241-1252.

Burrows, M., 1974, Modes of activation of motorneurons controlling ventilatory movements of the locust abdomen, *Phil. Trans. Roy. Soc. Lond. B.* 269:29-48.

Burrows, M., 1975, Co-ordinating interneurons of the locust which convey two patterns of motor commands: their connexions with ventilatory motorneurons, *J. Exp. Biol.* 63:735-753.

Chen, P. S., and Oechslin, A., 1976, Accumulation of glutamic acid in the paragonial gland of *Drosophila nigromelanica*, *J. Insect Physiol.* 22:1237-1243.

Chiu, Y. C., Fahmy, M. A. H., and Fukuto, T. R., 1973, Aryl *N*-hydroxy- and *N*-methoxy-*N*-methylcarbamates as potent reversible inhibitors of acetylcholinesterase, *Pestic. Biochem. Physiol.* 3:1-6.

Clements, A. N., and May, T. E., 1974a, Studies on locust neuromuscular physiology in relation to glutamic acid, *J. Exp. Biol.* 60:673-705.

Clements, A. N., and May, T. E., 1974b, Pharmacological studies on a locust neuromuscular preparation, *J. Exp. Biol.* 61:421-442.

Cull-Candy, S. G., 1975, Effect of denervation and local damage on extrajunctional L-glutamate receptors in locust muscle, *Nature* 258:530-531.

Cull-Candy, S. G., Donnellan, J. F., James, R. W., and Lunt, G. G., 1976, 2-amino-4-phosphonobutyric acid as a glutamate antagonist on locust muscle, *Nature* 262:408-409.

Daoud, A., and Usherwood, P. N. R., 1975, Action of kainic acid on a glutaminergic synapse, *Comp. Biochem. Physiol.* 52C:51-53.

Dowson, R. J., and Usherwood, P. N. R., 1972, The effect of low concentrations of L-glutamate and L-aspartate on transmitter release at the locust excitatory nerve-muscle synapse, *J. Physiol.* 229:13-14.

Dowson, R. J., Clements, A. N., and May, T. E., 1975, The action of some Harmala alkaloids on transmission at a glutamate-mediated synapse, *Neuropharmacol.* 14:235-240.

Evans, P. D., 1975, The uptake of L-glutamate by the central nervous system of the cockroach, *Periplaneta americana, J. Exp. Biol.* 62:55-67.

Fraser Rowell, C. H., and O'Shea, M., 1976, Neuronal basis of a sensory analyser, the acridid movement detector system. III. *J. Exp. Biol.* 65:617-625.

Gerschenfeld, H. M., 1973, Chemical transmission in invertebrate central nervous systems and neuromuscular junctions, *Physiol. Rev.* 53:1-119.

Granger, N. A., and Sehnal, F., 1974, Regulation of larval corpora allata in *Galleria mellonella, Nature* 251:415-417.

Holden, J. S., 1974, Glutamic acid and neuromuscular transmission in insects. Ph.D. dissertation, Dept. of Physiology and Biochemistry, Univ. of Southampton, England.

House, C. R., Ginsborg, B. L., and Silinsky, E. M., 1973, Dopamine receptors in cockroach salivary gland cells, *Nature, New Biol.* 245:63.

Hoyle, G., 1975, Evidence that insect dorsal unpaired median (DUM) neurons are octopaminergic, *J. Exp. Zool.* 193:425-431.

Irving, S. N., Osborne, M. P., and Wilson, R. G., 1976, Virtual absence of L-glutamate from the haemoplasm of arthropod blood, *Nature* 263:431-433.

Johnston, G. A. R., 1976, Physiologic pharmacology of GABA and its antagonists in the vertebrate nervous system. *in: GABA in Nervous System Function* (E. Roberts, T. N. Chase and D. B. Tower, eds.), pp. 395-411, Raven Press, New York.

Johnston, G. A. R., Stephanson, A. L., and Twitchin, B., 1976, Uptake and release of nipecotic acid by rat brain slices, *J. Neurochem.* 26:83-87.

Kerkut, G. A., and Walker, R. J., 1966, The effect of L-glutamate, acetylcholine and gamma-aminobutyric acid on the miniature end-plate potentials and contractures of the coxal muscles of the cockroach, *Periplaneta americana, Comp. Biochem. Physiol.* 17:435-454.

Lea, T. J., and Usherwood, P. N. R., 1973, The site of action of
    ibotenic acid and the identification of two populations of
    glutamate receptors on insect muscle fibers, *Comp. Gen.
    Pharmacol.* 4:333-350.
McDonald, T. J., 1972, Free radical mechanism for phenylhydrazine
    action on the retractor unguis muscle of the grasshopper,
    Romalea microptera, Comp. Gen. Pharmacol. 3:319-326.
McDonald, T. J., 1975, Neuromuscular pharmacology in insects,
    Ann. Rev. Ent. 20:151-166.
Miller, P. L., 1974, Rhythmic activities and the insect nervous
    system, *in: Experimental Analysis of Insect Behavior,* pp.
    114-138, Springer-Verlag, New York.
Miller, R., Leaf, G., and Usherwood, P. N. R., 1973, Blood gluta-
    mate in arthropods, *Comp. Biochem. Physiol.* 44A:991-996.
Miller, T. A., 1975, Neurosecretion and the control of visceral
    organs in insects, *Ann. Rev. Entomol.* 20:133-149.
Miller, T. A., 1976, Distinguishing between carbamate and organo-
    phosphate insecticide poisoning in house flies by symptomology,
    Pestic. Biochem. Physiol. 6:307-319.
Miller, T., and Kennedy, J. M., 1972, Flight motor activity of
    house flies as affected by temperature and insecticides,
    Pestic. Biochem. Physiol. 2:206.
Miller, T., and James, J., 1976, Chemical sensitivity of the hyper-
    neural nerve-muscle preparation of the American cockroach,
    J. Insect Physiol. 22:981-988.
Mulloney, B., 1976, Control of flight and related behaviour by the
    central nervous systems of insects, *in: Insect Flight* (R. C.
    Rainey, ed.), Wiley, New York.
Murdock, L. L., and Koidl, B., 1972a, Limited permeability and
    metabolism of L-glutamate in the locust gut wall, *J. Exp.
    Biol.* 56:781-794.
Murdock, L. L., and Koidl, B., 1972b, Blood metabolites after
    intestinal absorption of amino acids in locusts, *J. Exp.
    Biol.* 56:795-808.
Murdock, L. L., and Chapman, G. V., 1974, L-glutamate in arthropod
    blood plasma: physiological implications, *J. Exp. Biol.*
    60:783-794.
Neal, H., 1975a, Effects of L-glutamate and other drugs on some
    membrane properties of muscle fibers of Diptera, *J. Insect
    Physiol.* 21:1771-1778.
Neal, H., 1975b, Neuromuscular junctions and L-glutamate-sensitive
    sites in the fleshfly, *Sarcophaga bullata, J. Insect Physiol.*
    21:1945-1951.
Oertel, D., and Case, J. F., 1976, Neural excitation of the larval
    firefly photocyte: slow depolarization possibly mediated by
    a cyclic nucleotide, *J. Exp. Biol.* 65:213-227.
Osborne, N. N., and Neuhoff, V., 1974, Amino acid and serotonin
    content in the nervous system, muscle and blood of the cock-
    roach, *Periplaneta americana, Brain Res.* 80:251-264.

Robertson, H. T., and Juorio, A. V., 1976, Octopamine and some
    related noncatecholic amines in invertebrate nervous systems,
    Int. Rev. Neurobiol. 19:173-224.
Salpeter, M. M., and Faeder, I. R., 1971, The role of sheath cells
    in glutamate uptake by insect nerve-muscle preparations,
    Progr. Brain Res. 34:103-114.
Sehnal, F., and Granger, N. A., 1975, Control of corpora allata
    function in larvae of *Galleria mellonella*, *Biol. Bull.*
    148:106-116.
Shinozaki, H., and Shibuya, I., 1974, A new potent excitant, quis-
    qualic acid: effects on crayfish neuromuscular junction,
    Neuropharmacol. 13(7):665-672.
Smyth, T., Greer, M. H., and Griffiths, D. J. G., 1973, Insect
    neuromuscular synapses, *Am. Zool.* 13:315-319.
Starratt, A. N., and Brown, B. E., 1975, Structure of the penta-
    peptide proctolin, a proposed neurotransmitter in insects,
    Life Sci. 17:1253-1256.
Stevens, T. M., 1961, Free amino acids in the hemolymph of the
    American cockroach, *Periplaneta americana* L., *Comp. Biochem.
    Physiol.* 3:304-309.
Takeuchi, A., and Onodera, K., 1975, Effects of kainic acid on the
    glutamate receptors of the crayfish muscle, *Neuropharmacol.*
    14:619-625.
Usherwood, P. N. R., 1974, Nerve-muscle transmission, *in: Insect
    Neurobiology* (J. E. Treherne, ed.), pp. 245-305, Amsterdam,
    North Holland.
Usherwood, P. N. R., and Machili, P., 1968, Pharmacological pro-
    perties of excitatory neuromuscular synapses in the locust,
    J. Exp. Biol. 49:341-361.
Usherwood, P. N. R., and Cull-Candy, S. G., 1975, Pharmacology of
    somatic nerve-muscle synapses, *in: Insect Muscle* (P. N. R.
    Usherwood, ed.), Academic Press, New York.

Section II

Neurotoxic Actions
of Synthetic Insecticides
and Acaricides

NEUROTOXIC ACTIONS OF SYNTHETIC INSECTICIDES AND ACARICIDES

INTRODUCTION

R.M. Hollingworth

Purdue University

West Lafayette, Indiana 47907

The following seven chapters consider some current and novel classes of pesticides with attention to their actions on the nervous system. With the exception of the organophosphates and carbamates whose mode of action in insects is reasonably established to depend on inhibition of acetylcholinesterase, the detailed nature of the initial sites and modes of action of other long-established categories such as the cyclodienes, lindane, DDT and its analogs, and the pyrethroids remains relatively obscure. Almost nothing is known concerning the neurotoxicology of acaricides in mites and ticks. Further, as pointed out by Samaranayaka-Ramasamy in an earlier chapter, the lethal consequences of this initial attack on the nervous system in target species may be complex and are only now beginning to be understood.

The pyrethroids and DDT have been shown to have potent effects on the transient ionic conductance changes which develop the action potential across axonal membranes. This leads to disruption of axonal transmission (Narahashi, 1971, 1976), but the critical locus of these effects within the nervous system of insects is not known. From Narahashi's chapter below it is clear that the specific effects on ionic conductances are very dependant on molecular structure, and that a good isolated nerve preparation to study and predict the lethality of the pyrethroids is, as yet, lacking. Some of these matters have also been discussed recently by Miller and Adams (1977) and Narahashi et al. (1977).

Recently, it has been suggested that certain chlorinated hydrocarbons such as the cyclodienes, and possibly lindane, are

115

neurotoxic in a quite different manner from DDT and the
pyrethroids in that they act presynaptically causing the
excessive release of ACh (and conceivably other neurotransmitters)
into the synaptic cleft. This concept is supported in the work
of Uchida and his colleagues reported here, particularly with
reference to lindane and a range of lindane analogs. In
considering the actions of the various lindane isomers on the
nervous system, the marked structural specificity of neurotoxicity
is again apparent. The actual mechanisms by which transmitter
release may be facilitated by these organochlorines is unknown
and merits further study despite their declining significance
as pesticides.

Independent of our rather incomplete knowledge of the sites
and mechanisms of action of current pesticides on the nervous
system, novel chemicals acting on the nervous functions of
insects and acarines are regularly discovered. The nitromethylene
heterocycles described here for the first time by Soloway et al.
and by Reed and Erlam are one such group. Unfortunately their
environmental instability currently constitutes a barrier to
commercial useage. However, in view of their novel structures
and very rapid knockdown action, further study of their
mechanism of action is clearly worthwhile.

The formamidines, such as chlordimeform, were initially
discovered in the early 1960's, but in many ways they remain a
novel group whose mode of action on target species remains
mysterious. Lund et al. in their chapter present good evidence
that the mammalian lethality of the formamidines develops from
a local anesthetic-like action. However, further study has
shown that this probably is not related to their protective
effects against insects, mites, and ticks. Beeman and Matsumura's
article carefully catalogs the variety of actions which the
formamidines are known to exert on these organisms. The riddle
of the mode of action of formamidines such as chlordimeform has
stimulated research into several previously unexplored areas in
pesticide biochemistry e.g. monoamine oxidases, local anesthetics,
and prostaglandin synthetase (Holsapple et al., 1977). Perhaps
even more significant for the future are continuing studies of
the action of the formamidines on non-cholinergic sites in the
insect nervous system, and of the effect of these compounds on
insect behavior as the basis for their pestistatic actions.

A final theme in these chapters is the relationship of
metabolism to neurotoxicity. A particularly interesting
observation is reported by Benezet et al. who find increasing
potency and speed of action against vertebrates as N,N-dimethyl-
formamidines are sequentially N-demethylated. However, it remains
to be established that N-demethylation is an essential prerequisite
for intoxication by formamidines either in vertebrates or

invertebrates. Interestingly, certain toxic effects typical of
formamidines against cattle ticks (lethality and detachment from
the host) are known to be exerted with much greater potency by
N-demethyl chlordimeform than by chlordimeform itself, and the
effectiveness of chlordimeform in these actions is decreased by
treatment of the ticks with synergists which prevent N-demethylation (Stone et al., 1974).

REFERENCES

Holsapple, M. P., Blake, D. E., Hollingworth, R. M., and
    Yim, G. K. W., 1977, Prostaglandin synthetase inhibition
    by a formamidine pesticide, Pharmacologist 19:147.

Miller, T. A., and Adams, M. E., 1977, Central vs. peripheral
    action of pyrethroids on the housefly nervous system. In:
    Synthetic Pyrethroids (M. Elliott, ed.), ACS Symposium
    Series No. 42, American Chemical Society, Washington, D.C.,
    pp. 98-115.

Narahashi, T., 1971, Effects of insecticides on excitable
    tissues, Adv. Insect Physiol. 8:1.

Narahashi, T., 1976, Effects of insecticides on nervous
    conduction and synaptic transmission. In: Insecticide
    Biochemistry and Physiology , (C. F. Wilkinson, ed.),
    Plenum Press, New York, pp. 327-352.

Narahashi, T., Nishimura, K., Parmentier, J. L., Takeno, K.,
    and Elliott, M., 1977, Neurophysiological study of the
    structure-activity relation of pyrethroids. In: Synthetic
    Pyrethroids (M. Elliott, ed.), ACS Symposium Series No. 42,
    American Chemical Society, Washington, D.C., pp. 85-97.

Stone, B. F., Atkinson, P. W., and Knowles, C. O., 1974,
    Formamidine structure and detachment of the cattle tick
    Boophilus microplus, Pestic. Biochem. Physiol. 4:407.

NEUROPHYSIOLOGICAL STUDY OF THE STRUCTURE-ACTIVITY RELATIONS OF INSECTICIDES

Toshio Narahashi

Department of Pharmacology, Northwestern University

Medical School, Chicago, Illinois   60611

Structure-activity relationships of insecticides have been a subject of investigations for many years since the development of synthetic insecticides such as DDT and organophosphates. In most cases, these studies were based on the comparison of insect killing potencies of a variety of analogs and derivatives of a parent compound. However, since the action of an insecticide in killing insects is exerted as a result of a chain of reactions, it is difficult to relate such killing potencies to the chemical structures of the insecticide. The process of toxic action of an insecticide is summarized as follows.

After entering the insect body through the cuticle or other routes, an insecticide may be detoxified to non-toxic chemicals. For example, DDT is metabolized to DDE and DDA depending on the animal species used. Certain insecticides are converted into more toxic chemicals. A number of examples are known among organophosphate and carbamate insecticides. For instance, parathion is activated to paraoxon to inhibit cholinesterases. The activated compounds may also undergo detoxication. In any case the toxic component can eventually reach the target site which for many insecticides is the nervous system. Stimulation of the nerve as a result of the primary action of the active form of insecticide may lead to release of a toxic component from the nerve which in turn stimulates and paralyzes the nerve. These symptoms of poisoning of the nervous system cause the secondary and tertiary effects on the insect such as fatigue and metabolic exhaustion which in turn lead the insect to death. Therefore, the killing action involves a variety of reactions and the death is caused as a final product of this chain of reactions. Thus it is illogical to try to relate the killing potency to the chemical structure of the insecticide.

The structure-activity relationships are expected to be elucidated more clearly if the direct action of insecticides on the target site is compared. Thus the experiments would be straightforward
and relatively easy if the target site is clearly identified and
isolated in vitro. This is indeed the case for cholinesterases
which are major targets for organophosphate and carbamate insecticides. A large amount of data has been accumulated along this line
(Fukuto, 1971; Metcalf, 1971). Another example of such studies,
though not as extensive as the anticholinesterases, is seen with
rotenone. The potencies to inhibit glutamic dehydrogenase to block
nerve conduction and to kill insects were compared among a variety
of rotenone derivatives (Fukami et al., 1959). These three potencies ran parallel with each other.

However, for most other insecticides the target site is not
so well defined. Many insecticides such as DDT, lindane, cyclodienes and pyrethroids modify the nervous function, but the real
target site in the nervous system still remains to be seen. It is
likely that the target sites for these insecticides are not enzyme
systems, since most of them are known to directly interact with
nerve membrane ionic channels or synaptic junctions. Therefore,
the only practical way of comparing the direct action on the target
site would be to use the appropriate nerve preparations.

DDT AND ITS ANALOGS

DDT analogs have been studied extensively for their structure-
activity relationships (e.g. Holan, 1969, 1971a,b; Metcalf and
Fukuto, 1968; Fahmy et al., 1973). However, the major approach to
this problem has been to compare the potencies of various analogs
and derivatives in killing insects. As has been discussed in the
preceding section, several factors such as penetration of insecticides through the cuticle and metabolism of insecticides in the
animals have to be taken into consideration to interpret the
killing potency in the light of the molecular structure of the
insecticides. Then a question arises regarding the real target
site of DDT. There is no doubt that DDT acts primarily on the nervous system thereby causing a variety of disorders such as hyperexcitability, ataxia, convulsions and paralysis.

It has been well established that DDT causes repetitive discharges in various nerve tissues including certain sensory receptors and nerve fibers (see Narahashi, 1971, 1976 for comprehensive
literature). In the nerve fibers, repetitive activity is initiated
at least in part, as a result of an increase in negative (depolarizing) after-potential (Narahashi and Yamasaki, 1960). The increased and sustained depolarization that follows the action potential serves as a stimulus thereby triggering a train of action
potentials.

The mechanism underlying the increase in negative after-potential was studied by voltage clamp method (Narahashi and Haas, 1967, 1968; Hille, 1968; Pichon, 1969). This method permits measurements of membrane currents carried by sodium and potassium ions separately under the controlled membrane potential. From the observed membrane ionic currents and the membrane potential, the membrane conductances to sodium and potassium ions can be calculated separately. It has been demonstrated that DDT greatly prolongs the falling phase of thè sodium current through the inhibition of the sodium inactivation mechanism and partially inhibits the potassium activation mechanism. These two mechanisms are responsible for the falling phase of the action potential, so that the negative after-potential is augmented by DDT.

Crayfish have giant axons with diameters ranging from 100 to 200 μ. Because of the large diameter, the crayfish giant axons are among the excellent materials for intracellular recording of action potentials. It is also important that the nerves of the crayfish, being a member of the Phylum Arthropoda, have an insecticide sensitivity spectrum similar to that of insects. For example, the crayfish giant axons are as sensitive to DDT as the cockroach giant axons, whereas the squid giant axons are almost insensitive to DDT.

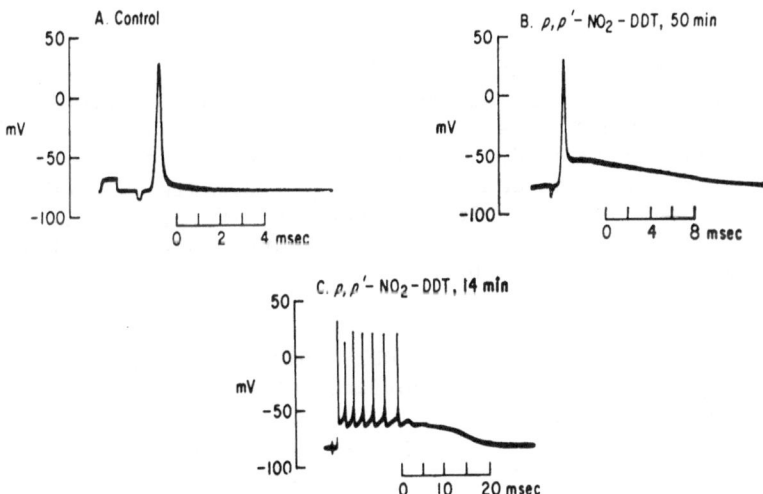

Fig. 1.   Excitatory action of p,p'-NO$_2$-DDT on the crayfish giant axon. Negative after-potential is increased and repetitive discharges are induced after application of 5 x 10^{-5}M (B) and 1 x 10^{-4}M (C) p,p'-NO$_2$-DDT (Wu et al., 1975).

The circumesophageal connectives were isolated from the crayfish, and their sheaths were removed. Action potentials were elicited by electrical stimulations via either a pair of silver wire
electrodes or a suction electrode, while recording was made by
means of an intracellular glass capillary microelectrode filled
with 3 M KCl solution. Under normal conditions, a single stimulus
elicited one action potential. Following application of p,p'-DDT
at a concentration of 1 x 10^{-4} M, the negative after-potential,
which was small in amplitude, increased substantially, eventually
giving rise to repetitive action potentials. Several DDT analogs
have been found to exert essentially the same effect as p,p'-DDT
(Wu et al., 1975). They were p,p'-NO_2-DDT (2,2-bis(p-nitrophenyl)-
1,1,1-trichloroethane), p,p'-CH_3O-DDT, p,p'-C_2H_5O-DDT, p,p'-C_3H_7O-
DDT, o,p'-DDT, p,p'-DDD and p,p'-C_2H_5-DDD. An example of such an
experiment with p,p'-NO_2-DDT is illustrated in Figure 1. Although
the action potential was slightly suppressed by some of these DDT
analogs after a prolonged exposure, there was no sign of potent
blocking action. It should be pointed out that p,p'-NO_2-DDT is
insecticidally inactive (Holan, 1969; Metcalf and Fukuto, 1968),
yet exerts the same effect on the isolated nerve as p,p'-DDT. This
group of DDT analogs may be called the excitatory group.

It is interesting to find the blocking action by certain DDT
analogs such as p,p'-NH_2-DDT and p,p'-OH-DDT. No repetitive discharges were produced by a single stimulus, and no increase in
negative after-potential was observed. The action potential was
simply blocked without any change in the resting membrane potential.
These analogs belong to the blocking group.

A third group of DDT analogs exerts both excitatory and blocking actions, and may be termed the dualist group. The first sign
of effect observed was an increase in negative after-potential
which occasionally gave rise to repetitive after-discharges. This
stage was followed by conduction block without any change in resting
membrane potential. The dualist group includes p,p'-CHO-DDT, 2,2-
bis(p-chlorophenyl)-1,1-dichlorocyclopropane (DCC), and 2,2-bis(p-
ethoxyphenyl)-3,3-dimethyloxetane (EDO). Two other analogs tested,
p,p'-CH_3CONH-DDT and p,p'-C_6H_5-DDT, were inactive on the crayfish
giant axon.

This study of the effects of DDT analogs on the crayfish giant
axons clearly illustrates the importance of comparing the direct
action on the target site for the purpose of elucidating the structure-activity relationship. Two points should be emphasized: One
is the fact that DDT analogs may exert qualitatively different
actions depending on the structure; the other is the fact that certain insecticidally inactive compounds are indeed active on the
nerve.

Excitatory and blocking actions, which are entirely different in nature, cannot be put together to relate to the chemical structure. These two actions must be the results of different interactions with nerve membrane components. Excitatory action is due to inhibitions of sodium inactivation and potassium activation, both of which cause an increase in negative after-potential which in turn gives rise to repetitive after-discharges. Blocking action is not due to depolarization, so that it must be brought about by inhibition of the sodium activation mechanism. This remains to be demonstrated. Dual action suggests that in certain DDT analogs there are two chemical groups which are responsible for excitatory and blocking actions. Further studies along this line are expected to identify the molecular architecture that is responsible for each type of action.

Three DDT analogs which are insecticidally inactive have been found effective on the isolated nerve preparation. They are p,p'-NO_2-DDT, p,p'-NH_2-DDT and p,p'-OH-DDT. One possible reason would be that they cannot effectively penetrate the cuticle. An alternative mechanism might be their high susceptibility for detoxication and excretion. No matter what the real mechanism responsible for their inability to kill insects may be, this result strongly emphasizes the need of comparing the direct action on the target site for the study of the structure-activity relationship. Furthermore, p,p'-NO_2-DDT causes excitation, whereas p,p'-NH_2-DDT and p,p'-OH-DDT cause blockade. Thus it would be misleading to relate the chemical structure to the activity by simple comparison of insecticidal potency. The actions on the target site must be carefully compared for elucidation of the true structure-activity relationships.

The available data are still insufficient to relate the molecular structure to the physiological action on the nerve membrane. Despite this, the present experimental results suggest the following mechanisms of action: (1) Hydrophobic side chains on the para positions and in appropriate sizes may be essential for excitatory action; (2) hydrophilic side chains capable of forming hydrogen bonds may be required for blocking action; and (3) restriction in rotation imposed by the grouping on the benzylic carbon may also cause blocking action.

NEW METHODS WITH CRAYFISH ABDOMINAL NERVE CORD

We have recently developed a method whereby potencies of a variety of insecticides in stimulating and blocking the nerve can be compared in an efficient way (Takeno et al., 1977). After comparing several nerve-muscle preparations including the crayfish abdominal nerve cord, the crayfish neuromuscular junction and the

frog neuromuscular junction, it was found that the abdominal nerve
cord of the crayfish is highly sensitive to various insecticides
and most convenient for quantitative estimate of relative potencies.

The abdominal nerve cord is isolated from the crayfish, Pro-
cambarus clarki or Orconestes virilis, and mounted in a Plexiglass
nerve chamber equipped with a pair of recording wire electrodes.
This preparation contains both synapses and nerve fibers. Under
normal conditions, the abdominal nerve cord discharges impulses
spontaneously at a frequency of approximately 100/sec for a period
of several hours. When a stimulating agent is applied, the frequency of spontaneous impulses increases. Figure 2 illustrates an
example of such an experiment with allethrin. The degree of frequency increase depends on the concentration of any particular
insecticide. In the case of allethrin, low concentrations ranging
from 10^{-8} M to 10^{-7} M simply increase the frequency, whereas
higher concentrations of 10^{-6} M or above increase and then decrease
the frequency (Fig. 3). Other insecticides such as DDT and toxa-
phene have also been shown to stimulate the crayfish abdominal
nerve cord in increasing the frequency of spontaneous discharges.
However, these chlorinated hydrocarbon insecticides do not cause
paralysis.

Since a large number of compounds have to be compared for
their nerve stimulating and/or blocking potencies, four abdominal
nerve cord preparations are handled at a time. Four preparations
are isolated and mounted in four independent chambers. Recording
of impulses is made from each preparation in succession using an
automatic switch. The recorded impulses are amplified and fed
into an oscilloscope, an audiomonitor and an electronic counter.

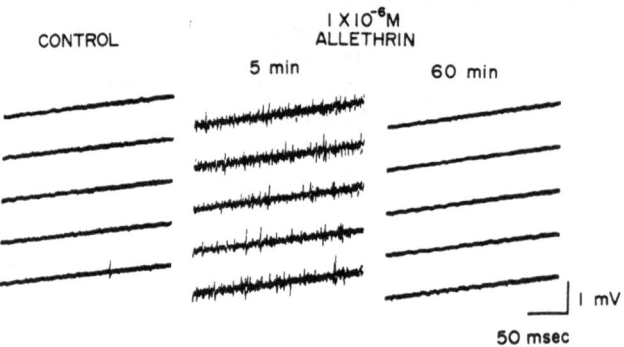

Fig. 2. Spontaneous impulse discharges from the crayfish abdominal
nerve cord before and after application of 1 x 10^{-6} M allethrin.
The nerve is first stimulated and then paralyzed (Takeno et al.,
1977).

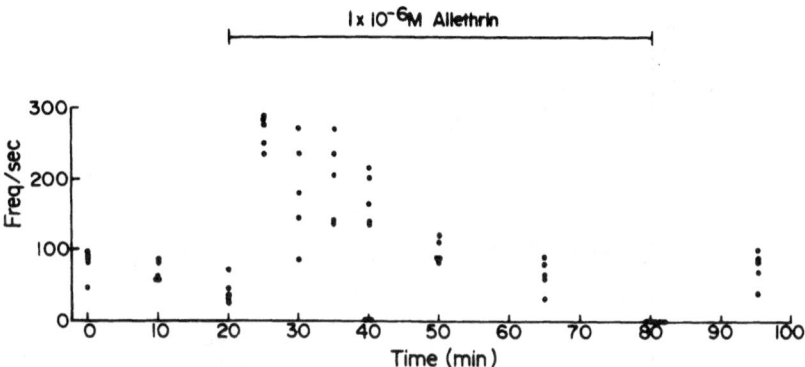

Fig. 3. Frequency of spontaneous impulse discharges from the cray-fish abdominal nerve cord as effected by 1×10^{-6} M allethrin (Takeno et al., 1977).

The counter displays the frequency in a digital form. The digital data can also be converted into an analog form via a digital-to-analog converter, and registered on a strip chart recorder as a function of time.

The actual protocol of measurements is as follows: The frequency of impulse discharges is counted from each nerve preparation for a period of one second 15 times at an interval of 1-2 seconds. This procedure is repeated three times every 10 minutes, giving the overall mean from the 45 measurements. This is the mean control frequency. Then a lowest concentration of the test compound is applied, and the frequency count is made 10, 20 and 30 minutes following application of the compound. After the last count, the concentration of the test compound is increased 10-fold, and the same procedure of frequency count is repeated. This procedure is repeated until the highest concentration of the compound is reached. The concentration range to be used depends on the potency of the compound. For pyrethroids, it usually ranges from 10^{-8} M to 10^{-5} M.

The data on impulse frequency thus obtained are plotted against the logarithm of the concentration as illustrated in Figure 4. The concentration at which the impulse frequency is increased to 200% of the control is termed NS_{200} (nerve stimulation to 200%). For certain insecticides such as pyrethroids, the frequency decreases as the concentration is further increased. Thus it is possible to obtain the concentration at which the frequency decreases back to the control level. This concentration is termed NB_{100} (nerve block to 100%). Further increase in concentration

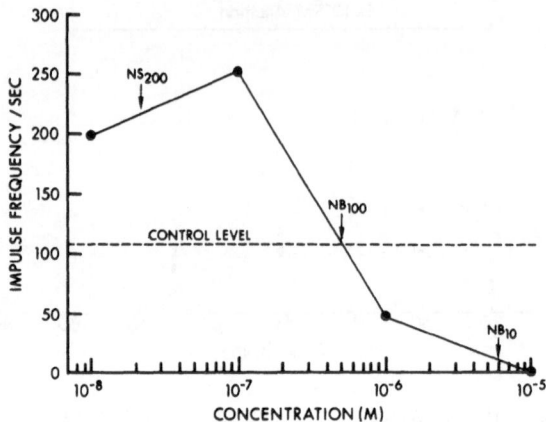

Fig. 4. Method of estimating NS_{200} (concentration to stimulate
the impulse frequency to 200% of the control), NB_{100} (concentration to block the frequency back to 100%), and NB_{10} (concentration
to block the frequency to 10%) using the crayfish abdominal nerve
cord. An example of an experiment with tetramethrin (Takeno et al.,
1977).

may decrease the frequency to a very low level permitting measure-
ment of NB_{10} (nerve block to 10%). Thus both nerve stimulating
and nerve blocking potencies can be estimated by this method.

STUDIES OF SYNTHETIC PYRETHROIDS

A number of synthetic pyrethroids have been compared for
their nerve stimulating and blocking potencies using the method
described in the preceding section. It has long been known that
natural pyrethrins and allethrin stimulate and then paralyze nerve
preparations (Lowenstein, 1942; Welsh and Gordon, 1947; Yamasaki
and Ishii, 1952; Narahashi, 1962; Burt and Goodchild, 1971;
Camougis and Davis, 1971; Camougis, 1973). Since these actions
of pyrethroids on the nerve are primarily responsible for producing
symptoms of poisoning, it would be appropriate to choose the
abdominal nerve cord of the crayfish for the purpose of comparing
the relative potencies of synthetic pyrethroids. The results
thus obtained can be compared with the data on their insecticidal
potencies.

Table 1. Potencies of tetramethrin and phenothrin in stimulating
the crayfish abdominal nerve cord and in killing house flies.

Compound	Isomer	NS_{200} $(\times10^{-8}M)$	NB_{100} $(\times10^{-8}M)$	LC_{50} $(\times10^{-4}M)$
Tetramethrin	(+)-trans	2.2	50	60.3
	(-)-trans	210	>1000	>151
	(+)-cis	6.0	630	66.4
	(-)-cis	130	>1000	>151
Phenothrin	(+)-trans	5.2	>1000	4.85
	(-)-trans	11.5	>1000	>143
	(+)-cis	6.8	>1000	5.71
	(-)-cis	102	>1000	144

Sixty-eight synthetic pyrethroids have been tested for their
potencies in stimulating and blocking the crayfish abdominal nerve
cord (Narahashi et al., 1977; Nishimura and Narahashi, 1977).
Several important and intriguing features were unveiled as a result
of comparison of the nerve potencies and the insecticidal potencies.
Some of the highlights of the finding will be discussed here. One
of the most important features is that the nerve potencies and the
insecticidal potencies do not necessarily run parallel with each
other. Certain pyrethroids were potent in stimulating the nerve,
yet relatively weak in killing insects. Some other pyrethroids
were not so potent in stimulating the nerve, yet relatively strong
in killing insects.

For various isomers of tetramethrin, the nerve stimulating
potency (reciprocal of NS_{200}) and the insecticidal potency (reciprocal of LC_{50}) show a good parallelism (Table 1). (+)-Isomer is
more potent than (-)-isomer in stimulating the nerve and killing
insects for both trans- and cis-tetramethrin. However, the situation is more complicated for phenothrin (Table 1). Although (-)-
trans form is only slightly less active on the nerve than (+)-trans
form, the former is much less active insecticidally than the latter. A good parallelism is seen between the nerve and insecticidal
potencies for (+)-cis and (-)-cis phenothrin.

The data of Table 1 also illustrate some qualitative difference between tetramethrin and phenothrin in their actions on the
nerve. (+)-Trans tetramethrin has a nerve blocking as well as a
nerve stimulating action. (+)-Cis tetramethrin can also block the
nerve but to a lesser extent than (+)-trans form. However, (+)-
trans and (+)-cis phenothrin do not block the nerve effectively
despite their almost equivalent nerve stimulating action to the
corresponding tetramethrin isomers. Furthermore, (+)-trans and
(+)-cis phenothrin are much more potent than the corresponding
(-)-isomers in their insecticidal potencies. These differences
suggest that the mechanisms of action on the nerve are different
between tetramethrin and phenothrin and that factors other than
the actions on the nerve are responsible for the difference in
insecticidal potency between tetramethrin and phenothrin.

Striking differences have been found between (+)-trans and
(-)-trans permethrin (Fig. 5). Although (+)-trans form does not
stimulate nor block the nerve at a concentration of 1 x 10^{-5} M, it
shows a potent insecticidal activity. On the contrary, (-)-trans
permethrin is potent in stimulating the nerve with a NS_{200} of 1.5
x 10^{-8} M, yet 170 times weaker as an insecticide than (+)-trans
form. Similar comparison can be made with bioresmethrin (Fig. 6)
and its analog with a 2,2-dichlorovinyl side chain. Bioresmethrin
effectively stimulates the nerve with a NS_{200} of 5 x 10^{-8} M, whereas
its dichloro derivative does not stimulate the nerve even at 1 x 10^{-5}
M despite the fact that they show an equipotent insecticidal activity.

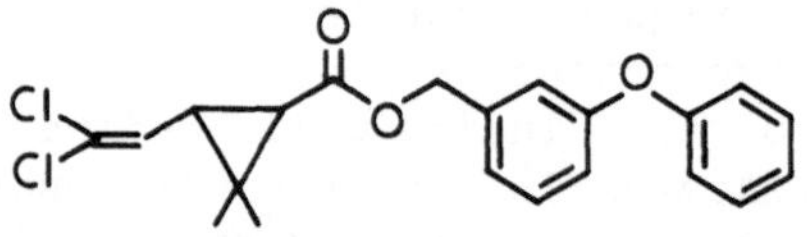

Fig. 5.   Structure of permethrin.

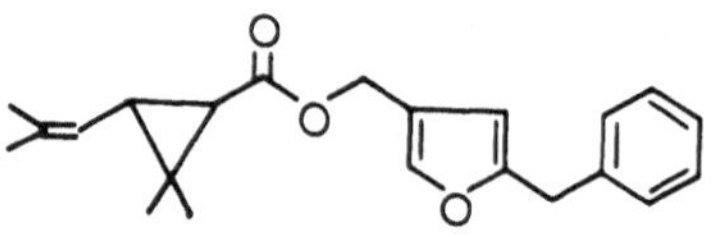

Fig. 6.   Structure of bioresmethrin.

Three possible factors are conceivable for the difference in nerve potency and insecticidal potency. If the rate of penetration of a compound through the cuticle is exceedingly slow, it may not exert a potent killing action even though it is active on the nerve because the compound could be detoxified by the time it reaches the target site. However, since all the pyrethroids tested are fairly lipid soluble, it is unlikely that this factor contributes greatly to the observed difference between the nerve potency and the insecticidal potency.

Secondly, the rate of detoxication may be drastically different between the isomers or compounds in question. This factor is likely to be an important factor responsible for the large difference between the nerve potency and insecticidal potency.

The third possible factor is species difference. The sensitivity of the crayfish abdominal nerve cord to the pyrethroids may not necessarily represent the sensitivity of the insect nerve. However, it is unlikely that there is a large difference in the sensitivity to various pyrethroids between the crayfish nerve and the insect nerve, because both the preparations have been found to be extremely sensitive to the insecticidally active pyrethroids such as allethrin and pyrethrin I (Takeno et al., 1977; Narahashi et al., 1977; Burt and Goodchild, 1971). Both crayfish and insect belong to the Phylum Arthropoda, and exhibit a similar spectrum of nerve sensitivity for insecticides such as pyrethroids and DDT, whereas squid which belongs to the Phylum Mollusca has a different nerve sensitivity spectrum (Narahashi, 1971).

CONCLUSIONS

These studies of DDT analogs and synthetic pyrethroids illustrate the importance of comparing the direct actions on the target site for the purpose of elucidating the true structure-activity relationship. Mere comparison of insecticidal potencies could lead to erroneous conclusions because factors other than the potency on the target site are generally involved in determining the killing activity. The methods described in this paper are expected to be utilized more extensively in order to clarify the relationship between the chemical structure and the primary action on the target site.

REFERENCES

Burt, P.E., and Goodchild, R., 1971, The site of action of pyrethrin I in the nervous system of the cockroach Periplaneta americana L., Entomol. Exp. Appl. 14:179.

Camougis, G., 1973, Mode of action of pyrethrin on arthropod
    nerves, in: Pyrethrum, The Natural Insecticide (J.E. Casida,
    ed.), pp. 211–222, Academic Press, New York.
Camougis, G., and Davis, W., 1971, A comparative study of the
    neuropharmacological basis of action of pyrethrins, Pyre-
    thrum Post 11:7.
Fahmy, M.A.H., Fukuto, T.R., Metcalf, R.L., and Holmstead, R.L.,
    1973, Structure–activity correlations in DDT analogs, J.
    Agr. Food Chem. 21:585.
Fukami, J., Nakatsugawa, T., and Narahashi, T., 1959, The relation
    between chemical structure and toxicity in rotenone deriva-
    tives, Japan. J. Appl. Entomol. Zool. 3:259.
Fukuto, T.R., 1971, Relationships between the structure of organo-
    phosphorus compounds and their activity as acetylcholinester-
    ase inhibitors, Bull. World Health Org. 44:31.
Hille, B., 1968, Pharmacological modifications of the sodium
    channels of frog nerve, J. Gen. Physiol. 51:199.
Holan, G., 1969, New halocyclopropane insecticides and the mode
    of action of DDT, Nature (London) 221:1025.
Holan, G., 1971a, Rational design of insecticides, Bull. World
    Health Org. 44:355.
Holan, G., 1971b, Rational design of degradable insecticides,
    Nature (London) 232:644.
Lowenstein, O., 1942, A method of physiological assay of pyre-
    thrum extract, Nature (London) 150:760.
Metcalf, R.L., 1971, Structure–activity relationships for insecti-
    cidal carbamates, Bull. World Health Org. 44:43.
Metcalf, R.L., and Fukuto, T.R., 1968, The comparative toxicity
    of DDT and analogs to susceptible and resistant houseflies
    and mosquitos, Bull. World Health Org. 38:633.
Narahashi, T., 1962, Effect of the insecticide allethrin on mem-
    brane potentials of cockroach giant axons, J. Cell. Comp.
    Physiol. 59:61.
Narahashi, T., 1971, Effects of insecticides on excitable tissues,
    in: Advances in Insect Physiology, Vol. 8 (J.W.L. Beament,
    J.E. Treherne, and V.B. Wigglesworth, ed.), pp. 1–93,
    Academic Press, London and New York.
Narahashi, T., 1976, Effects of insecticides on nervous conduc-
    tion and synaptic transmission, in: Pesticide Biochemistry
    and Physiology (C.F. Wilkinson, ed.), pp. 327–352, Plenum
    Press, New York.
Narahashi, T., and Haas, H.G., 1967, DDT: Interaction with
    nerve membrane conductance changes, Science 157:1438.
Narahashi, T., and Haas, H.G., 1968, Interaction of DDT with
    the components of lobster nerve membrane conductance, J.
    Gen. Physiol. 51:177.
Narahashi, T., and Yamasaki, T., 1960, Mechanism of increase in
    negative after-potential by dicophanum (DDT) in the giant
    axons of the cockroach, J. Physiol. (London) 152:122.

Narahashi, T., Nishimura, K., Parmentier, J.L., Takeno, K., and
    Elliott, M., 1977, Neurophysiological study of the struc-
    ture-activity relation of pyrethroids, in: Synthetic
    Pyrethroids (M. Elliott, ed.), pp. 85-97, Symposium Series No.
    42, American Chemical Society, Washington, D. C.
Nishimura, K., and Narahashi, T., 1977, Structure-activity
    relationships of pyrethroids based on direct action on
    nerve, Pesticide Biochem. Physiol. In press.
Pichon, Y., 1969, Effets du D.D.T. sur la fibre nerveuse isolée
    d'insecte. Etude en courant et en voltage imposés, J.
    Physiol. (Paris) 61 (Suppl. 1):162.
Takeno, K., Nishimura, K., Parmentier, J., and Narahashi, T.,
    1977, Insecticide screening with isolated nerve preparations
    for structure-activity relationships, Pesticide Biochem.
    Physiol. In press.
Welsh, J.H., and Gordon, H.T., 1947, The mode of action of cer-
    tain insecticides on the arthropod nerve axon, J. Cell.
    Comp. Physiol. 30:147.
Wu, C.H., van den Bercken, J., and Narahashi, T., 1975, The
    structure-activity relationship of DDT analogs in crayfish
    giant axons, Pesticide Biochem. Physiol. 5:142.
Yamasaki, T., and Ishii, T. (former name of T. Narahashi), 1952,
    Studies on the mechanism of action of insecticides, IV, The
    effects of insecticides on the nerve conduction of insect,
    Oyo-Kontyu (J. Nippon Soc. Appl. Entomol.) 7:157.

TOXICITIES OF γ-BHC AND RELATED COMPOUNDS

Matazaemon Uchida, Toshio Fujita, Norio Kurihara, and
Minoru Nakajima
Department of Agricultural Chemistry, Kyoto University
Kyoto, Japan 606

INTRODUCTION

There are eight diastereoisomers of BHC (Benzene hexachloride,
1,2,3,4,5,6-hexachlorocyclohexane). Structural variations in
these isomers have been known to cause remarkable changes in
physiological effects against insects and mammals as shown in
Table 1. Observation of the poisoning symptoms in insects shows
that γ-BHC (lindane) is characterized as a potent excitant, while
δ-BHC is a typical depressant (Mullins, 1955). Thus, BHC isomers
have a dual activity and there seems to be a strict stereospecificity in their physiological effects.

Table 1.   Physiological Effect of BHC Isomers[a]

BHC Isomer	Configuration	Physiological Effect
α	*a a e e e e*	weak excitant
β	*e e e e e e*	inert or weak depressant
γ	*a a a e e e*	strong excitant
δ	*a e e e e e*	strong depressant
ε	*a e e a e e*	not insecticidal
η	*a e a a e e*	not insecticidal
θ	*a e a e e e*	unknown
ι	*a e a e a e*	unknown

[a]Mullins (1955)

133

Among α-, β-, γ- and δ-BHC, γ-BHC is the most toxic against
not only insects, but also mammals (Metcalf, 1955). In their
toxicity to higher plants and microorganisms, however, δ-BHC is
the most effective among the isomers (Lyr, 1967; Rohwer, 1949).
The biological actions of BHC isomers can be classified into two
groups as shown in Table 2: the group 1 type where the γ-isomer is
the most potent, and the group 2 type in which δ-BHC is most
effective. The excitant and depressant effects of BHC isomers,
which seem to have different physiological causes, belong to
groups 1 and 2, respectively. This work attempts to establish
the difference in their modes of action.

Table 2.   Biological Activities of BHC Isomers

Group 1	
Insecticidal action[a]	γ > α > δ > β
Mammalian toxicity[b]	γ > δ > α > β
Group 2	
Toxicity against higher plants[c]	δ > γ ≃ α ≃ β
Toxicity against microorganisms[d]	δ > γ > α ≃ β

a) Mullins (1955), b) Metcalf (1955), c) Lyr (1967),
and d) Rohwer (1949)

THE DEPRESSANT-LIKE ACTIONS OF BHC ISOMERS

We measured the inhibitory potencies of BHC isomers against
a beef cerebral Na+-K+-ATPase preparation, yeast (Saccharomyces
cerevisiae) growth, and nerve conduction in the American cockroach (Periplaneta americana (L.)). The inhibitory activities
against ATPase and yeast growth were obtained as the -log of the
molar concentration required for 50% inhibition (pI_{50}). The
neurodepressing activity was determined as -log of the minimum
molar concentration blocking nerve conduction (-log MIC), using
external electrode techniques and isolated nerve cords of
American cockroaches (Uchida et al., 1974b). The biological
data and a physicochemical constant (log P) are given in Table 3.
Partition coefficients (P) determined with the 1-octanol-water
system have been widely used for structure-activity studies
(Hansch, 1971; Hansch and Glave, 1971; Leo et al., 1971). According to Leo et al. (1971), log P is an excellent parameter
of the lipophilic property of a molecule. The partition
coefficients of BHC isomers were determined by electron capture
gas chromatography (Kurihara et al., 1973). The log P values
of DDT and DFDT (2,2-bis(4-fluorophenyl)-1,1,1-trichloroethane)
were calculated by means of the additivity rule with the use of
a radioisotopically determined log P value of ^{3}H-methoxychlor,
4.30 (Leo et al., 1971).

Table 3. The Effect of Various Inhibitors on ATPase, Yeast Growth and Nerve Conduction.

Inhibitor	log P^a	pI_{50}ATPase Observed	Calcd.	pI_{50}yeast Observed	Calcd.	-log MIC Observed	Calcd.
Methanol	-0.66	-0.23[b]	0.02[c]	-0.06[b]	-0.08[d]	-- [b]	-0.41[e]
Ethanol	-0.16	0.43	0.41	0.44	0.39	-0.01	0.04
1-Propanol	0.34	0.72	0.79	0.93	0.85	0.41	0.50
1-Butanol	0.84	1.10	1.18	1.23	1.31	1.05	0.96
1-Pentanol	1.34	1.55	1.57	1.77	1.77	1.55	1.41
1-Hexanol	2.03	2.40	2.10	2.36	2.40	2.08	2.05
1-Heptanol	2.59	2.78	2.53	2.84	2.92	2.71	2.56
1-Octanol	3.15	3.05	2.96	3.32	3.44	2.92	3.07
L-Menthol	3.07	2.87	2.90	3.21	3.36	2.80	3.00
Thymol	3.30	3.22	3.08	3.69	3.57	3.52	3.21
α-BHC	3.81	--	3.46	--	4.04	--	3.66
β-BHC	3.79	--	3.44	--	4.03	--	3.65
γ-BHC	3.72	3.35	3.40	4.00	3.96	3.40	3.59
δ-BHC	4.14	4.09	3.73	4.51	4.35	4.00	3.97
DDT	5.76*	4.80	4.97	--	5.78	--	5.43
DFDT	4.62*	3.60	4.09	--	4.76	--	4.39
Ether	0.77	--	1.12	--	1.24	0.82	0.89

a) Taken from Uchida et al., (1974b), Leo et al. (1971) and Hansch and Glave (1971), except for values with asterisk. The log P of 1-heptanol was calculated as the mean of log $P_{1-hexanol}$ and log $P_{1-octanol}$.

b) The values are the means of those obtained from at least three replicates. The SE is estimated as ±0.01 log unit.

c, d and e) Calculated by Eqs. [1], [2], and [3], respectively.

δ-BHC inhibited the Na+-K+-ATPase, yeast growth and the conduction of the cockroach nerve cords more than the γ-isomer. For α- and β-BHC, precise inhibitory potencies could not be obtained because of their limited solubilities. The water solubility at 28°C has been shown to be 69.7, 6.9, 254 and 540 x 10^{-7} mole/1 for α-, β-, γ-, and δ-BHC, respectively. The addition of a small amount of a protein such as bovine serum albumin (BSA) to an aqueous solution containing the isomer increased solubility 20-50 times (Kurihara et al., 1973). Thus, we feel that the increased solubility of γ- and δ-BHC in our experimental systems should be sufficient to give a true index of inhibitory activity due to the presence of proteinaceous materials in varying amounts. This is not the case, however, for α- and β-BHC. Other compounds such as aliphatic alcohols, DDT analogs, menthol, and thymol also inhibited the same biological systems (Table 3). Each of the inhibitory activities shown by such structurally unrelated compounds, is best correlated by a

single parameter, log P. Figure 1 shows the correlation between
the inhibitory potency against Na+-K+-ATPase and log P. The
correlations for the above three inhibitory activities with log P
are shown as Eqs. [1], [2] and [3], respectively. The slopes
and the intercepts are determined by the method of least squares.

$$pI50_{ATPase} = 0.77(\pm 0.08)\log P + 0.53(\pm 0.23)$$
$$n = 14, \; r = 0.988, \; s = 0.237 \qquad [1]$$

$$pI_{50yeast} = 0.92(\pm 0.04)\log P + 0.53 \; (\pm 0.11)$$
$$n = 12, \; r = 0.998, \; s = 0.101 \qquad [2]$$

$$-\log MIC = 0.91(\pm 0.08)\log P + 0.19(\pm 0.19)$$
$$n = 12, \; r = 0.993, \; s = 0.162 \qquad [3]$$

In these and following equations, n is the number of compounds
studied, r is the correlation coefficient, and s is the standard
deviation. The figures in parentheses are the 95% confidence
limits. It seems reasonable to consider that for each of the
inhibiting actions a common critical step, which is governed
solely by the hydrophobicity of the molecule, is shared by
such a diverse set of compounds as BHC isomers, aliphatic
alcohols and other neutral compounds. Stereochemistry of the

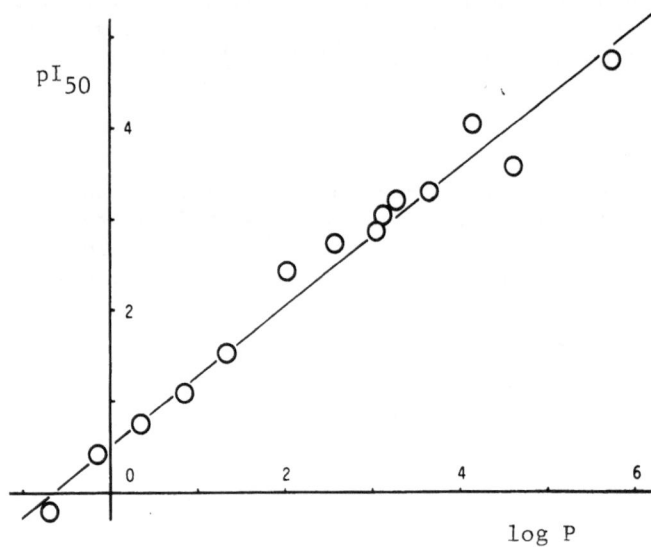

Figure 1. Correlation of log P with Inhibitory Potency
against Na+-K+-ATPase

BHC isomers does not play any role as such. Considering that the
log P values of α- and β-BHC are 3.81 and 3.79, their activities
might lie between those of γ- and δ-isomer, should they be
sufficiently soluble.

A number of biological effects shown by various series of
compounds have been correlated with log P. Hansch (1972) has
found that the linear relationships can be broadly placed into
two groups according to the slope. One group shows slopes lying
between 0.5 and 0.85. In most of the biological actions showing
the slope in this range more or less isolated proteins play a
significant role. The mean value of the slopes for this group
of actions, 0.74 ± 0.09, coincides with that observed for 1-to-1
binding of neutral compounds to protein. The other group shows
slopes lying between 0.85 and 1.20. The structure-activity
relationships for hemolytic, narcotic, and antibacterial
activities of various sets of compounds are classified in this
group. The critical step of these activities has been suggested
to be membrane perturbation.

The relationship expressed by Eq. [1] with the slope of 0.77
belongs to the first group classified by Hansch. The critical
process of Na^+-K^+-ATPase inhibition seem to involve the hydrophobic interaction of inhibitor molecules with the enzyme protein,
perhaps with the K^+-site of the ATPase. The K^+-site has been
considered to be the site of competitive inhibition of the enzyme,
and it would be surrounded by lipophilic constituents of the
enzyme (Israel et al., 1965; Israel and Salazar, 1967).

The slopes observed in Eqs. [2] and [3] of 0.92 and 0.91
suggest that the inhibition of yeast growth and the cockroach
nerve conduction is governed by a critical step involving membrane perturbation. The inhibition of nerve conduction seems to
be the direct cause of the depressant or narcotic action exerted
by BHC isomers. The narcotic activity in term of the minimum
effective concentration (MIC, mole/l) of a variety of neutral
compounds against frog heart has been expressed by Eq. [4]
(Hansch and Glave, 1971), which is very similar to Eq. [3].

$$-\log MIC = 0.93 \log P + 0.11$$
$$n = 28, \ r = 0.973, \ s = 0.182 \qquad [4]$$

Lyr (1969) and Batterton et al. (1972) have found that the
growth inhibition of yeast and algae by BHC isomers and DDT
are accompanied by a concomitant inhibition of Na^+-K^+-ATPase.
They assumed that the critical process of growth inhibition
involved Na^+-K^+-ATPase inhibition. Since the yeast Na^+-K^+-ATPase
inhibition seems also to be due to a hydrophobic interaction, it
is reasonable that this action shows a similar dependence on
log P of inhibitors as demonstrated in Eq. [1]. However, as

described above, the yeast growth inhibition is correlated to log P of the inhibitors with a different sensitivity. Lyr's observation does not necesarily mean that the growth inhibition can be attributed solely to Na^+-K^+-ATPase inhibition.

Matsumura and Patil (1964) have reported that the Na^+-K^+-ATPase inhibition by DDT and analogs is related to their lethal action on mosquito larvae. As described above, Na^+-K^+-ATPase inhibition is governed only by the hydrophobicity of the inhibitor. On the other hand, the lethal effect shown by γ-BHC and DDT analogs is mainly due to their excitatory action on the nervous system. This in turn has been found to be governed not only by the hydrophobicity but also by the steric parameter (Fahmy et al., 1973; Kiso et al., 1977). Therefore, their work should not be taken as a direct evidence for a relationship between insecticidal action and ATPase inhibition. In fact, the poisoning symptoms of insects intoxicated with a specific Na^+-K^+-ATPase inhibitor, ouabain, are quite different from those caused by γ-BHC and DDT.

THE NEUROEXCITATORY ACTIONS OF BHC ISOMERS

γ-BHC is characterized as a contact poison (Mullins, 1955). In order to arrive at the site of action, γ-BHC has to penetrate the insect integument. Passive penetration through the integument has been considered to be one of the crucial factors in the mode of action of insecticides. Armstrong et al. (1951) have reported that grainweevils exposed to deposits of α-, β-, γ- and δ-BHC, accumulated the γ-isomer about 50 times more rapidly than the others. However, our recent studies (Kurihara et al., 1974) with American cockroaches showed different results. Penetration rates of BHC isomers into cockroaches decreased in the order of δ > γ > α > β and the penetration as well as the translocation processes were dependent on the physicochemical properties of the molecules such as log P and "adsorption equilibrium constant" to such macromolecules as nylon 6 and BSA from the aqueous phase. Therefore, the penetration of BHC isomers does not seem to be the crucial process governing the stereospecificity of their mode of insecticidal action. BHC isomers appear to exert their stereospecificity only after they arrive at the site of action.

The insects intoxicated by γ-BHC show violent quiverings of the body, particularly in their legs, accompanied by abnormal flutterings. These poisoning symptoms of γ-BHC suggest that its insecticidal activity is due to its excitatory action against the insect nervous system. In the nervous system of insects γ-BHC has been known to cause excessive after-discharges (Narahashi, 1971).

We examined the relationship between the activity which produces after-discharges in insect nerves and that which induces convulsions in intact insects by using 13 γ-BHC analogs besides α- and γ-BHC in male adult American cockroaches. The lindane analogs used, the structures of which are shown in Table 4, were prepared according to reported methods (Sanemitsu et al., 1972, 1975; Tanaka et al., 1975; Kiso et al., 1975a, 1975b, 1975c). For the assay of neuroexcitatory activity, external electrode techniques were used with isolated nerve cords of American cockroaches (Uchida et al., 1975). Each insecticide at a concentration higher than a certain value caused after-discharges in the cockroach ventral nerve cord. The minimum molar concentration (MEC_{AD}) of each insecticide which produced after-discharges within 2 hours at 20°C was determined. The values of the -log MEC_{AD} of these lindane analogs are shown in Table 4.

Table 4   Neuroexcitatory, Convulsive and Lethal Activities of Lindane Analogs against *Periplaneta americana* (L.)

Compound No.	Substituents 1	2	3	4	5	6	-log MEC_{AD}[a] (mole/1)	-log MEC_{CA}[b] (μmole/insect)	-log HLD[c] (μmole/insect)
1(γ-BHC)	Cl	Cl	Cl	Cl	Cl	Cl	7.3(±0.15)[d]	2.3(±0.15)[d]	1.7(±0.15)[d]
2	Cl	Cl	Br	Cl	Cl	Cl	6.5	1.7	1.7
3	Cl	Cl	OCH₃	Cl	Cl	Cl	6.2	1.6	1.3
4	Cl	Cl	SCH₃	Cl	Cl	Cl	5.7	1.0	0.7
5	Cl	Cl	Cl	H	Cl	Cl	6.3	1.4	1.1
6	F	Cl	Cl	Cl	Cl	Cl	7.4	2.4	1.8
7	Br	Cl	Cl	Cl	Cl	Cl	6.4	1.8	0.9
8	CH₃	Cl	Cl	Cl	Cl	Cl	6.0	1.4	0.8
9	OCH₃	Cl	Cl	Cl	Cl	Cl	6.9	2.0	1.1
10	OC₂H₅	Cl	Cl	Cl	Cl	Cl	5.5	1.3	0.4
11	F	Br	Cl	Cl	Cl	Cl	6.4	1.8	1.5
12	Br	Br	Cl	Cl	Cl	Cl	6.0	1.3	0.7
13	Br	Cl	Cl	Cl	Cl	Br	5.5	0.9	0.6
14	CH₃	Cl	Cl	CH₃	Cl	Cl	5.0	0.9	0.3
15 (α-BHC)	Cl[e]	Cl	Cl	Cl	Cl	Cl	4.6	0.6	0.0

a) Neuroexcitatory activity.
b) Convulsive activity.
c) Lethal activity.
d) Mean value of two or three runs.
e) The configuration of this substituent is represented by 1'.

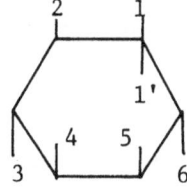

In order to assay convulsive and insecticidal activities, a certain amount of methanol solution containing various amounts of

insecticide was injected into the ventral side of the abdomen of
male adult cockroaches with a microsyringe. When more than a
threshold dose of each insecticide was applied, the insects
showed uncoordinated quivering movements in their legs and wings.
These poisoning symptoms were similar for all the compounds.
From observations of the symptoms of injected cockroaches the
minimum effective dose (or concentration), MEC_{CA}, of the lindane
analogs was expressed as the dose required to produce convulsions
within 3 hours after injection. The 50% lethal dose (HLD) was
also estimated from the number of dead cockroaches found within
24 hours after injection at 25°C. The values of the $-\log MEC_{CA}$
and $-\log$ HLD are shown in Table 4.

Lindane analogs exert an excitatory effect which produces
after-discharges in the central nervous system of American cockroaches as shown in Figure 2. The most active compound among
the lindane analogs is the 1-fluoro analog (6) which is as active
as lindane (1). The α-isomer (15) also exhibits after-discharges,
although it required a higher concentration (2.5×10^{-5}M) than any
lindane analog in Table 4. β- and δ-BHC were inactive up to a
concentration of 5×10^{-5}M.

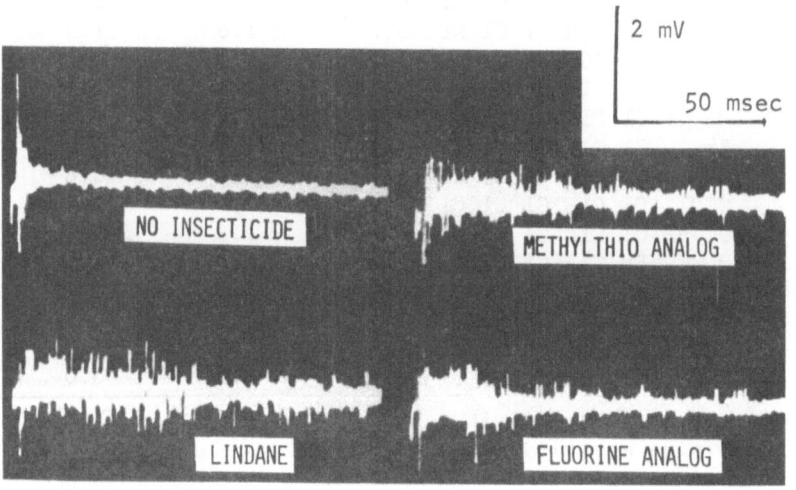

Figure 2. After-Discharges Caused by Lindane Analogs in
Cockroach Isolated Nerve Cord.
The stimulus was applied after 2 hours immersion in a saline containing: no insecticide, lindane (5×10^{-8}M), 3-methylthio analog
(4) (2×10^{-6}M), and 1-fluoro analog (4×10^{-8}M).

The neuroexcitatory activity of lindane analogs against American
cockroach nerves decreases in the order of 1-fluoro analog ≃ lindane > 1-methoxy analog (9) > 3-bromo analog (2) > 1-bromo analog
(7) ≃ 1-fluoro-2-bromo analog (11). Each of the neuroexcitatory
lindane analogs was toxic against intact cockroaches. Table 4
shows that the convulsive and insecticidal activities of lindane
analogs decrease almost in the same order.

As shown in Figure 3, the neuroexcitatory activity of lindane analogs which causes the after-discharges is directly
related to their convulsant action. Figure 3 also shows that
the lethal effect of lindane analogs against American cockroaches
is related to the ability to produce after-discharges in the
central nervous system. Using the method of least squares for
15 compounds, such good correlations can be expressed as Eqs.
[5] and [6].

$$-\log \text{MEC}_{CA} = 0.65(\pm 0.10)(-\log \text{MEC}_{AD}) - 2.46(\pm 0.64)$$
$$n = 15, \ r = 0.966, \ s = 0.140 \qquad [5]$$

$$-\log \text{HLD} = 0.64(\pm 0.17)(-\log \text{MEC}_{AD}) - 2.94(\pm 1.07)$$
$$n = 15, \ r = 0.911, \ s = 0.235 \qquad [6]$$

The coincidence in the slopes of these two equations
emphasizes that the neuroexcitatory action responsible for after-
discharges probably causes convulsions and the lethal effect in
the same manner. The small difference in the intercepts may be
attributed mainly to the metabolic loss of toxicants. With few
exceptions, the metabolic degradation of lindane analogs having
different substituents seems to occur almost to a similar extent,
at least for the present periods. If not, the correlations such
as Eqs. [5] and [6] could not be obtained. A study of the
effect of structural variation on the metabolism of lindane
analogs conducted in this laboratory will be published elsewhere
(Kiso et al., 1977).

Another study from this laboratory (Tanaka et al., 1976)
shows that hexadeuterio-γ-BHC exhibits various degrees of isotope
effect in its toxicity against various biological systems. A
large isotope effect (the ratio: lindane/d_6-lindane=6.82±1.18),
was observed for the metabolic rate from γ-BHC to γ-pentachloro-
cyclohexene. Interestingly, there is no isotope effect in the
neuroexcitatory action against cockroach nerves. The ratios in
the minimum doses (lindane/d_6-lindane) causing convulsions and
having insecticidal effects aginst P. americana, 2.0 and 8.0
respectively, seem to indicate the difference in the degrees of
metabolic degradation during the different periods required for
these tests. The difference between intercept values of Eqs.

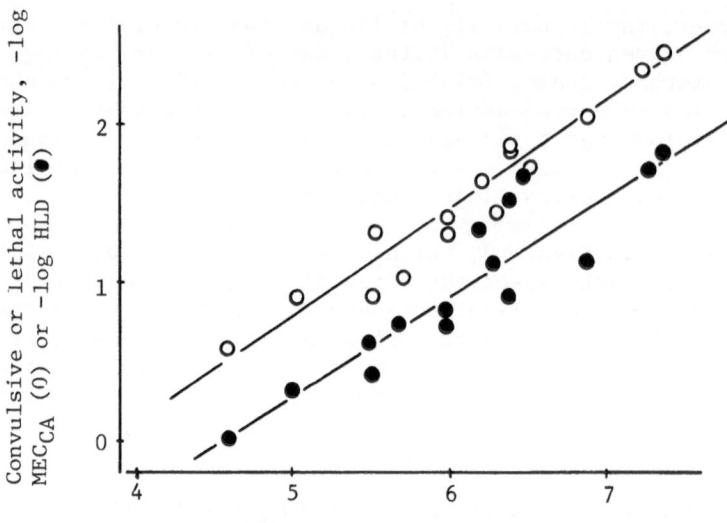

Figure 3.   Relationships among the Neuroexcitatory, Convulsive, and Lethal Activities of Lindane Analogs.

[5] and [6], 0.48, corresponds to the log value of the ratio of the two isotope effects, $\log(8.0/2.0) = 0.6$. The lindane analogs used here seem to be subject to metabolic degradation to a similar extent to each other.

   As discussed above, the neuroexcitatory activity of γ-BHC causes poisoning symptoms which are well characterized by convulsions and resulting death. Recently, we found that the repetitive firing caused by a set of DDT analogs is well related to their convulsive and insecticidal actions (Uchida et al., 1974a). The symptoms of DDT poisoning on the cockroaches are different from those of lindane. The onset of γ-BHC poisoning is slow and it causes abnormal movements in wings, whereas DDT produces a slightly faster onset and uncoordinated leg movements. The difference in the symptoms between lindane and DDT is explained by the difference in the neuroexcitative patterns i.e. after-discharges and repetitive firings. Although the latent period was considerably longer, dieldrin (HEOD) and aldrin also produced after-discharges similar to those of lindane analogs (Table 5). Trans-aldrindiol exerted the same symptoms on American cockroaches more quickly than HEOD or aldrin as reported by Wang et al. (1971).

Table 5   Neuroexcitatory, Convulsive and Lethal Activities
of Aldrin, Dieldrin and Trans-aldrindiol.

Compound	Neuroexcitatory activity[a]	Convulsive activity[b]	Lethal activity[c]
aldrin	--[d]	2.3	1.7
dieldrin	--[d]	2.4	2.0
trans-aldrindiol	5.0	0.7	0.4

a) $-\log \text{MEC}_{AD}$(mole/l), b) $-\log \text{MEC}_{CA}$(μmole/insect), c) $-\log$
HLD(μmole/insect), d) Latent period was too long.

THE EFFECTS OF NEREISTOXIN ON THE NEUROEXCITATORY
ACTION OF INSECTICIDES

The after-discharges caused by lindane analogs, as well
as such chlorinated cyclodiene insecticides as HEOD, aldrin, and
trans-aldrindiol, were quickly suppressed by the addition of more
than 1×10^{-6}M of nereistoxin (NTX) as shown in Figure 4. The
threshold concentration of NTX agrees with that obtained by
Sakai (1967) for blockage of synaptic transmission of the sixth
abdominal ganglion of American cockroaches, 2×10^{-6}M. Since NTX
is an antagonist of acetylcholine (ACh), the after-discharges
induced by these chlorinated hydrocarbon insecticides seem to be
due to an accumulation of ACh. Neither γ-BHC nor HEOD seems to
act as a cholinomimetic agent on the postsynaptic membrane since
they are able to induce after-discharges first. If they would
act as cholinomimetics, they should first display spontaneous
firing. Considering that γ-BHC and HEOD do not inhibit acetylcholinesterase (AChE) (Hartley and Brown, 1955), it is probable

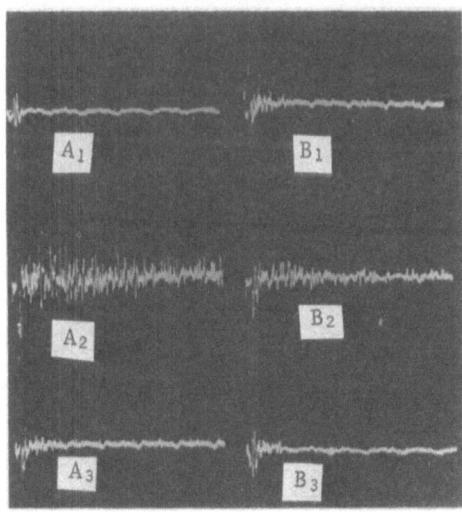

Figure 4. After-Discharges
Caused by γ-BHC and HEOD and
their Suppression by NTX. A_1:
Before treatment, A_2: 60 min
after the treatment with γ-BHC
(2×10^{-8}M), A_3: 10 min after the
following addition of NTX
(1×10^{-6}M), B_1: Before treatment,
B_2: 90 min after treatment with
HEOD (1×10^{-5}M), and B_3: 10 min
after the following addition of
NTX (1×10^{-6}M).

10 mV

100 msec

that the accumulation of ACh is due to an enhanced release of ACh
from the presynaptic membrane. The mechanism by which HEOD causes
after-discharges has been recently studied by Shankland and
Schroeder (1973). Their observations, using other ACh-antagonists
such as atropine and d-tubocurarine, agree with the present
results.

In order to confirm the above discussion further, we used an
anti-AChE agent: m-isopropylphenyl N-methylcarbamate (18). This
carbamate insecticide inhibits AChE resulting in the accumulation
of ACh in the nervous system. As shown in Figure 5, the carbamate
($6x10^{-7}M$) was able to induce after-discharges which continued for
a few hours and resulted in spontaneous discharges. Under these
conditions blockage of synapses was not observed. It has been
shown that AChE inhibitors such as demeton, methyldemeton, and
diazoxon elicit prolonged after-discharges by a single stimulus
followed by synaptic blockage (Metcalf et al., 1968; Narahashi
and Yamazaki, 1960). Burt et al.(1966) found that the lower
the concentration of diazoxon, the longer the time required for
blocking nerve conduction. The present experimental conditions
correspond to this situation. The after-discharges caused by the
carbamate seem to be the result of ACh accumulation in synapses.
These after-discharges were suppressed effectively by the
addition of NTX ($1x10^{-6}M$). However, the after-discharges re-
appeared about half an hour after the initial blocking by NTX.
Inhibition of AChE may result in an accumulation of ACh sufficient
to overcome $1x10^{-6}M$ of NTX competitively. The minimum concentration of the carbamate which causes after-discharges in the
cockroach nerve, $6x10^{-7}M$, is of the same order as the I_{50}
concentration ($3.4x10^{-7}M$) obtained by Metcalf et al. (1968) for
inhibition of fly-head AChE. The sensitivity to NTX suggests
that the neuroexcitatory actions of γ-BHC and HEOD share a common
process with those of carbamates i.e. a high level of ACh

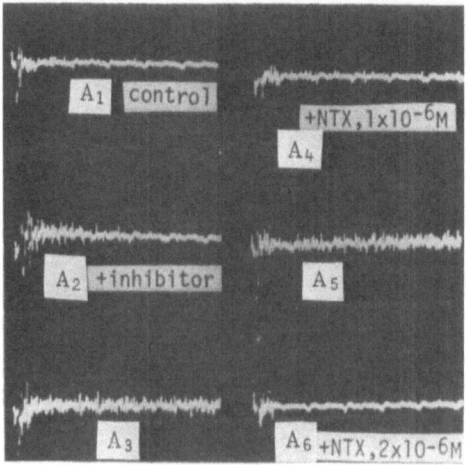

Figure 5. After-Discharges
Induced by m-Isopropylphenyl N-
Methylcarbamate ($6x10^{-7}M$). A_1:
Before treatment, A_2: 6 min after the treatment with the carbamate, A_3: 10 min after the
treatment, A_4: 6 min after the
following addition of NTX (1x
$10^{-6}M$) to A_3, A_5: 30 min after
the addition of NTX, and A_6: 10
min after the further addition
of NTX ($2x10^{-6}M$).

10 mV

100 msec

accumulates which results in after-discharges. The symptoms of
insects poisoned with γ-BHC, HEOD, and anti-AChE are similar to
one another.

When nerve cords were pretreated with NTX ($1-2 \times 10^{-6}$M) for
more than 20 min γ-BHC and HEOD caused no electrophysiological
effects. The conduction not mediated by the cholinergic synapses
in the NTX-poisoned nerves was unaffected by lindane analogs and
HEOD under these conditions. Thus, the present results suggest
that the most important aspect of the insecticidal action of γ-
BHC and HEOD seems to be an enhanced release of ACh from presynaptic membranes of cholinergic synapses.

The ability of DDT and 2,2-bis(4-bromophenyl)-1,1,1-
tricholoroethane (DBrDT) to produce the repetitive discharges
was unaffected by the addition of NTX. DDT and DBrDT showed
repetitive activity even on nerve preparations treated with
4×10^{-5}M of NTX for 20 min (Figure 6). Since all the cholinergic
synapses of the poisoned nerve cords are blocked, the repetitive
responses must be conducted through those connected without ACh-
mediated synapses. Narahashi (1971) considered that DDT activated
the axonal membrane to cause prolongation of the negative after-
potential (NAP). The resulting NAP was believed to initiate
repetitive firings. Thus, the present observations, together
with our previous report (Uchida et al., 1974a), seem to support
the idea that the repetitive effect on the noncholinergic axonal
membrane may be the most important aspect of the insecticidal
action of DDT analogs. The site of action of DDT and DBrDT,
which are insensitive to NTX, is distinguishable from those of
γ-BHC and HEOD, which are sensitive to NTX.

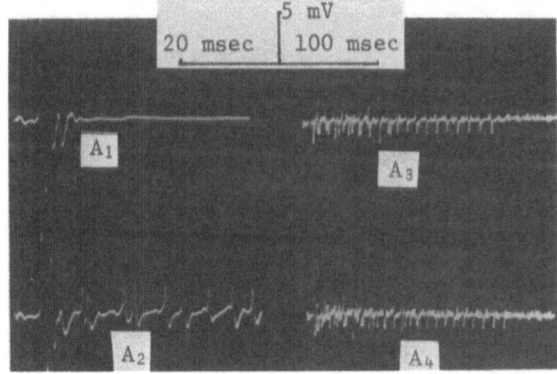

Figure 6. The Activi-
ty of DDT and DBrDT on a
Nerve Preparation Pre-
treated with NTX. A_1:
After pretreatment with
NTX (4×10^{-5}M), A_2 and A_3:
20 min after the
addition of DDT (1×10^{-6}M),
A_4: 20 min after the
addition of DBrDT (4×10^{-6}M).

Table 6　　　　　Neuroexcitatory, Convulsive, Insecticidal and
Anti-AChE Activities of Carbamate Insecticides.

Compound No.	R_1	R_2	Neuroexcitatory activity $-\log MEC_{AD}{}^{a}$	Convulsive activity $-\log MEC_{CA}{}^{b}$	Lethal activity $-\log HLD^{c}$	Anti-AChE activity	
						$pI_{50}{}^{d}$	$\log ki^{e}$
16	CH_3	H	6.1^{f}	1.6^{f}	1.2^{f}	4.85	3.57
17	C_2H_5	H	6.4	2.1	1.8	5.32	4.54
18	$CH(CH_3)_2$	H	7.2	2.6	2.3	6.47	5.72
19	CH_3	CH_3	4.4	0.4	0.1	--	2.15
20	C_2H_5	CH_3	5.0	0.8	0.8	--	2.52
21	$CH(CH_3)_2$	CH_3	6.1	1.7	1.7	4.30	3.37

a) mole/l, against *P. americana*.
b,c) mole/insect, against *P. americana*.
d) From Metcalf et al. (1968),
　 against fly-head AChE.
e) From Nishioka et al. (1976, 1977, and
　 unpublished), on bovine erythrocyte AChE.
f) The SE is estimated as ±0.15 log unit.

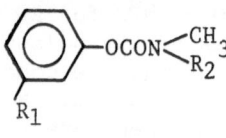

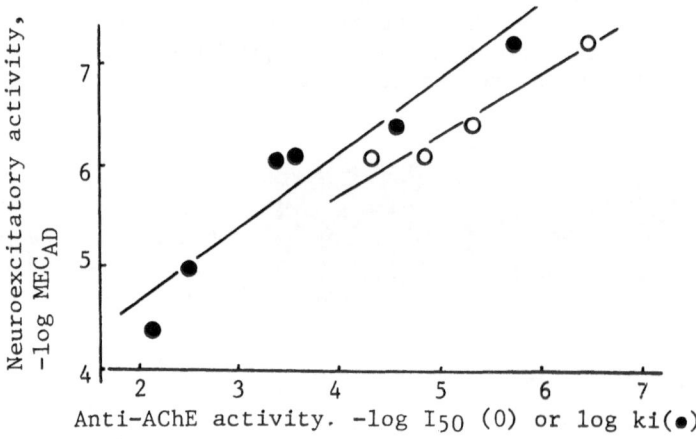

Figure 7.　Relationship between the Neuroexcitatory and Anti-
AChE Activities of Carbamate Insecticides.

ANTIACETYLCHOLINESTERASE AND NEUROEXCITATORY ACTIVITIES
OF CARBAMATE INSECTICIDES

The carbamate insecticides in Table 6, which inhibit AChE to various degrees, also exhibit after-discharges sensitive to NTX. In Figure 7 the relation between anti-AChE and the neuroexcitatory activities of these carbamates is shown. The higher the anti-AChE activity of the carbamate, the stronger its neurotoxic effect. Thus, the inhibition of AChE and the resulting ACh accumulation cause after-discharges in the central nervous system. A similar result was obtained by Metcalf et al. (1968) who studied the activity of carbamates in causing spontaneous firing in the ventral nerve cords of American cockroaches. Although the after- and spontaneous discharges are distinguishable from each other, both seem to be attributable to a common factor, i.e., excessive ACh accumulation.

Interestingly, the plots between neuroexcitatory and convulsive activities for the carbamates fall on a line close to the line for lindane analogs (Figure 8). Therefore, the convulsions probably occur regardless of whether a high level of ACh is brought about by its excessive release from the presynaptic region or by AChE inhibition. The convulsions caused by lindane analogs as well as by carbamates were suppressed when 2 μl of NTX solution (1×10^{-3}M) were injected. The after-discharges in the central nervous system are likely to be the direct cause of convulsions and the similarity in the poisoning symptoms of γ-BHC and carbamates are understandable on this basis.

The effect of carbamates in producing after-discharges is also closely related with the lethal activity. The regression analyses gave Eqs. [7] and [8] for the correlations in the

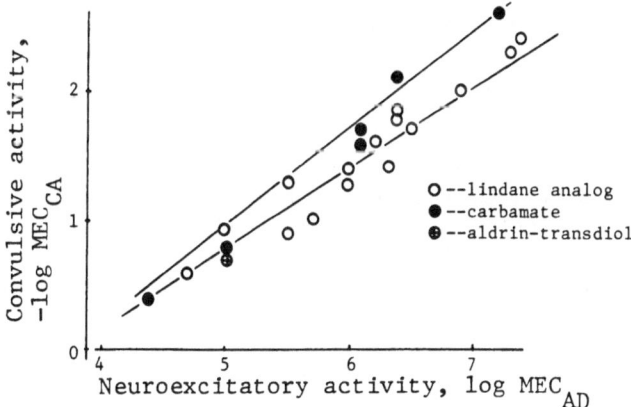

Figure 8.   Relationship between the Convulsive and Neuro-
            excitatory Activities of Insecticides.

biological activites of carbamates in Table 6. The similarity
between Eqs. [7] and [8] means that the convulsions caused by

$$-\log \text{MEC}_{CA} = 0.80(\pm 0.12)(-\log \text{MEC}_{AD}) - 3.18(\pm 0.71)$$
$$n = 6, \; r = 0.994, \; s - 0.097 \tag{7}$$

$$-\log \text{HLD} = 0.76(\pm 0.25)(-\log \text{MEC}_{AD}) - 3.15(\pm 1.49)$$
$$n = 6, \; r = 0.973, \; s = 0.204 \tag{8}$$

carbamates are intimately connected with the resulting death.
There seems to be no significant loss of carbamates used here
during their lethal actions in vivo.

CONCLUSION

BHC has both depressant and excitant effects against
insects and mammals. The first, as well as the other depressant-
like actions of BHC isomers, has been shown to be determined
solely by hydrophobicity. These actions are well characterized
as physical toxicities. The weak insecticidal activity of δ-BHC
should be due to its depressant action or secondary effect
associated with it.

The neuroexcitatory effect producing after-discharges in the
nervous system of insects, where γ-BHC is the most potent isomer,
is shown to be the main cause of insecticidal action. Pharmacological evidence suggests that the neuroexciting action of γ-
BHC (lindane) is exerted by the abnormal release of ACh from the
presynaptic membranes. This concept of the mode of action of
γ-BHC is supported by the similarity in poisoning symptoms to
those of anti-AChE agents such as carbamates.

REFERENCES

Armstrong, G., Bradbury, F., and Standen, H., 1951, The penetra-
    tion of insect cuticle by isomers of benzene hexachloride,
    Ann. Appl. Biol. __38__:555.
Batterton, J. C., Boush, G. M., and Matsumura, F., 1972, DDT:
    Inhibition of sodium chloride tolerance by the blue-green
    alga, *Anacystis nidulans, Science* __176__:1141.
Burt, P. E., Gregory, G. E., and Molloy, F. M., 1966, A histo-
    chemical and electrophysiological study of the action of
    diazoxon on cholinesterase activity and conduction in ganglia
    of the cockroach, *Periplaneta americana* (L.), *Ann. Appl.
    Biol.* __58__:341.
Fahmy, M.A.H., Fukuto, T.R., Metcalf, R.L., and Holmstead, R.L.,
    1973, Structure-activity correlations in DDT analogs,
    J. Agr. Food Chem. __21__:585.
Hansch, C., 1971, Quantitative structure-activity relationships in
    drug design. In: *Drug Design* Vol. 1. (E. J. Ariëns, ed.),
    Academic Press, New York, pp. 271-342.

Hansch, C., 1972, A computerized approach to quantitative biochem-
    cal structure-activity relationships, *Adv. Chem. Series*,
    No. 114, (R. F. Gould, ed.). American Chemical Society,
    Washington, D.C., pp. 20-40.
Hansch, C., and Glave, W. R., 1971, Structure-activity relation-
    ships in membrane perturbing agents, *Mol. Pharmacol.* 7:337.
Hartley, J. B., and Brown, A.W.A., 1955, The effects of certain
    insecticides on the American cockroach, *J. Econ. Entomol.* 48:
    265.
Israel, Y., and Salazar, I., 1967, Inhibition of brain microsomal
    adenosine triphosphatase by general depressants, *Arch. Bio-
    chem. Biophys.* 122:310.
Israel, Y., Kalant, H., and Langer, I., 1965, Effect of ethanol on
    Na$^+$-K$^+$-Mg^{2+}-stimulated microcosmal ATPase activity, *Biochem.
    Pharmacol.* 14:1805.
Kiso, M., Irie, Y., Sanemitsu, Y., Kurihara, N., and Nakajima, M.,
    1975a, Syntheses and PMR studies of pentachlorocyclohexanecar-
    bonitrile, pentachloromethylcyclohexane and tetrachlorodi-
    methylcyclohexane, *Agr. Biol. Chem.* 39:451.
Kiso, M., Maeda, M., Kurihara, N., and Nakajima, M., 1975b, Synthe-
    ses of α- and γ-BHC alkylthio analogs, *Agr. Biol. Chem.*
    39:459.
Kiso, M., Tanaka, K., Sanemitsu, Y., Yoshida, M., Kurihara, N.,
    and Nakajima, M., 1975c, Syntheses of γ-BHC alkoxy analogs,
    Agr. Biol. Chem. 39:443.
Kiso, M., Nohta, M., Tanaka, K., Kurihara, N., Fujita, T., and
    Nakajima, M., 1977, Insecticidal activity and microsomal
    metabolism of biooxidizable lindane analogs, *Pestic. Biochem.
    Physiol.* (in press).
Kurihara, N., Uchida, M., Fujita, T., and Nakajima, M., 1973,
    Studies on BHC isomers and related compounds. V. Some
    physicochemical properties of BHC isomers, *Pestic. Biochem.
    Physiol.* 2:383.
Kurihara, N., Uchida, M., Fujita, T., and Nakajima, M., 1974,
    Studies on BHC isomers and related compounds. VI. Penetration
    and translocation of BHC isomers in the cockroach and their
    correlation with physicochemical properties, *Pestic. Biochem.
    Physiol.* 4:12.
Leo, A., Hansch, C., and Elkins, D., 1971, Partition coefficients
    and their uses, *Chem. Rev.* 71:525.
Lyr, H., 1967, On the mechanism of action of δ-HCH in fungi, *Z.
    Allg. Mikrobiol.* 7:373.
Lyr, H., 1969, Zum Wirkungsmechanismus von Hexachlorocyclohexan
    Isomeren in Hefezellen, *Z. Allg. Mikrobiol.* 9:545.
Matsumura, F., and Patil, K. C., 1964, Adenosine triphosphatase
    sensitive to DDT in synapses of rat brain, *Science* 166:121.
Metcalf, R.L., 1955, *Organic Insecticides*, Interscience, New
    York.

Metcalf, R.L., Gruhn, W.B., and Fukuto, T.R., 1968, Electrophysio-
    logical action of carbamate insecticides in the central ner-
    vous system of American cockroach, *Ann. Entomol. Soc. Amer.*
    61:618.
Mullins, L.J., 1955, Structure-toxicity in hexachlorocyclohexane
    isomers, *Science* 122:118.
Narahashi, T., 1971, Effects of insecticides on excitable tissues,
    Adv. Insect Physiol. 8:1.
Narahashi, T., and Yamazaki, T., 1960, Nervous and cholinesterase
    activities in the cockroach as affected by demeton and
    methyldemeton, *J. Appl. Entomol. Zool.* 4:64.
Nishioka, T., Kitamura, K., Fujita, T., and Nakajima, M., 1976,
    Kinetic constants for the inhibition of the acetylcholines-
    terase by phenyl carbamates, *Pestic. Biochem. Physiol.* 6:320.
Nishioka, T., Fujita, T., Kamoshita, K., and Nakajima, M., 1977,
    Mechanism of inhibition reaction of acetylcholinesterase by
    phenyl N-methylcarbamates. Separation of hydrophobic,
    electronic, hydrogen bonding and proximity effects of aromatic
    substituents, *Pestic. Biochem. Physiol.* 7:107.
Rohwer, S. A., 1949, Effect of individual BHC isomers on plants,
    Agr. Chem. 4:75.
Sakai, M., 1967, Studies on the insecticidal action of nereistoxin,
    V. Blocking action on the cockroach ganglion, *Botyu-Kagaku*
    32:21.
Sanemitsu, Y., Kurihara, N., Nakajima, M., McCasland, G.E.,
    Johnson, L.F., and Carey, L.C., 1972, Syntheses and proton
    magnetic resonance studies at 300 MHz of two new bromopen-
    tachlorocyclohexanes and three new bromotrichlorocyclohexenes,
    Agr. Biol. Chem. 36:845.
Sanemitsu, Y., Minamite, Y., Kurihara, N., and Nakajima, M.,
    1975, Syntheses of 1,2,3,4,5,6-hexaheterohalocyclohexanes:
    fluorine- and bromine-containing lindane analogs, *Agr. Biol.
    Chem.* 39:223.
Shankland, D.L., and Schroeder, M.E., 1973, Pharmacological evi-
    dence for a discrete neurotoxic action of dieldrin (HEOD) in
    the American cockroach, *Periplaneta americana* (L.), *Pestic.
    Biochem. Physiol.* 3:77.
Tanaka, K., Kiso, M., Yoshida, M., Kurihara, N., and Nakajima, M.,
    1975, Syntheses and PMR studies of 1,2,3,4,5-pentachlorocyclo-
    hexane isomers, tetrachloromonomethoxycyclohexane isomers
    and related compounds, *Agr. Biol. Chem.* 39:229.
Tanaka, K., Kurihara, N., and Nakajima, M., 1976, Comparative
    insecticidal activities and metabolic rates of lindane and its
    hexadeuterio-analog, *Pestic. Biochem. Physiol.* 6:386.
Uchida, M., Naka, H., Irie, Y., Fujita, T., and Nakajima, M.,
    1974a, Insecticidal and neuroexciting actions of DDT analogs,
    Pestic. Biochem. Physiol. 4:451.
Uchida, M., Kurihara, N., Fujita, T., and Nakajima, M., 1974b,
    Inhibitory effects of BHC isomers on Na^+-K^+-ATPase, yeast
    growth, and nerve conduction, *Pestic. Biochem. Physiol.* 4:260.

Uchida, M., Irie, Y., Kurihara, N., Fujita, T., and Nakajima, M., 1975, The neuroexcitatory, convulsive and lethal effects of lindane analogs on *Periplaneta americana* (L.), *Pestic. Biochem. Physiol.* 5:258.

Wang, C.M., Narahashi, T., and Yamada, M., 1971, The neurotoxic action of dieldrin and its derivatives in the cockroach, *Pestic. Biochem. Physiol.* 1:84.

NITROMETHYLENE HETEROCYCLES AS INSECTICIDES

S. B. Soloway, A. C. Henry, W. D. Kollmeyer, W. M. Padgett[a], J. E. Powell, S. A. Roman, C. H. Tieman, R. A. Corey and C. A. Horne

Shell Development Company

Modesto, California 95350

Nitrogen heterocycles substituted in the 2-position by a nitromethylene group are generally insecticidal. Affecting the level of activity principally are (1) the number and character of heteroatoms in the ring, (2) the ring size, and (3) the nature of substitution on (a) nitrogen, (b) the nitromethylene side chain, and (c) the ring carbons. The interplay of these structural variations results in compounds ranging from the inactive to the extraordinarily potent. The compound with highest activity to corn earworm, seventeen times that of parathion, is tetrahydro-2-(nitromethylene)-2H-1,3-thiazine.

INTRODUCTION

In quest of new classes of insecticides acting by heretofore unrecognized mechanisms, we examined a variety of heterocycles substituted with a nitromethyl group. Whereas aromatic systems afforded low levels of activity at best, some saturated heterocycles substituted with a nitromethylene group have provided compounds of extraordinary potency. Patent applications for these compounds have been filed in this and other countries and some patents have issued. Some of the main features of the nitromethylene heterocycles are presented here in terms of structure-activity relationships and properties. Full descriptions of chemical synthesis and biological testing will appear elsewhere.

---

a) Present address: Drake Chemical Company, P.O. Box 26, Lock Haven, Pennsylvania 17745.

STRUCTURE—ACTIVITY RELATIONSHIPS

The aromatic heterocycles examined are shown in Table 1. Of the fourteen heterocyclic systems, insecticidal activity was found only in the case of pyridine. Some of the more active members are presented in Table 2 together with their corn earworm activity, shown in parenthesis, relative to that of parathion taken as equal to 100. These compounds are depicted in their tautomeric, nitro-methylene structures as they appear to exist in water. The value of an alkyl group, particularly methyl on nitrogen, is noteworthy. Indeed, the desmethyl homologue of Compound 1 is inactive. The effect of groups larger than methyl, however, is detrimental as shown by Compounds 2 and 4.

Table 1.   Aromatic heterocycles with nitromethyl substitution.

Pyridine	Quinoline
Imidazole	Isoquinoline
Pyrimidine	1,2,5-Oxadiazole
Pyrazine	Benzothiazole
Furan	Benzoxazole
Thiophene	Benzimidazole
Cinnoline	Quinoxaline

Table 2.   2-(Nitromethyl)pyridines.

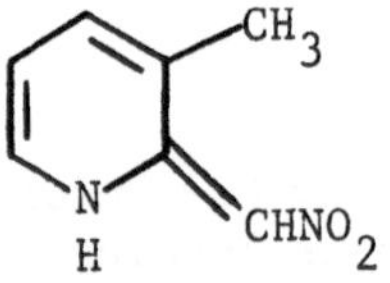

(12)

Compound 1

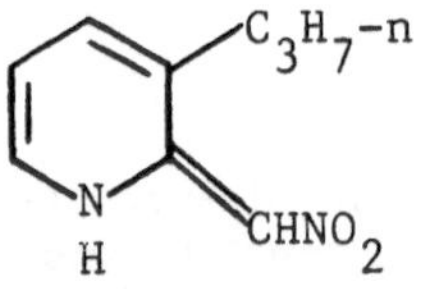

(3)

Compound 2

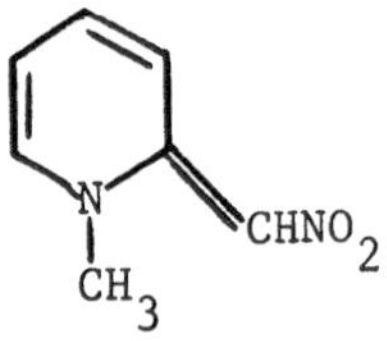

(40)

Compound 3

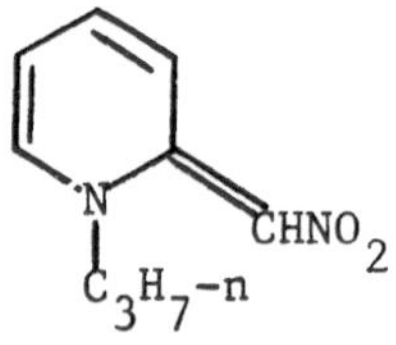

(20)

Compound 4

   Surpassing the nitromethyl pyridines in activity are a number
of similarly constituted saturated systems of which the principal
examples are shown in Table 3 together with their corn earworm
activity relative to parathion. The prime member of the group is
the tetrahydrothiazine Compound 15 with an activity seventeen times
that of parathion.

   The effect of number and character of heteroatoms and of ring
size on insecticidal activity is profound. For example, the next
smaller and next larger ring homologues (Compounds 14 and 16) of
Compound 15 are much less active. Even more adverse to activity is
the presence of oxygen in place of sulfur in the ring (Compounds
11 and 12; Compound 13 was not tested). Methyl-substituted nitrogen
in place of sulfur, however, still affords highly active compounds
(Compounds 8 and 9).

Table 3. Structure and relative activity, in parenthesis, of
          principal nitromethylene heterocycles.

Compound 5 (90)	Compound 6 (160)	Compound 7 (10)
Compound 8 (300)	Compound 9 (140)	Compound 10 (30)
Compound 11 (0)	Compound 12 (60)	Compound 13 (-)
Compound 14 (8)	Compound 15 (1700)	Compound 16 (40)

The role of methyl substitution on nitrogen in affecting
insecticidal activity is varied and conflicting. Whereas the
mono-methyl Compounds 8 and 9 are highly active, their N,N'-un-
substituted parents are less active by more than one order of
magnitude. Entirely detrimental is the effect of N,N'-dimethyl
substitution, the resulting homologues of Compounds 8 and 9 being
essentially inert. This effect of two methyl radicals on either
side of the nitromethylene group is also shown by the 3-methyl
homologue of Compound 3, which is inactive. A different picture
emerges among the mono-nitrogen ring compounds. N-methyl substitution in Compound 5 does not alter activity, whereas it effects
a six-fold reduction with Compound 6. Similarly to the effect of
larger alkyl groups noted for the compounds in Table 2, N-ethyl
substitution in Compound 6 reduces activity by a factor of twelve.
This adverse effect of N-substitution is mimicked in the N-methyl
homologue of Compound 15 with an activity one-twelfth that of its
parent.

Properties of Tetrahydro-2-(Nitromethylene)-
2H-1,3-Thiazine (Compound 15)

The physical nature of the nitromethylene insecticides is
exemplified by the properties listed for Compound 15 in Table 4.
A pale yellow solid of moderately low volatility, Compound 15 is
highly soluble in water and chlorinated hydrocarbons, moderately
in acetone, and only slightly in hydrocarbons. These solubilities
are reflected in the partition coefficients showing a preference
for water over octanol and chloroform over water.

With respect to chemical breakdown, Compound 15 is generally
reactive. Hydrolysis occurs rapidly in acidic solutions, moderately
in basic solutions, but sluggishly at physiological pH. In both
water and methylene chloride, Compound 15 has a half-life of minutes
upon irradiation with 350 nanometer lamps.

In laboratory testing, Compound 15 has shown a broad spectrum
of insecticidal activity as indicated by the values shown in Table 5,
being particularly active against lepidopterous larvae on plants.
It is essentially inactive, however, towards the two-spotted spider
mite on bean plants, and to mosquito larvae (Anopheles albimanus)
in water. Systemic activity towards corn earworm was evidenced when
third instar larvae were placed on foliage of bean plants whose
roots were held in water; the LC_{50} value was 0.4 ppm, which is about
one-fiftieth that of AZODRIN[R] Insecticide. Additionally, solutions
of Compound 15 poured on soil of potted cotton, cabbage, and corn
plants controlled corn earworm, cabbage looper, and black cutworm.
Besides controlling foliage insects by direct or root application,
Compound 15 applied to soil was active towards soil-inhabiting
insects, larvae of western spotted cucumber beetle, and black
cutworm, feeding on corn plants.

Table 4. Physical and Chemical Properties of
Tetrahydro-2-(Nitromethylene)-2H-1,3-Thiazine
(Compound 15)

Physical Form	- Pale yellow needles from isopropanol
Melting Point, °C	- 78
Vapor Pressure, mm @ 25°	- 4.2×10^{-7}
Solubility, %w/v	- Water, 20
	Acetone, 7
	Xylene, < 1
	Chloroform, 30
Partition Coefficient	- Octanol/water, 0.4
	Chloroform/water, 7.0
Hydrolytic Stability, $t_{1/2}$	- 3 hrs at pH 1.1
	> 3 months at pH 7.0
	13 days at pH 9.1
Photochemical Stability, $t_{1/2}$	- 10 min, water
	1 min, methylene chloride

Table 5. Insecticidal Activity of Compound 15[a]

House Fly	160
Pea Aphid	20
Corn Earworm	1700
Cabbage Looper	130
Black Cutworm	800
Lygus spp.	130

a) Activity relative to parathion equal to 100,
    except for Lygus where AZODRIN Insecticide
    is the standard equal to 100.

Table 6. Activity of Compounds 6 and 15 to Higher Animals

Compound 15

    Rat, acute oral LD_{50} - 300 mg/kg

    Rabbit, percutaneous LD_{50} - 2000 mg/kg

    Rainbow trout, LC_{50} - 150 ppm @ 48 hours

Compound 6

    Mouse, acute oral LD_{50} - 400 mg/kg

    Chicken, acute oral LD_{50} - > 1000 mg/kg

Although highly active against insects, the nitromethylene
compounds (6 and 15) are much less so to higher animal forms as
indicated by the data in Table 6. Moderate activity is indicated
for mice and rats by oral administration, and slight to rabbits
by skin application. Both to fish (rainbow trout) and to chickens,
these compounds show little effect.

CONCLUSION

As exemplified by Compound 15, the nitromethylene heterocycles
are extraordinarily active towards insects, especially lepidopterous
larvae, moderately with respect to rodents, and slightly to chickens
and fish. Chemically, these compounds are subject to rapid degradation under both hydrolytic and photochemical conditions. This
combination of chemical and biological properties provides a novel
class of potent insecticides that appear to be environmentally non-
persistent and ecologically safe.

THE HOUSE FLY METABOLISM OF NITROMETHYLENE INSECTICIDES

W.T. Reed and G.J. Erlam

Shell Development Company, Modesto, California, USA

and Shell Biosciences Lab., Sittingbourne, Kent, UK

The insect metabolism of some nitromethylene insecticides has been examined in house flies (Musca domestica) using ^{14}C radiolabeled materials and gas-liquid chromatography. Preliminary results indicate that metabolism occurs most likely by an oxidative pathway with the primary site of attack being at the nitromethylene carbon. Depending upon the analog involved, the metabolism may result in the formation of a carbonyl compound with the elimination of CO_2 or the carbon bearing the nitro group can be converted to a carboxylic acid. In addition, some unidentified polar materials were formed. In the case of a highly polar analog, the parent compound was excreted without modification. Oxidative detoxication was involved in the methylenedioxyphenyl synergism of these compounds although the levels of synergism could not be accounted for by the changes in detoxication rates alone.

INTRODUCTION

Certain nitromethylene heterocyclic compounds represent an interesting new class of insecticide (Soloway et al., 1978). A study of the house metabolism of selected analogs was undertaken in the hope of contributing to an understanding of their toxicity to insects, especially as related to synergism by methylenedioxyphenyl synergists.

159

METHODS AND MATERIALS

Toxicity measurements were made by injecting groups of 20
adult, female, three-day-old house flies (susceptible NAIDM strain)
with the toxicant dissolved in 0.2 μl acetone/DMSO, 50/50. The
equipment included an Isco Model M micro-applicator fitted with an
250 μl Tamac syringe and a 27-gauge needle. Mortality was observed at
24 hours. With synergist pretreatment, 10 μg of sesamex was applied
topically to the dorsum of the flies in 1 μl of acetone 4 hours prior
to injection. Knockdown measurements were made by spraying 100
one-day-old mixed-sex house flies in a wind-tunnel with the toxicant
dissolved in kerosene/acetone, 80/20 at a concentration of
0.1% (w/v).

Knockdown observations were made at one-minute intervals. KT_{50}
and LD_{50} figures were calculated by Least Squares Analysis.

The toxicants used were technical grade (>95% pure):

  SD 33420   Piperidine, 2-(nitromethylene)-.

  SD 33690   Piperidine, 1-ethyl-2-(nitromethylene)-.

  SD 34064   Pyridinium, 1-methyl-2-(aci-nitromethyl)-
                   -hydroxide, inner salt.

  SD 34145   Pyridinium, 1-propyl-2-(aci-nitromethyl)-
                   -hydroxide, inner salt.

The metabolism studies were done with materials radiolabeled
with ^{14}C at the nitromethylene carbon with the exception of SD 33690
which was analyzed by GLC.

Flies injected with SD 33690 (1μg/fly) were incubated for up
to 16 hours in glass petri dishes at 22°C. At the end of each
incubation period, the flies were anesthetized with CO_2 (in many
cases, this was not necessary as the flies were moribund, however,
they were not dead during this time period) and homogenized in 4 ml
acetone and 0.5 gm sodium sulfate in a Potter-Elvehjem tissue
grinder. Extraction was accomplished by adding 4 ml physiological
saline plus 4 ml acetone and the resulting precipitated protein
was removed by centrifugation (105,000 g max). The resulting supernatant was decanted and combined with 15 ml redistilled benzene and
enough sodium sulfate to saturate the aqueous phase. This was mixed
thoroughly and the upper (benzene and acetone) layer was decanted.
The extraction was repeated three additional times using 10 ml
benzene aliquots. Saturation of the aqueous phase was maintained
with additional sodium sulfate. The resulting benzene plus acetone
phase contained essentially all of the SD 33690 and was dried with
magnesium sulfate prior to analysis.

The analysis was done using a Micro-Tek MT-220 gas-liquid chromatograph with a high temperature ^{63}Ni electron capture detector. A 24" x 1/4" o.d. column packed with 2% Reoplex 400 on Gas Chrom Q (100-200 mesh) was used for separation with a nitrogen carrier gas flow rate of 80 milliliters per minute. The column oven was maintained at 185°C, the detector at 245°C, and the transfer lines at 210°C. The power supply to the detector was set at 35 volts in the DC mode. The recovery was determined by relative peak heights.

For SD 33420 where radiolabeled material was available (specific activity: 50.7μCi/mg), injected flies (1μg/fly) were incubated in 50 ml Erlenmeyer flasks for 0, 1/2, 1, 2, 4, 6, and 16 hours. At the end of these periods the external surface of the flies was rapidly rinsed with acetone to remove any compound that may have migrated to the outside of the cuticle. The insects were then homogenized in acetone and sodium sulfate in a Potter-Elvehjem tissue grinder. The radiation in the supernatant was quantitated using a Nuclear-Chicago thin window gas flow G-M counter. The identity of the radioactive components was determined by TLC using precoated silica gel (0.25 mm) plates. The mobile phase was 19% isopropyl alcohol, 76% ethyl acetate, and 5% water. In this system, SD 33420 had an R_f of 0.42.

The chromatograms were scanned with a Nuclear-Chicago 2 pi G-M gas flow strip scanner and the quantitation of the compounds present was recorded by a digital printer. The incubation flasks were rinsed three times with acetone, counted, chromatographed and the TLC's scanned with the 2 pi scanner. The insoluble fly residue, remaining after the acetone homogenization, was ashed and the resultant carbon dioxide was captured in benzylamine-toluene scintillation fluid and counted in a Packard Tri-Carb Liquid Scintillation Spectrometer.

The gases respired by the insects were captured by purging the 50 ml incubation flask with air (flow rate - 50 ml/min) which was subsequently bubbled through a benzylamine-toluene cocktail packed in ice. This test, however, would have been insufficient to determine the identity of the vapor. Carbon dioxide, the probable result of an oxidative degradation, or nitromethane, the probable product of reductive metabolism, would both have been trapped in the scintillation cocktail. In order to differentiate between the two, the respired vapors were bubbled through 50 ml of saturated aqueous barium hydroxide and then through 50 ml of chilled benzylamine-toluene scintillation fluid. Treated flies were incubated in this manner for 16 hours, after which the benzylamine trap was replaced with fresh solution and 6 ml concentrated HCl was injected into the barium hydroxide solution. As soon as all visible traces of barium carbonate had disappeared (about ten minutes), the second benzylamine-toluene trap was removed. Both samples were then

counted in the liquid scintillation counter. Any carbon dioxide
present in the respired vapor reacted with the barium hydroxide to
form barium carbonate. Upon acidification, the barium carbonate
reverted to carbon dioxide, which was captured in the benzylamine
cocktail. To demonstrate that nitromethane would not be held and
released under these circumstances, the experiment was repeated
except that no SD 33420-treated flies were used; instead, 4.8 µg of
^{14}C nitromethane was added to the barium hydroxide solution prior
to acidification. Here, the radiation was not released by acidification as it was with ^{14}C CO_2.

   In a separate set of experiments with SD 33420 to determine
the nature of some of the metabolites found, large numbers of flies
were sprayed with ^{14}C SD 33420. The flies were then washed three
times with ethanol which was combined with the ethanolic cage
washings, homogenized in water (2.5g flies per 50 ml water) and
the homogenate filtered and treated with sufficient ethanol to
precipitate protein and eye pigment. The precipitate was removed
by centrifugation and the supernatant was extracted with $CHCl_3$
(3 x 50 ml). The aqueous phase remaining was lyophilized and
redissolved in the minimum volume of water. Each extract was
counted in a liquid scintillation counter and examined by paper
chromatography. The remains of the flies and the centrifugation
pellet were combusted and the CO_2 collected and counted. The
aqueous extract was chromatographed on paper using butanol/acetic
acid/water, 44/25/20.

   Flies injected with SD 34064 (specific activity of 9.6 µCi/mg
and SD 34145 (specific activity of 9.0 µCi/mg) were treated in a
similar manner to those injected with SD 33420. The flies were
homogenized in acetone with sodium sulfate in a Potter-Elvehjem
tissue grinder. The insoluble fraction was removed by centrifugation at (105,000 g max) for 10 minutes. The identity of some of
the components of the supernatant was determined by TLC using precoated silica gel (0.25 mm thickness) plates. The mobile phase was
40% tetrahydrofuran, 10% H_2O, and 50% methanol. The resultant
chromatograms were scanned with a 2 pi G-M gas flow strip scanner
with an integrator. Total radiation in the samples was determined
using liquid scintillation. In order to determine more about the
nature of the acetone insoluble fraction, the acetone precipitated
pellet resulting from centrifugation was resuspended in H_2O and
centrifuged again. This procedure was repeated twice. An aliquot
of the water sample was counted using an ethanol-toluene scintillation cocktail while another was repeatedly extracted with diethyl
ether and counted. The radioactivity contained in all of the
insoluble plugs formed by centrifugation was determined by ashing
the samples and counting the resulting CO_2. In order to quantitate
the entire amount of radioactive carbon associated with the flies,
whole, treated flies were incubated, frozen and ashed, and the
resulting CO_2 counted.

RESULTS

The knockdown, toxicity, and synergism for each of the toxicants used are represented in Table 1.

The detoxication of SD 33690, with and without synergist pretreatment, is summarized in Figure 1. Without synergist, the compound rapidly degraded until there was none remaining at three hours. Following synergist pretreatment, no metabolism took place for one hour after which the compound was degraded, although not completely.

The detoxication of SD 33420, with and without synergist pretreatment, is represented in Figure 2. The distribution of the radiolabel following injection of SD 33420 into house flies, is summarized in Table 2. The radiation in the external rinse, the material that moved from inside the insect to the external surface, was SD 33420 as determined by TLC. The radiation in the soluble fraction of the homogenate was also principally SD 33420. No SD 33420 was excreted; this fraction was composed principally of two more polar materials with R_f's of 0.33 and 0.21 compared to SD 33420 which had an R_f of 0.42. The radioactivity in the insoluble fraction of the homogenate was removed from the soluble fraction following denaturation of the protein with acetone and centrifugation, implying a protein complex. The radiolabeled respired gases were exclusively carbon dioxide; no nitromethane was present.

Following a more comprehensive examination of the internal metabolites using large numbers of flies, at least four different radiolabeled materials were found present after paper chromatography using butanol/acetic acid/ water as a mobile phase with R_f's of 0, 0.75, 0.81, and 0.86. The second metabolite (R_f equal 0.75) had the same R_f in the paper chromatographic system as pipecolic acid.

The results pertaining to the rate of degradation of SD 34145 are summarized in Figure 3. It was evident that the injected SD 34145 was slowly converted to an acetone insoluble, centrifugable fraction. No radiolabeled vapors were respired. No radioactivity was excreted. That all of the radioactivity was retained inside the fly was verified by the whole fly ashings when all of the applied radioactivity was recovered after 16 hours incubation. The TLC's indicated that essentially all of the acetone soluble material recovered from the homogenate was the parent compound, SD 34145, (R_f equals 0.7). At the six hour incubation period, 85% of the acetone insoluble fraction redissolved in water of which only 4% partitioned into ether. The remaining 15% was found upon ashing the H_2O insoluble plug formed after centrifugation of the H_2O suspension.

TABLE 1

Insect toxicity of selected nitromethylene heterocycle insecticides.

Compound	Structure	Knockdown (KT50, Min)	House fly injection Unsynergized LD50 (μg/Fly)	Synergized LD50 (μg/Fly)	Synergism Factor
SD 33420		2.0	0.35	0.018	19x
SD 33690		0.7	>2	0.0026	>770x
SD 34064		>30	2	0.3	7x
SD 34145		4.4	0.16	0.0007	230x

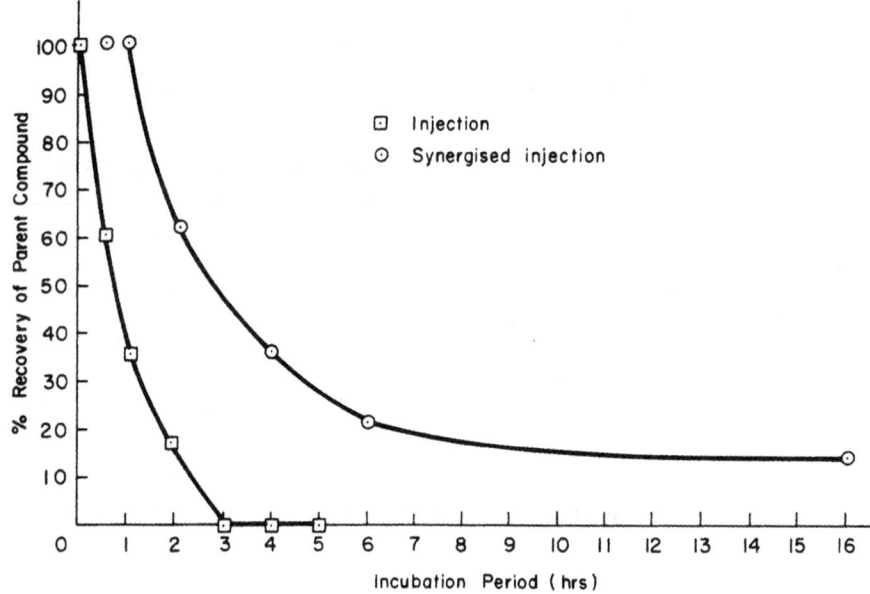

Figure 1. In vivo degradation of SD 33690 in house flies.

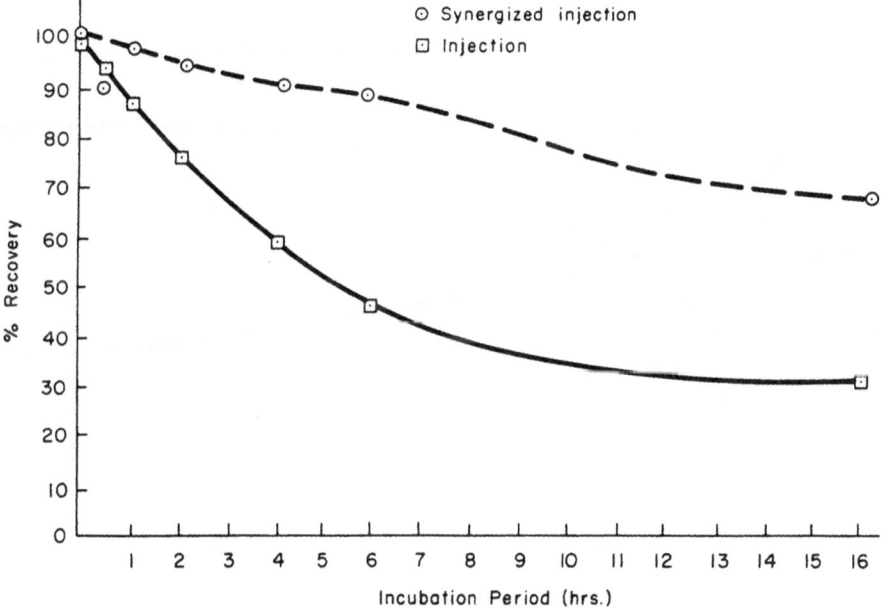

Figure 2. In vivo detoxification of SD 33420 in house flies.

TABLE 2

The Metabolic Fate of SD 33420 in House Flies in terms
of Percent Recovery of the Applied Dose

	Incubation period (hours)						
	0	1/2	1	2	4	6	16
Homogenate	97	91	84	71	49	36	21
External Rinse (SD 33420)	3	3	3	5	10	10	12
Insoluble Fly Residue	1	5	8	9	12	14	13
Excretion	0	2	2	?	4	6	13
Carbon Dioxide	0	1	4	7	12	13	30
Total	101	102	101	94	87	79	89

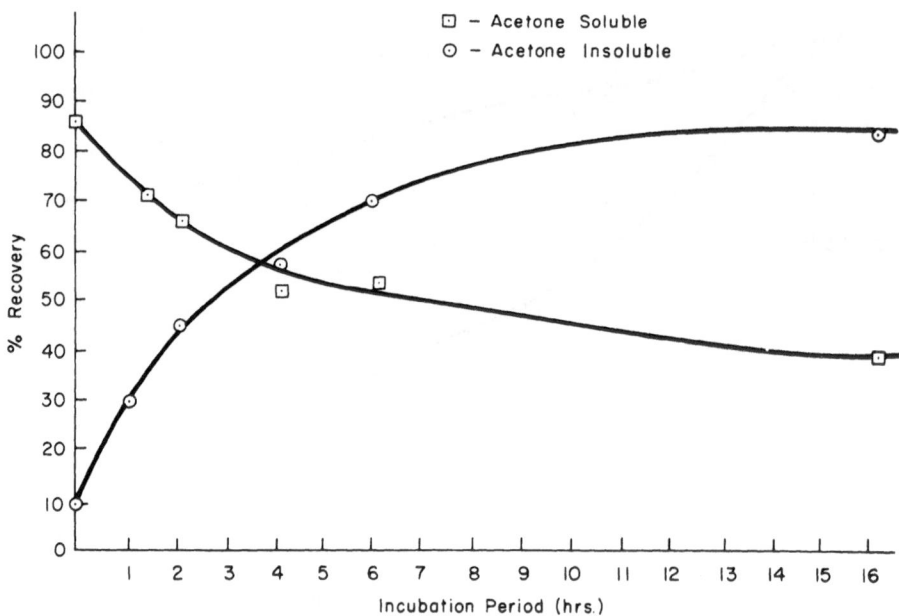

Figure 3. In vivo house fly degradation of SD 34145.

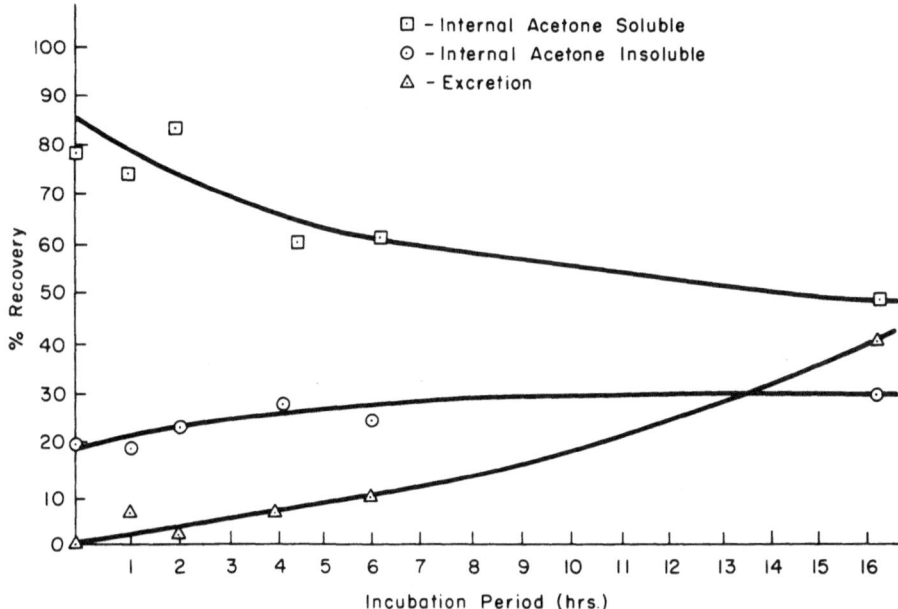

Figure 4. In vivo house fly degradation of SD 34064.

The distribution of radiation following injection of SD 34064 is represented in Figure 4. The acetone soluble fraction decreased with the concurrent increase of an acetone insoluble fraction (centrifuged out at 10,000 RPM for ten minutes) and excreted material. This acetone soluble fraction, by TLC analysis, was principally SD 34064 (R_f of 0.57) in addition to a metabolite appearing at the longer incubation periods with an R_f of 0.33. Homarine, (pyridinium, 2-carboxyl-1-methyl-hydroxide, inner salt) the corresponding carboxylic acid, was demonstrated to be a chemical oxidation product of SD 34064 (Henry, 1975, unpublished) and had an R_f of 0.33. Based on this, the observed metabolite was theorized to be homarine. A TLC analysis of the excreted radioactivity at 16 hours indicated the presence of the parent compound, SD 34064, (86%) and homarine (14%). No radiolabeled CO_2 was respired. When the acetone insoluble centrifugate was extracted with water, all of the radioactivity moved into the water phase . When this in turn was extracted with diethyl ether, essentially all of the radioactivity stayed in the water phase, indicating that the radioactivity was associated with soluble proteins and not phospholipids.

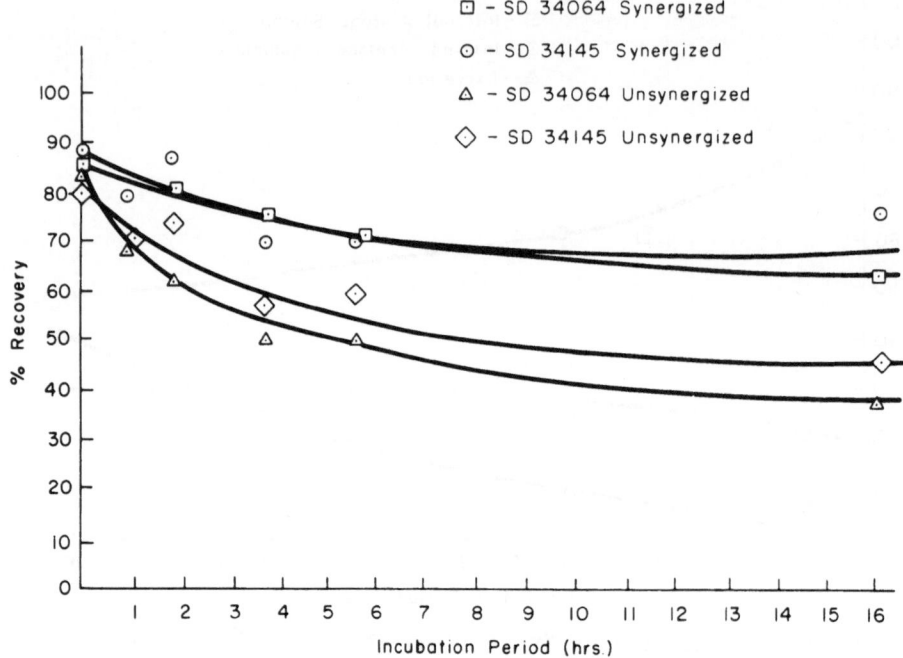

Figure 5.   Comparative synergized and unsynergized house fly
            detoxification rates of SD 34064 and SD 34145.

     The difference in the rate of metabolism of SD 34064 and
SD 34145 resulting from synergist pretreatment is represented in
Figure 5.

DISCUSSION

     It is apparent from these results that each of the nitromethy-
lene insecticides studied is metabolized by house flies, most likely
by an oxidative pathway. The use of methylenedioxyphenyl synergists
slows this process. While the decreased detoxication is apparently
a factor in the compounds' synergism, it most likely is not the sole
factor responsible. The metabolic changes are too small to account
for the relatively large synergism factors (e.g., >770x for
SD 33690).

     The metabolism of SD 33420 appears to proceed via at least two
pathways, both involving oxidative attack at the nitromethylene
carbon. One pathway leads to carbon dioxide and most likely
2-piperidone. The other leads to 2-pipecolic acid. None of these
materials are toxic at 2μg/fly injected, indicating that the nitro
methylene insecticides are most likely active in their own right

and not because of an oxidative activation. The possibility exists
that one of the other unidentified metabolites is toxic; however,
since they are found in relatively small quantities and since the
nitromethylene insecticides are synergized rather than antagonized
by sesamex, the oxidative formation of a more toxic material seems
unlikely. This theory is supported by the fact that some of these
materials have extremely rapid knockdown activity (Table 1) such
that it does not seem that there is time for an adequate amount of
an active metabolite to be formed to produce the observed biological effect.

    The more polar aci-nitropyridinium analog, SD 34064, seemed
also to be metabolized to the corresponding carboxylic acid,
homarine. Flies excrete SD 34064 unchanged as well as its metabolic product homarine, whereas nothing was excreted following
injection with SD 34145. The type of metabolism that took place
was possibly similar for both compounds, the oxidative degradation
to the corresponding acid. The metabolite(s) from SD 34145 appeared
to be more tightly bound to the protein than was homarine inasmuch
as none of the materials were found in the soluble fraction. Instead, the metabolite(s) seemed to form a loose association with
soluble proteins as the radioactivity was precipitated by acetone
denaturation and centrifugation. The radioactive fraction was
resuspendible in water and would not partition into ether, indicating that the radioactive metabolite was associated with soluble
proteins rather than phospholipids. Additional studies in this
area are being pursued.

REFERENCE

Soloway, S.B., Henry, A.C., Kollmeyer, W.D., Padgett, W.M., Powell,
J.E., Roman, S.A., Tieman, C.H., Corey,R.A., and Horne, C.A., 1978.
Nitromethylene heterocycles as insecticides. In: Pesticide and
Venom Neurotoxicity (D.L. Shankland, R.M. Hollingworth and T. Smyth,
Jr., eds.) Plenum Press, New York, pp. 153-158.

THE CARDIOVASCULAR TOXICITY OF CHLORDIMEFORM:

A LOCAL ANESTHETIC-LIKE ACTION

Albert E. Lund, George K. W. Yim and Daniel L. Shankland

Department of Entomology, Purdue University

West Lafayette, Indiana 47907

INTRODUCTION

Chlordimeform (CDM) is a formamidine pesticide with interesting and unusual biological activities (Hollingworth, 1976). It is moderately toxic to mammals (mouse oral LD_{50}=195-310 mg/kg; Hollingworth, 1976). It has little action on cholinergic transmission in insects or mammals (Dittrich, 1966; Beeman and Matsumura, 1973), although a decrease in acetyl choline receptor sensitivity has been observed in frog muscle following large doses of CDM (Wang et al., 1975; Watanabe et al., 1975). CDM and related compounds inhibit monoamine oxidase in rat and mouse liver (Beeman and Matsumura, 1973; Aziz and Knowles, 1973) and uncouple oxidative phosphorylation and electron transport in rat liver mitochondria (Abo-Khatwa and Hollingworth, 1974). Although each of these authors suggested that such actions could be involved in acute toxicity, no one has satisfactorily related these biological actions to toxicity. Furthermore, certain poisoning symptoms such as the rapid onset of tremors and convulsions could not be explained readily by either of these biochemical sites of action (Neumann and Voss, 1977; Lund l et al., 1977). Thus the cause of death and the physiological mechanisms underlying some symptoms remain unknown.

Beeman and Matsumura (1974) showed that 200 mg/kg CDM given i.p. decreased the mean arterial blood pressure in the rabbit, but they did not further investigate the mechanism of the hypotensive action. The purpose of this investigation was to study the action of CDM on the mammalian cardiovascular system and contribution of such actions to the lethal effects of CDM.

171

METHODS

Arterial blood pressure and heart rate were monitored in 7-12 kg dogs anesthetized with pentobarbital. Right ventricular contractile force was measured with a strain gauge sewn onto the heart while the animals were artificially respired. Peripheral vascular resistance was measured by perfusing a hind limb at a constant flow rate (27 ml/minute) with blood taken from the femoral artery and monitoring changes in the perfusion pressure. Drugs were administered via the cephalic vein or the femoral artery (hind limb perfusion experiments only).

RESULTS AND DISCUSSION

Chlordimeform at doses of 1-30 mg/kg i.v. caused initial decreases in mean arterial blood pressure and cardiac contractility within one minute, followed by secondary increases above predrug levels (Figure 1). These parameters returned to control levels within one hour. There was relatively little effect on the heart rate. Hyperventilation, tremors and occasional clonic convulsions were associated with the transition from the depressor to the pressor responses in lightly anesthetized dogs.

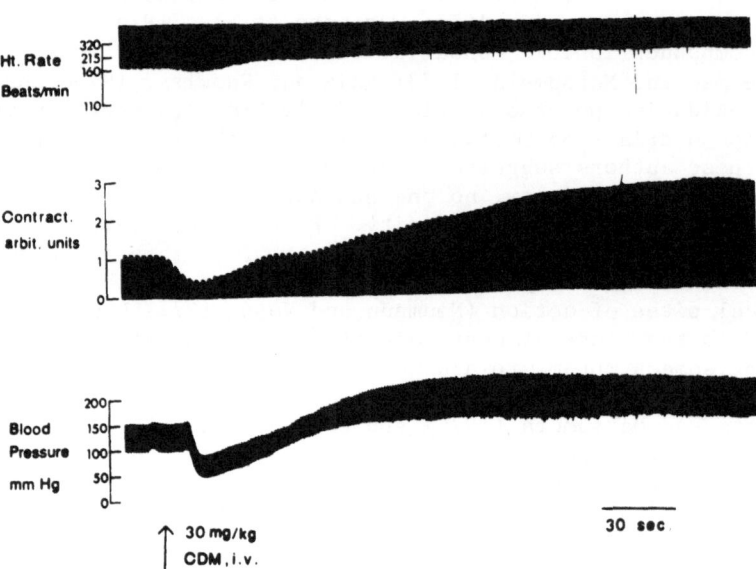

Fig. 1. Response of heart rate, cardiac contractility and blood pressure to 30 mg/kg CDM i.v. Arbit. units=Arbitrary units.

Deep anesthesia antagonized both tremors and the hypertension but not the initial depressor actions on blood pressure and cardiac contractility. After lethal doses of CDM ($\geq$50 mg/kg, i.v.), cardiac contractility was severely depressed and arterial blood pressure rapidly fell to zero. Although respiratory arrest occurred simultaneously, cardiovascular collapse is assumed to be the primary cause of death since artificial respiration did not protect the animals. This has been confirmed with conscious animals also. Figure 2 shows that in addition to causing cardiac depression CDM decreased vascular resistance when injected into a perfused hind limb. These results suggest that the lethal hypotension is the combined result of both myocardial depression and vasodilation.

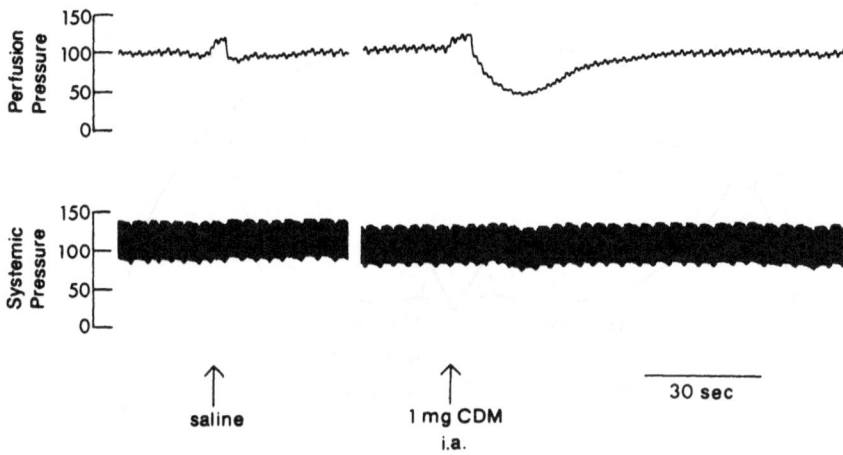

Fig. 2. Response of hind limb perfusion pressure and systemic arterial pressure to 1 mg CDM i.a. Scales in mm Hg.

The possible sites of action of CDM can be summarized by considering a simplified outline of the autonomic control of the arterial blood pressure (Figure 3). Blood pressure is produced when blood is forced to flow against a resistance. Blood flow is a function of cardiac contractility and heart rate, and resistance is a function of vascular tone. Stimulation of the parasympathetic nervous system depresses both the heart and peripheral vasculature via muscarinic synapses and therefore decreases blood pressure. The sympathetic nervous system after nicotinic synapses in the paravertebral ganglia, makes adrenergic contact with the cardiovascular system. β-Adrenergic stimulation

increases the heart rate and contractility and dilates the
peripheral vessels whereas α-adrenergic stimulation constricts
the vasculature. The response to sympathetic stimulation is thus
usually (but not necessarily) hypertension. Obviously, the blood
pressure is determined by the interaction between the parasympathetic and sympathetic nervous systems. In addition to these
autonomic effects, histaminergic stimulation can produce hypotension as a result of vasodilation. Thus the possible sites of
action of a drug producing cardiovascular toxicity are numerous.
The mechanisms of the secondary hypertension and initial hypotension caused by CDM were investigated using pharmacological and
surgical techniques.

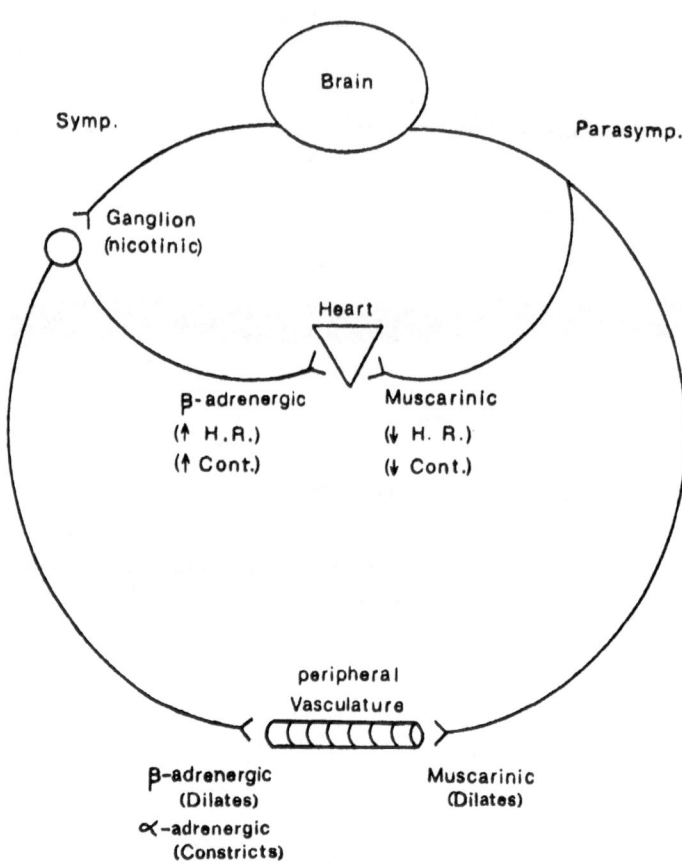

Fig. 3. Diagramatic representation of autonomic control of the
cardiovascular system. See text for explanation. ↑H.R.=increase
heart rate, ↑Cont.=increase cardiac contractility, Symp.=
sympathetic, Parasymp.= parasympathetic.

The secondary increase in cardiac contractility which accompanied the secondary pressor response (Fig. 1) was blocked by the β-adrenergic antagonist propranolol, the ganglionic blocker hexamethonium, and the central sympathetic blocker diazepam. A secondary increase in peripheral resistance was observed accompanying the pressor response after intravenous injections of CDM. This does not show in Figure 2 where administration was intra-arterial (local rather than systemic). The increase in peripheral resistance was abolished by ligation of the femoral and sciatic nerves, by hexamethonium i.v. and by the α-adrenergic blocker phentolamine i.a.. These findings suggest that the secondary hypertension caused by CDM results from myocardial and vascular stimulation by sympathetic activity of central origin.

The initial depressor action of CDM arises by a different mechanism. Bilateral vagotomy (parasympathectomy) or the muscarinic blocker atropine had no effect on the cardiac depression caused by CDM, and atropine or the histaminergic blocker tripelennamine i.a. had no effect on the CDM-induced vasodilation. Likewise, CDM had no effect on the increases in heart rate and cardiac contractility caused by the ganglionic stimulant DMPP or by the β-adrenergic agonist isoproterenol. Chlordimeform also had no effect on the vasoconstriction caused by the α-adrenergic agonist norepinephrine. These findings suggest that the CDM-induced hypotension is not the result of interference with the autonomic nervous system but rather the result of a direct depressant action of CDM on cardiac and vascular smooth muscle.

Although the precise biochemical mechanism for the cardiovascular depression remains unproved, a plausible hypothesis is suggested by the observation that CDM possesses local anesthetic activity with a potency similar to that of procaine when applied to a frog sciatic nerve (Chinn et al., 1976). The structural requirements for a local anesthetic are quite broad, but three features are believed to be necessary: (a) a hydrophobic aromatic ring, (b) a hydrophilic group, usually a substituted amine group, and (c) a 6-9 Å chain separating these two groups (Buchi and Perlia, 1971). The structure of CDM is compatible with this structural pattern (Figure 4), and certain local anesthetics such as holocaine and guanicaine are amidines. The effects of intravenously administered local anesthetics on the cardiovascular system have been well studied (de Jong 1972, Covino and Vassallo 1976) and they are qualitatively identical and quantitatively similar to those described for CDM in this report. Further comparisons made in this laboratory between the effects of the local anesthetic lidocaine and CDM on cardiac contractility and vascular resistance show great similarities and further suggest that a mechanism of action common to that of local anesthetics may be found for CDM. More detailed results will be published elsewhere.

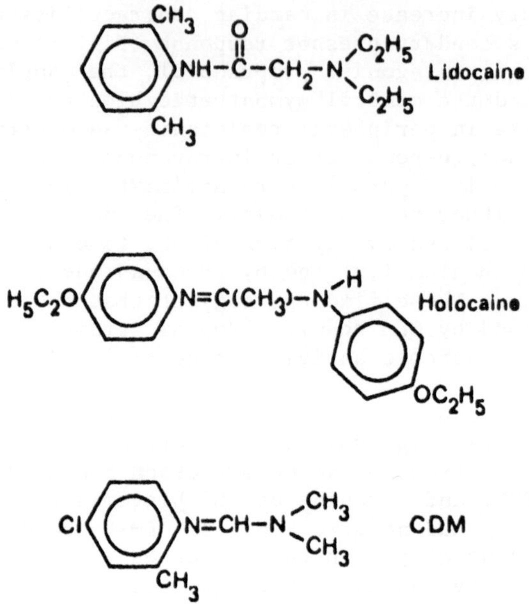

Fig. 4.   Structures of the local anesthetics lidocaine and holocaine and CDM.

REFERENCES

Abo-Khatwa, N. and Hollingworth, R. M., 1974, Pesticidal chemicals affecting some energy-linked functions of rat liver mito-chondria in vitro. Bull. Environ. Contam. Tox. 12(4):446-454.

Aziz, S. A. and Knowles, C. O., 1973, Inhibition of monoamine oxidase by the pesticide chlordimeform and related compounds. Nature 242:417-418.

Beeman, R. W. and Matsumura, F., 1973, Chlordimeform: A pesticide acting upon amine regulatory mechanisms. Nature 242:273-274.

Beeman, R. W. and Matsumura, F., 1974, Studies on the action of chlordimeform in cockroaches. Pest. Biochem. Physiol. 4:325-336.

Buchi, J. and Perlia, X., 1971, Structure-activity relations and physicochemical properties of local anesthetics. In: Local Anesthetics, Vol. 1. International Encyclopedia of Pharmacology and Theraputics, (P. Lechat, ed.), Pergamon Press, Oxford, pp. 39-130.

Chinn, C., Pfister, W. R., and Yim, G. K. W., 1976, Local anes-
    thetic-like actions of the pesticide chlordimeform.
    Federation Proceedings 35:729.
Covino, B. G. and Vassallo, H. G., 1976, Local Anesthetics:
    Mechanisms of Action and Clinical Use. Grune and Stratton,
    N.Y., 173 pp.
de Jong, R. H., 1972, Physiology and Pharmacology of Local Anes-
    thesis. Charles C. Thomas, Springfield, 267 pp.
Dittrich, V., 1966, N-(2-methyl-4-chlorophenyl)-N',N'-dimethyl-
    formamidine (C-8514/Schering 36268) evaluated as an
    acaricide. J. Econ. Entomol. 59:889-893.
Hollingworth, R. M., 1976, Chemistry, biological activity, and
    uses of formamidine pesticides. Environ. Health Perspect.
    14:57-69.
Lund, A. E., Shankland, D. L., Chinn, C., and Yim, G. K. W.,
    1977, Similar cardiovascular toxicity of lidocaine and
    the pesticide chlordimeform. Toxicol. Appl. Pharmacol.
    (In Press).
Neumann, R. and Voss, G., 1977, MAO inhibition, an unlikely mode
    of action for chlordimeform. Experientia 33:23-24.
Wang, C. M., Narahashi, T., and Fukami, J., 1975, Mechanism of
    neuromuscular block by chlordimeform. Pestic. Biochem.
    Physiol. 5:119-125.
Watanabe, H., Tsuda, S., and Fukami, J., 1975, Effects of
    chlordimeform on rectus abdominis muscle in frog. Pestic.
    Biochem. Physiol. 5:150-154.

FORMAMIDINE PESTICIDES-ACTIONS IN INSECTS AND ACARINES

Richard W. Beeman and Fumio Matsumura

Department of Entomology, University of Wisconsin

Madison, Wisconsin 53706

The formamidines are a novel group of acaricide-insecticides, unique both in chemical structure and in their range of biological activities. No general agreement exists concerning their mechanisms of action. The biological and pharmacological activities of the formamidine pesticides have recently been reviewed (Hollingworth, 1976; Matsumura and Beeman, 1976). This report will attempt to reassess the problem of formamidine pesticidal mechanisms, and to define future research needs.

The aryl formamidines are toxic to a broad spectrum of organisms including species of plants, animals, and bacteria (Hollingworth, 1976). In addition to their biocidal properties, members of this class exert a wide variety of biochemical and pharmacological actions. Included among the formamidines are respiratory uncouplers (Abo-Khatwa and Hollingworth, 1972, 1973), monoamine oxidase (MAO) inhibitors (Beeman and Matsumura, 1973; Aziz and Knowles, 1973), local anesthetics (Chinn et al., 1976), cholinomimetics (Mitsov, 1966), cholinolytics (Vlakhov, 1966a, 1966b; Wang et al., 1975; Watanabe et al., 1975), adrenomimetics (Matsumura and Beeman, 1976), and adrenolytics (Vlakhov, 1966b).

If we consider only the insecticidal, acaricidal, and ovicidal effects of the formamidines, multiplicity of action continues to be manifest. The nature and mechanisms of these actions are the subject of this paper. In view of the unusual complexity of the insecticidal actions of the formamidines, and the variety of biochemical mechanisms which be invoked to explain them, special

effort is required to isolate each behavioral and biochemical
effect from others and to clearly define it, both conceptually and
experimentally.

IN VIVO EFFECTS OF FORMAMIDINES ON INSECTS AND ACARINES

Chlordimeform, the single most important formamidine insecticide, has two distinct actions, ovicidal and insecticidal. In
general the ovicidal action of pesticides can be classified into
two types, namely a chemosterilant effect, and a direct toxic
effect on fertile eggs. Chlordimeform is toxic only to older
eggs, and death does not occur until the time of eclosion in
contrast to many ovicides (Hirano et al., 1972; Salkeld and Potter,
1953). The apparant ovicidal action of chlordimeform may really
be a special case of larvicidal action, a possibility which has
been emphasized recently by several observers (Hollingworth,
1976; Gemrich et al., 1976a).

The insecticidal and acaricidal actions of chlordimeform must
also be itemized. The first is its direct killing action. This
is most potent against early instar larvae of most pests including
the well known cases among lepidopterous insects, but is sometimes
significant against adults, particularly acarines. Greater sensitivity of early instar larvae is a general phenomenon for many
insecticides (e.g., Harris and Gore, 1971), but is particularly
conspicuous with chlordimeform (Hirano et al., 1972; Gemrich et
al., 1976 b).

The sublethal effects of chlordimeform also play an important
role in pest suppression. Indeed, for a commercial insecticide,
chlordimeform in many cases has remarkably low acute toxicity.
Hyperactivity, seen at lethal and sublethal doses of chlordimeform,
has been observed in cockroaches, mites, ticks, and lepidoptera.
In cases of acute toxicity, this symptom may be related to the
cause of death. An opposite effect, inactivation, is seen in
tick larvae immediately after treatment with formamidines
(Atkinson and Knowles, 1974).

Another prominent sublethal effect of chlordimeform is a
potent repellent action, revealed by laboratory choice bioassays
(Dittrich, 1971; Hirano et al., 1972; Doane and Dunbar, 1973) and
by lab and field observations (Doane and Dunbar, 1973; Gemrich
et al., 1976b). Most of the remaining sublethal effects of
chlordimeform can be described as repellent-like. For example,
chlordimeform inhibits feeding in plant-sucking insects (Hirata
and Sogawa, 1976), and causes detachment of feeding ticks (Gladney
et al., 1974; Stone et al., 1974). Finally, chlordimeform causes
colony dispersal in gregarious species. This has been observed
with larvae of insects (lepidoptera, hymenoptera) and ticks
(Atkinson and Knowles, 1974).

The effects of chlordimeform and related formamidines on
insects and acarines (direct lethality, hyperexcitation, inactivation, repellency, antifeeding, tick detachment, and colony
dispersal) may arise via different mechanisms. In order to
progress towards a comprehension of the mechanisms of action of
formamidines it will be necessary to isolate each distinct behavioral effect in "pure" form, and ultimately to correlate them with
specific biochemical lesions.

For example, Stone et al. (1974) have suggested that prolonged hyperactivity and detachment of feeding ticks are two
distinct behavioral phenomena, since they could be separated with
appropriate doses of formamidines. Detachment occurred only with
low doses of chlordimeform and N-desmethylchlordimeform. In
contrast, at high doses, hyperactivity continued to be observed
while the ticks remained attached.

Furthermore, Stone et al. (1974) were successful in demonstrating that a synergist can modify the tick detachment potency
of formamidines: when sesamex was used as a synergist the detachment effect of chlordimeform was antagonized, whereas that of
N-desmethylchlordimeform was synergized. Since irritation of
sensory nerve endings, the presumed cause of any simple repellent
action, should be immune from metabolic mediation, the above data
suggest that tick detachment behavior may not reflect simple
repellency. Furthermore, detachment was not immediate, but continued over a two-hour period.

Atkinson and Knowles (1974) distinguished two types of colony
dispersal behavior in cattle ticks, namely immediate and delayed.
They demonstrated that these two behavioral phenomena arise via
different mechanisms, by finding formamidines which specifically
produced only one or the other of the two forms of dispersal.

We have recently been able to clearly differentiate the antifeeding effect of chlordimeform from its repellency effect in
cockroaches. For our purposes, we define antifeeding as "rejection
of untreated food by chlordimeform-treated insects" and repellency
as "rejection of treated food by untreated insects" (e.g. as
revealed by a choice bioassay). In order to avoid any repellency
effect chlordimeform and other amines are given to the cockroach
via abdominal injection. Thus there is little chance that these
compounds come in contact with chemoreceptors on the antennae
and other parts of the body. Also the doses were selected so as
not to cause hyperexcitation. Using this approach, we found that
chlordimeform has a potent antifeeding or anorectic effect in
cockroaches (Table 1). Even at a low dose level of 5 µg/roach
the amount of food ingestion was reduced by 96%. This effect was
not shared by another MAO inhibitor of similar acute toxicity

Table 1.   Anorectic Action of Chlordimeform and Several Other
Neuroactive Amines in American Cockroaches.[a]

Compound[b]	Dose (μg/insect)	Feeding Response Average amount eaten (μg)	No. tested
Control (H$_2$O)	–	15.9	80
Chlordimeform	0.5	9.6	10
	1	3.0	15
	5	0.5	31
	20	0.3	13
	80	0.4	12
Tranylcypromine	100	12.0	17
	200	4.7	17
Phenelzine	10	20.1	5
	100	9.4	4
Tryptamine	100	12.3	12
	200	1.8	8
CDMT	50	7.5	15
	160	0.2	8

[a] To measure the effect of these amines on appetite, adult male
Periplaneta *americana* were held in battery jars in groups of ten,
and starved for 11 days (H$_2$O only). Cannibalism sometimes occurred,
and the insects involved were discarded. Five μl of an aqueous solution of the test compound (as its hydrochloride or sulfate salt)
was injected intra-abdominally into each cockroach, and the insects
were held for 2 hours. Then they were isolated in 1 pint card-
board ice-cream cartons, each containing a pre-weighed dog food
pellet (30-50 mg). After 5 hours the insects were removed, the
pellets again weighed, and the amount eaten was calculated. Values
given are the means of 4-80 determinations.

[b] Compounds used were chlordimeform (N-(4-chloro-o-tolyl)-N',N'-di-
methylformamidine hydrochloride), tranylcypromine (trans-2-
phenylcyclopropylamine sulfate), phenelzine (2-phenylethylhydra-
zine sulfate), tryptamine hydrochloride, and CDMT (5-chloro-N,N-
dimethyltryptamine hydrochloride). The latter compound was
synthesized in our laboratory. The others were obtained commer-
cially or as gifts.

tranylcypromine, which did not produce anorexia, even at 100 µg/
roach. In contrast, Stone et al. (1974) found that MAO inhibitors
caused tick-detachment behavior, although they were somewhat less
effective than chlordimeform.

Repellency has been confused not only with antifeeding, but
with direct lethality. Non-feeding which results from repellency
or appetite loss may lead to death by starvation, particularly in
rapidly developing first instar larvae. Thus the striking stage-
selectivity of chlordimeform referred to earlier may in part
reflect stage differences in resistance to food-deprivation, and
may not be a simple case of selective acute toxicity. This possibility has not always received due consideration in the literature.
For example, Hirano et al. (1972) reported an enormous difference
in the toxicity of chlordimeform to second and third instar larvae
of the rice stem borer. No mention was made of the possibility of
starvation, although data are presented in the same paper showing
that first instar larvae of this species are strongly repelled
(choice bioassay) by comparable concentrations of chlordimeform.
Even in adult insects it has been clearly demonstrated that the
antifeeding effect of chlordimeform can lead to death by starvation
(Hirata and Sogawa, 1976).

BIOCHEMICAL LESIONS AND ELECTROPHYSIOLOGICAL EFFECTS

Having recognized the lethal and behavioral effect of formamidines, the problem of their biochemical mechanisms of action
remains. Our research group has pointed out that chlordimeform
has several types of effects on non-cholinergic amine regulatory
systems in insects and mites (Matsumura and Beeman, 1976).
Chlordimeform inhibits MAO from cheese mites and tryptamine-N-
acetyl transferase from cockroaches in vitro, alters the normal
metabolic patterns of exogenous amines in vivo, and is a potent
cardio-accelerator in cockroaches. In addition we have shown that
chlordimeform inhibits coupling between octopamine and cyclic AMP
synthesis in cockroach ganglia. However, at this point it is not
possible to infer any causative relationships between these biochemical effects and the behavioral effects of chlordimeform.

Uncoupling of oxidative phosphorylation was shown to contribute to the acute toxicity of chlordimeform to cockroaches, but
cannot account for the range of behavioral effects of this pesticide (Abo-Khatwa and Hollingworth, 1972). Although symptoms of
hyperactivity in insects poisoned with organophosphates, carbamates,
and chlorinated hydrocarbons have been correlated with actions on
the cholinergic nervous system, so far this has not been demonstrated with chlordimeform.

Wang et al. (1975) and Watanabe et al. (1975) reported that chlordimeform showed cholinergic blocking action at the frog neuromuscular junction. However, we showed that acute symptoms of hyperexcitation in affected cockroaches are accompanied by neurophysiological symptoms of excitation in the central nervous system (Beeman and Matsumura, 1974). Furthermore, we found that transmission through the (cholinergic) cercal synapse in the cockroach sixth abdominal ganglion is not blocked by chlordimeform. Thus, so far there is no evidence for a cholinergic action of chlordimeform in insects. Also, it is not certain whether acute symptoms of excitation in chlordimeform-treated cockroaches are related to MAO inhibition, since not all MAO inhibitors are excitants in this species (e.g. phenelzine, Table 2).

Among the MAO inhibitors and amines tested, tranylcypromine was the only compound which caused similar in vivo and electrophysiological excitation symptoms to chlordimeform (Table 2 and unpublished observations). Both tryptamine analogs induced opposite effects (i.e. depression) while phenelzine had no effects at all. An interesting observation is that local anaesthetics, which have been shown to cause similar vasorelaxation effects to chlordimeform in a mammalian system (Chinn et al., 1976) were not toxic to cockroaches (Table 2 and unpublished observations), and furthermore caused depressant symptoms, indicating that the local anaes-

Table 2.   Acute Toxicity and Associated Behavioral Effects of Chlordimeform and Other Neuroactive Amines in Cockroaches.

Compound	Acute LD_{50} (24 hr) ($\mu g/g$)[a]	Behavioral Effects
Chlordimeform	500[b]	excitant
Tranylcypromine	700[b]	strong excitant
Phenelzine	>700[c]	none
Tryptamine	>830[c]	weak depressant
CDMT	400-700[c,d]	strong depressant
Phenacaine[f]	<420[c,e]	strong depressant

[a]intra-abdominal injection

[b]Beeman, R. W. MS Thesis, 1974.

[c]LD_{50}'s are estimations based on observation of 10-20 insects for each compound.

[d]LD_{50} for knockdown. Recovery was slow and incomplete.

[e]LD_{50} for knockdown. Recovery was rapid and complete.

[f]N,N'-bis(p-ethoxyphenyl)acetamidine hydrochloride; Holocaine.

thetic effect of chlordimeform does not play a significant role in acute poisoning of cockroaches.

The biochemical cause of repellency has not been studied. MAO inhibition, a potent action of chlordimeform in mites and ticks (Matsumura and Beeman, 1976; Atkinson et al., 1974), has not been shown to be related to the colony dispersal and toxic actions of formamidines in ticks (Stone et al., 1974), or to the anorectic effect of chlordimeform in cockroaches described here. Attempts to correlate MAO inhibition with detachment activity of formamidines in feeding ticks have also failed (Stone et al., 1974).

No mechanisms can yet be postulated for the anorectic effect of chlordimeform in cockroaches. However, in the rat, monoaminergic mechanisms may be involved in the anorectic actions of several neuroactive amines. For example, amphetamine, fenfluramine, and MAO inhibitors all produce anorexia in rats. In the case of amphetamine, this effect has been correlated with adrenergic receptor stimulation in the brain (Holtzman and Jewett, 1971). Analogous mechanisms may exist in insects. For example, the two tryptamine analogs tested produced a considerable degree of anorexia in cockroaches (Table 1). Thus, the possibility that chlordimeform induces anorexia via stimulation of indoleamine receptors must be considered.

CONCLUSION

It is apparent from the preceding discussion that the effects of chlordimeform are diverse and complex, and that several different "pestistatic" mechanisms may be operating. In this paper, we have attempted to clearly separate the phenomena of anorexia, repellency, excitation, local anaesthesia, acute toxicity, and others. As an example, we have reported our observation of a potent effect of chlordimeform in insects, anorexia which can be studied apart from other in vivo effects. Clear perception and differentiation of a particular in vivo effect is an essential prelude to a search for the causative biochemical lesion.

REFERENCES

Abo-Khatwa, N., and Hollingworth, R. M., 1972, Chlordimeform: The
    relation of mitochondrial uncoupling to toxicity in the
    German cockroach, Life Sci. 11, part 2: 1181-1190.

Abo-Khatwa, N., and Hollingworth, R. M., 1973, Chlordimeform:
    Uncoupling activity against rat liver mitochondria, Pestic.
    Biochem. Physiol. 3: 358-369.

Atkinson, P. W., and Knowles, C. O., 1974, Induction of hyperacti-
    vity in larvae of the cattle tick Boophilus microplus by
    formamidines and related compounds, Pestic. Biochem. Physiol.
    4: 417-424.

Atkinson, P. W., Binnington, K. C., and Roulston, W. J., 1974,
    High monoamine oxidase activity in the tick Boophilus micro-
    plus, and inhibition by chlordimeform and related pesticides,
    J. Austr. Entomol. Soc. 13: 207-210.

Aziz, S. A., and Knowles, C. O., 1973, Inibition of monoamine
    oxidase by the pesticide chlordimeform and related compounds,
    Nature 242: 417-418.

Beeman, R. W., and Matsumura, F., 1973, Chlordimeform: a pesti-
    cide acting upon amine regulatory mechanisms, Nature 242: 273-
    274.

Beeman, R. W., and Matsumura, F., 1974, Studies on the action of
    chlordimeform in cockroaches, Pestic. Biochem. Physiol. 4:
    325-336.

Chinn, C., Pfister, W. R., and Yim, G. K. W., 1976, Local anaesthe-
    tic-like actions of the pesticide chlordimeform (CDM), Fed.
    Proc. 35: 729.

Dittrich, V., 1971, Biological action of chlorphenamidine, Report
    to FAO/WHO.

Doane, C. C., and Dunbar, D. M., 1973, Field evaluation of insecti-
    cides against the gypsy moth and the elm spanworm and repel-
    lent action of chlordimeform, J. Econ. Entomol. 66: 1187-1189.

Gemrich, E. G., II, Kaugars, G., and Rizzo, V. L., 1976a, Insecti-
    cidal and miticidal activity of arylthioformamidines, J. Agric.
    Food Chem. 24: 593-595.

Gemrich, E. G., II, Lee, B. L., Tripp, M. L., and VandeStreek, E.,
1976b, Relationship between formamidine structure and
insecticidal, miticidal, and ovicidal activity, J. Econ.
Entomol. 69: 301-306.

Gladney, W. J., Ernst, S. E., and Drummond, R. O., 1974, Chlordimeform: a detachment-stimulating chemical for three-host
ticks, J. Med. Entomol. 11: 569-572.

Harris, C. R., and Gore, F., 1971, Toxicological studies on cut-
worms. VIII. Toxicity of three insecticides to the various
stages in the development of the darksided cutworm, J. Econ.
Entomol. 64: 1049-1050.

Hirano, T., Kawasaki, H., Shinohara, H., Kitagaki, T., and
Wakamori, S., 1972, Studies on some biological activities of
N-(2-methyl-4-chlorophenyl)-N',N'-dimethylformamidine (Gale-
corn) to the rice stem borer, Chilo suppressalis Walker,
Botyu-Kagaku (Bull. Inst. Insect Control) 37: 135-41.

Hirata, M., and Sogawa, K., 1976, Antifeeding activity of chlordimeform for plant-sucking insects, Appl. Entomol. Zool. 11:
94-99.

Hollingworth, R. M., 1976, Chemistry, biological activity, and uses
of formamidine pesticides, Environ. Health Perspect. 14:
57-69.

Holtzman, S. G., and Jewett, R. E., 1971, The role of brain norepinephrine in the anorexic effects of dextroamphetamine and monoamine oxidase inhibitors in the rat, Psychopharmacol. 22:
151-161.

Matsumura, F., and Beeman, R. W., 1976, Biochemical and physiological effects of chlordimeform, Environ. Health Perspect. 14:
71-82.

Mitsov, V., 1966, Pharmacological assaying of some compounds of
the formamidine group, Nauch. Tr. Vissh. Med. Inst. Sofia
45(5): 61-67.

Salkeld, E. H., and Potter, C., 1953, The effect of the age and
stage of development of insect eggs on their resistance to
insecticides, Bull. Entomol. Res. 44: 527-580.

Stone, B. F., Atkinson, P. W., and Knowles, C. O., 1974, Formamidine structure and detachment of the cattle tick Boophilus
microplus, Pestic. Biochem. Physiol. 4: 407-416.

Vlakhov, V., 1966a, The effect of drug preparation no. 31 on the
    vegetative nervous system, Nauch. Tr. Vissh. Med. Inst.
    Sofia 45(5): 43-49.

Vlakhov, V., 1966b, Influence of drug preparation no. 18 on the
    cardiovascular system, Nauch. Tr. Vissh. Med. Inst. Sofia
    45(5): 51-59.

Wang, C. M., Narahashi, T., and Fukami, J., 1975, Mechanism of
    neuromuscular block by chlordimeform, Pestic. Biochem.
    Physiol. 5: 119-125.

Watanabe, H., Tsuda, S., and Fukami, J., 1975, Effects of chlor-
    dimeform on rectus abdominus muscle of frog, Pestic. Biochem.
    Physiol. 5: 150-154.

FORMAMIDINE PESTICIDES - METABOLIC ASPECTS OF NEUROTOXICITY

Herman J. Benezet, Kuo-Mei Chang and Charles O. Knowles

Department of Entomology, University of Missouri

Columbia, Missouri 65201

Formamidines are a relatively new class of agricultural chemicals, and within this group there exist diverse types of pesticidal activity. For example, compounds active as herbicides,
fungicides, nematocides, bactericides, insecticides, and acaricides
have been discovered. The insecticide and acaricide $\underline{N}$'-(4-chloro-
$\underline{o}$-tolyl)-$\underline{N},\underline{N}$-dimethylformamidine or chlordimeform has received the
most attention from a toxicological standpoint since it has been
used extensively for insect and acarine control (Knowles, 1976).

The known biochemical effects of chlordimeform in mammals were
recently reviewed (Hollingworth, 1976; Knowles, 1976; Matsumura and
Beeman, 1976). We have been most interested in the interaction of
chlordimeform with biogenic amine regulatory mechanisms (Knowles,
1976). Our approach has been to study the biochemical effects of
known mammalian metabolites of chlordimeform as well as those of
the parent compound. This paper describes the toxicity and symptomology of several formamidines to mice and rats as well as their
interaction with certain components of the biogenic amine system.
Emphasis is given to the neurotoxic effects of chlordimeform and
its metabolites.

MATERIALS AND METHODS

Animals and Compounds

Male Swiss-Webster strain mice weighing about 20 g each were
obtained from National Lab., O'Fallon, Mo., and male Sprague Dawley
rats weighing about 150 g each were obtained from Charles River

Breeding Lab., Wilmington, Mass. The sources and properties of the formamidines and related compounds listed in Table 1 were reported by Chang and Knowles (1977).

Toxicity and Symptomology

The toxicity to mice of the compounds in Table 1 was investigated. Depending upon its solubility properties, the compound was dissolved in distilled water, 0.01N HCl, acetone, or corn oil to yield a concentration of 20 mg/ml. Three mice were injected intraperitoneally with each compound at a dosage of 100 mg/kg, and mortality was recorded at 24 hr.

Rats were injected intraperitoneally, subcutaneously, and intraventricularly with various doses of chlordimeform and its known metabolites to determine toxicity and symptomology. For intraperitoneal and subcutaneous treatment the hydrochloride salts of the formamidines and 4-chloro-o-toluidine were dissolved in distilled water; 4'-chloro-o-formotoluidide was dissolved in dimethyl sulfoxide. For intraventricular injection the technique of Noble et al. (1967) was used. Rats were anesthetized with ether, and the formamidines (base forms) and 4'-chloro-o-formotoluidide in dimethyl sulfoxide solution were injected into the lateral ventricle of the brain at a maximum rate of 1 μl/second. The total volume for injection never exceeded 30 μl. Following injection the rats were administered oxygen for about 5 min.

Symptoms of poisoning were observed, and the time interval between treatment and death was recorded.

MAO Inhibition In Vitro

Mouse brains were removed and homogenized in 1.15% KCl to yield a concentration of 50 mg of tissue/ml. The homogenate was centrifuged at 1200 g for 5 min, and the supernatant was used as the monoamine oxidase (MAO) source.

The radiochemical technique of Wurtman and Axelrod (1963) as described by Nagatsu (1973) was used to assay for MAO. The standard 0.3-ml incubation mixture contained 0.1 ml of MAO preparation, 0.1 ml of phosphate buffer (0.5M, pH 7.4), 0.05 ml of radiolabeled substrate (tryptamine-^{14}C) and 0.05 ml of nonradioactive tryptamine. The final substrate concentration was 7.5 x 10^{-5}M. Incubation was carried out for 30 min with shaking at 37°C, and the reaction was stopped with 2N HCl. Toluene was added, and the mixture was shaken vigorously to extract the deaminated metabolites. Following a brief centrifugation an aliquot of the toluene extract was radioassayed by liquid scintillation spectrometry.

Appropriate blanks were run to correct for nonenzymatic degradation and for any of the original substrate that partitioned into
the toluene.

To determine the potency of formamidines as MAO inhibitors,
various amounts of acetone solutions of the compound were added
to reaction tubes. The acetone was evaporated under a stream of
nitrogen. The assay was conducted as described above with no
deliberate preincubation of inhibitor with enzyme prior to the
addition of substrate. The percentage of MAO inhibition at the
inhibitor concentration of 1×10^{-4}M was determined. I_{50} values
were determined for those compounds giving greater than 50% inhibition at the concentration of 1×10^{-4}M.

MAO Inhibition In Vivo

Male rats were treated intraperitoneally with sublethal doses
of chlordimeform (25, 50, and 75 mg/kg), and the degree of inhibition of brain MAO 1 hr following injection was determined. Rats
were treated in a similar way with a lethal dose of chlordimeform
(125 mg/kg), and the MAO activity was determined at death. In
another study rats were injected intraperitoneally with chlordimeform (75 mg/kg), demethylchlordimeform (60 mg/kg), 4'-chloro-
o-formotoluidide (150 mg/kg), harmaline (40 mg/kg), and tranylcypromine (30 mg/kg). The MAO activity in rat brain was determined
at 0, 1, 2, 4, and 8 hr post-treatment.

The brains were removed, quick-frozen, and stored at -20°C until
analyzed. Brains were homogenized in 1.15% KCl solution (0°C) at
a concentration of 50 mg tissue/ml. The homogenate was centrifuged
at 1200 g for 5 min, and the supernatant was used as the MAO
source.

The residual MAO activity was measured as described for in
vitro studies with tryptamine-^{14}C and tyramine-^{14}C as substrates.

Brain Levels of Serotonin and Dopamine

Male rats were injected subcutaneously with chlordimeform
(150 mg/kg), demethylchlordimeform (100 mg/kg), 4'-chloro-o-formo-
toluidide (175 mg/kg), and harmaline (40 mg/kg). Rats were
sacrificed at 1, 2, 4, 8, and 24 hr post-treatment. Brains were
removed, quick-frozen, and stored at -20°C.

Tissue was extracted and assayed for amines on the same day
using a procedure slightly modified from Schlumpf et al. (1974).
The frozen brains were weighed and homogenized in 10 ml of HCl-
butanol (0.85 ml HCl/1000 ml n-butanol). The homogenate was

centrifuged for 10 min at 2000 g, and the supernatant was removed
and added to a reaction tube containing 20 ml of heptane and 4 ml
of 0.1M HCl. The tube was shaken vigorously (Vortex mixer) for
10 min. The mixture was centrifuged, and the acid phase was used
for serotonin and dopamine assay.

For serotonin determinations 0.25 ml of o-phthalaldehyde
reagent (20 mg % HCl) were added to 1.5 ml of the HCl brain extract. The solution was made to 4 ml with 5N HCl. The fluorophore was developed at 100°C for 5 min. The tubes were equilibrated
to room temperature, and the fluorescence was read on a Turner
fluorometer at 360 (7-60) - 470 (48) nm. Blanks were prepared
with all reagents, but the fluorophore was not developed.

For dopamine assay 1 ml of the acid brain extract (adjusted
to about pH 6.0) was diluted with 1 ml of 0.1M phosphate buffer
(pH 6.5). One ml of 4% EDTA solution was added followed exactly
2 min later with 0.1 ml of iodine solution (4.8 g KI and 0.25 g
iodine in 50 ml water). After 2 min 0.5 ml of alkaline sulfite
solution (5 ml 12.6% Na_2SO_3 made to 25 ml with 5N NaOH) were
added followed in 2 min by 0.6 ml of 5N acetic acid. All of the
above procedures were carried out at room temperature. Fluorophore was developed at 100°C for 5 min. Tubes were cooled in ice,
equilibrated to room temperature, and the fluorescence was determined at 325 (7-60 + 110-855)-405 (405) nm. Blanks were prepared
with all reagents except that the order of addition for the iodine
solution and alkaline sulfite solution was reversed.

Sleep Time

Male mice were injected intraperitoneally with a 30% solution
of ethanol in saline at a dosage of 0.017 ml/g (4 mg/g). Mice were
placed on a metal ring, and sleep time measurements were initiated
when the mice lost their ability to balance on the ring. They
were placed upside down on a "V" board (125°), and sleep time was
terminated when the mice were able to right themselves.

Mice were injected intraperitoneally at 0, 30, and 60 min
prior to administering the alcohol with the following compounds:
chlordimeform (50 mg/kg), demethylchlordimeform (50 mg/kg),
didemethylchlordimeform (5 mg/kg), 4'-chloro-o-formotoluidide
(100 mg/kg), harmaline (50 mg/kg), SKF-525A (50 mg/kg), and
triazole (500 mg/kg).

RESULTS

The toxicity to mice of chlordimeform and four of its known
mammalian metabolites is given in Table 1. When injected intraperitoneally at 100 mg/kg it appeared that didemethylchlordimeform
was the most toxic followed by demethylchlordimeform and chlordimeform; 4'-chloro-o-formotoluidide and 4-chloro-o-toluidine were
not toxic at this dosage level.

Table 1 also presents the toxicity to mice of other formamidines and related compounds. In addition to chlordimeform,
N'-(3-chloro-p-tolyl)-N,N-dimethylformamidine was the only chloro-
tolyl dimethylformamidine showing toxicity at 100 mg/kg. In the
xylyl dimethylformamidines toxicity to mice at 100 mg/kg was observed with the 2,4-xylyl, 3,4-xylyl, and 3,5-xylyl derivatives.
N'-(2,4-xylyl)-N-methylformamidine (BTS-27271) also was toxic.
With the two diaryltriazapentadienes the 4-chloro-o-tolyl derivative (BTS-23376) was toxic, but no toxicity was evident with the
2,4-xylyl derivative (amitraz). The other two formamidines
(U-42558 and U-42564) and 2,4-formoxylidide and 2,4-xylidine were
not toxic to mice when injected at a dosage of 100 mg/kg (Table 1).

The toxicity to rats of chlordimeform, demethylchlordimeform,
didemethylchlordimeform, 4'-chloro-o-formotoluidide, and 4-chloro-
o-toluidine following intraperitoneal, subcutaneous, and intraventricular injection is given in Tables 2, 3, and 4, respectively. Chlordimeform and its two formamidine metabolites were more
toxic by intraperitoneal treatment (Table 2) than by subcutaneous
treatment (Table 3). Chlordimeform also was more toxic by intraperitoneal injection (Table 2) than by intraventricular injection
(Table 4). However, demethylchlordimeform and especially didemethylchlordimeform were appreciably more toxic when injected
directly into the brain (Table 4) as compared to intraperitoneal
(Table 2) and subcutaneous injection (Table 3). With the three
formamidines toxicity decreased in the order didemethylchlordimeform > demethylchlordimeform > chlordimeform for each mode of
treatment (Tables 2, 3, and 4). 4'-Chloro-o-formotoluidide was
not toxic to rats when administered subcutaneously at 400 mg/kg
(Table 3) and intraventricularly at 66.6 mg/kg (Table 4); however,
50% mortality of rats was obtained when the compound was administered intraperitoneally at 400 mg/kg (Table 2). The toxicity
to rats of 4-chloro-o-toluidine was not examined by subcutaneous
and intraventricular routes. Following intraperitoneal injection
of 4-chloro-o-toluidine at a dosage of 500 mg/kg 75% mortality
was observed (Table 2).

The symptoms manifested by rats poisoned with chlordimeform
following intraperitoneal and subcutaneous injection were similar.
A marked hyperexcitability, which increased in intensity with time,
with a sensitivity to external stimuli ensued about 20 min

Table 1. Toxicity to Mice of Formamidines and Related Compounds and Potency as Inhibitors of Mouse Brain Monoamine Oxidase In Vitro

Compound[a]	Toxicity[b] Number Alive/Dead at 24 Hr (n=3)	Monoamine Oxidase % Inhibition at 1×10^{-4} M	I_{50}, M
Chlordimeform and Metabolites			
Cl-4,CH$_3$-2-Ph-N=CH-N(CH$_3$)$_2$ (Chlordimeform)	2/1	43.0	$> 1 \times 10^{-4}$
Cl-4,CH$_3$-2-Ph-N=CH-NHCH$_3$ (Demethylchlordimeform)	1/2	56.3	8.2×10^{-5}
Cl-4,CH$_3$-2-Ph-N=CH-NH$_2$ (Didemethylchlordimeform)	0/3	49.3	$> 1 \times 10^{-4}$
Cl-4,CH$_3$-2-PhNHCHO (4'-Chloro-$\underline{o}$-formotoluidide)	3/0	74.0	2.8×10^{-5}
Cl-4,CH$_3$-2-PhNH$_2$ (4-Chloro-$\underline{o}$-toluidine)	3/0	20.0	$> 1 \times 10^{-4}$
Other Formamidines and Related Compounds			
Cl-6,CH$_3$-2-Ph-N=CH-N(CH$_3$)$_2$	3/0	31.7	$> 1 \times 10^{-4}$
Cl-5,CH$_3$-2-Ph-N=CH-N(CH$_3$)$_2$	3/0	51.7	8.4×10^{-5}
Cl-3,CH$_3$-2-Ph-N=CH-N(CH$_3$)$_2$	3/0	28.8	$> 1 \times 10^{-4}$
Cl-3,CH$_3$-4-Ph-N=CH-N(CH$_3$)$_2$	2/1	72.8	4.5×10^{-5}
CH$_3$-2,3-Ph-N=CH-N(CH$_3$)$_2$	3/0	57.5	8.0×10^{-5}
CH$_3$-2,4-Ph-N=CH-N(CH$_3$)$_2$	2/1	48.2	$> 1 \times 10^{-4}$
CH$_3$-2,5-Ph-N=CH-N(CH$_3$)$_2$	3/0	35.3	$> 1 \times 10^{-4}$
CH$_3$-2,6-Ph-N=CH-N(CH$_3$)$_2$	3/0	51.3	9.1×10^{-5}
CH$_3$-3,4-Ph-N=CH-N(CH$_3$)$_2$	0/3	48.1	$> 1 \times 10^{-4}$
CH$_3$-3,5-Ph-N=CH-N(CH$_3$)$_2$	2/1	19.1	$> 1 \times 10^{-4}$

CH_3-2,4-Ph-N=CH-NHCH$_3$ (BTS-27271)	0/3	33.3	$> 1 \times 10^{-4}$
(Cl-4,CH$_3$-2-Ph-N=CH)$_2$NCH$_3$ (BTS-23376)	0/3	61.8	4.4×10^{-5}
(CH$_3$-2,4-Ph-N=CH)$_2$NCH$_3$ (Amitraz)	3/0	20.8	$> 1 \times 10^{-4}$
Cl-4,CH$_3$-2-Ph-N=CH-N(CH$_3$)(SPh) (U-42558)	3/0	29.0	$> 1 \times 10^{-4}$
CH$_3$-2,4-Ph-N=CH-N(CH$_3$)(SPh) (U-42564)	3/0	25.0	$> 1 \times 10^{-4}$
CH$_3$-2,4-PhNHCHO (2,4-Formoxylidide)	3/0	45.0	$> 1 \times 10^{-4}$
CH$_3$-2,4-PhNH$_2$ (2,4-Xylidine)	3/0	7.8	$> 1 \times 10^{-4}$

[a] In this column phenyl is abbreviated Ph.

[b] Mice were injected intraperitoneally with compounds at a dosage of 100 mg/kg.

Table 2.   Toxicity to Rats Following Intraperitoneal Injection
of Chlordimeform and Metabolites

Compound (no. rats tested)	Dosage, mg/kg	% Mortality, 24 Hr
Chlordimeform (10)	75	0
	125	80
Demethylchlordimeform (12)	60	0
	75	25
	100	100
Didemethylchlordimeform (5)	10	0
	25	75
4'-Chloro-o-formotoluidide (12)	100	0
	200	0
	400	50
4-Chloro-o-toluidine (4)	500	75

following subcutaneous injection of a lethal dose (200 mg/kg).
Stimulation caused rapid running and intense escape behavior.
Prostration with hyperextension of hind legs occurred at later
stages of poisoning. Death occurred between 50 and 143 min post-
injection (Table 3). Following subcutaneous injection of rats
with a lethal dose of demethylchlordimeform (150 mg/kg) symptoms
elicited were qualitatively similar to those with chlordimeform
but were more intense. Hyperexcitation began about 5 min post-
injection and death occurred between 17 and 50 min following
treatment (Table 3). When rats were injected subcutaneously with
a lethal dose of didemethylchlordimeform (35 mg/kg) hyperexcitability began within 3 to 4 min posttreatment and by 5 to 6 min
convulsions were evident. Rats died between 9 and 10 min post-
injection (Table 3). Symptoms from intraventricular treatment of
rats with the formamidines were similar to those from subcutaneous
treatment. However, symptoms following intraventricular injection
of didemethylchlordimeform began immediately following treatment,
whereas those from chlordimeform and demethylchlordimeform occurred
after a latent period. Rats treated with 4'-chloro-o-formotoluidide
were asymptomatic following subcutaneous and intraventricular treatment at the highest dosages employed. When administered intraperitoneally at 400 mg/kg a sedative action was apparent followed in
about 15 min by a condition in which the rats failed to respond to
external stimuli (anesthetic effect). A similar anesthetic condition, which ensued about 1 min following treatment, was observed
when rats were injected intraperitoneally with 4-chloro-o-toluidine
at 500 mg/kg.

Table 3. Toxicity to Rats Following Subcutaneous Injection of Chlordimeform and Metabolites

Compound (no. rats tested)	Dosage, mg/kg	Time until Death, Min Mean (Range)		% Mortality, 24 Hr
Chlordimeform (6)	150	-		0
	200	83	(50-143)	100
Demethylchlordimeform (6)	100	-		0
	150	31	(17- 50)	100
Didemethylchlordimeform (5)	25	-		0
	35	9.7	(9- 10)	100
4'-Chloro-o-formotoluidide (6)	175	-		0
	400	-		0

Table 4. Toxicity to Rats Following Intraventricular Injection of Chlordimeform and Metabolites

| Compound (no. rats tested) | Dosage | | % Mortality, 24 Hr |
	mg/rat	mg/kg	
Chlordimeform (15)	10	66.6	0
	25	166.6	60
	30	200.0	100
Demethylchlordimeform (14)	5	33.3	0
	10	66.6	57
	25	166.6	100
Didemethylchlordimeform (11)	0.1	0.6	0
	0.5	3.3	0
	1.0	6.6	80
4'-Chloro-o-formotoluidide (4)	10	66.6	0

MAO Inhibition In Vitro

Of chlordimeform and its metabolites the most potent inhibitor
of mouse brain MAO in vitro was 4'-chloro-o-formotoluidide followed
by demethylchlordimeform, didemethylchlordimeform, chlordimeform,
and 4-chloro-o-toluidine (Table 1).

The other formamidines and related compounds also inhibited
mouse brain MAO, but none was as potent as 4'-chloro-o-formotolui-
dide (Table 1).

MAO Inhibition In Vivo

Inhibition of rat brain MAO in vivo by chlordimeform was dose
dependent. When rats were injected with chlordimeform at sublethal
dosages of 25, 50, and 75 mg/kg and MAO activity was determined
after 1 hr the percentage inhibition of tyramine and tryptamine
oxidative deamination was 13.2% and 12.8%, 21.4% and 14.6%, and
31.4% and 18.6%, respectively. When rats were injected with chlordimeform at the lethal dose of 125 mg/kg and MAO activity assayed
at the time of death the percentage inhibition of tyramine and
tryptamine was 24.1% and 15.6%, respectively.

Chlordimeform and its metabolites inhibited rat brain MAO in
vivo even after 8 hr (Tables 5 and 6). In all cases the deamination of tyramine (Table 5) was inhibited to a greater extent than
was the deamination of tryptamine (Table 6).

The classical MAO inhibitors harmaline and tranylcypromine
were much more potent than chlordimeform or any of its metabolites
(Tables 5 and 6).

Brain Levels of Serotonin and Dopamine

Chlordimeform, demethylchlordimeform, and 4'-chloro-o-formo-
toluidide each effected an increase in rat brain levels of
serotonin (Table 7) and dopamine (Table 8) following subcutaneous
injection; however, they were not as effective as harmaline.

Sleep Time

Chlordimeform, demethylchlordimeform, 4'-chloro-o-formotolui-
dide, SKF-525A, and triazole prolonged ethanol-induced sleep in
mice (Table 9). Didemethylchlordimeform and harmaline appeared to
decrease ethanol sleep time (Table 9).

Table 5. Inhibition of Tyramine Oxidative Deamination by Brain
Monoamine Oxidase Following Intraperitoneal Injection of Rats
with Chlordimeform (75 mg/kg), Demethylchlordimeform
(60 mg/kg), 4'-Chloro-o-formotoluidide (150 mg/kg),
Harmaline (40 mg/kg), and Tranylcypromine (30 mg/kg)

Compound	% Inhibition at Indicated Hr Following Injection[a]			
	1	2	4	8
Chlordimeform	31.0 ± 2.7	38.3 ± 3.9	34.7 ± 3.8	34.9 ± 5.3
Demethyl-chlordimeform	45.1 ± 5.4	34.6 ± 9.9	33.2 ± 4.1	28.0 ± 4.5
4'-Chloro-o-formotoluidide	49.3 ± 2.2	43.3 ± 3.5	51.5 ± 5.0	34.7 ± 4.6
Harmaline	67.5 ± 2.0	66.3 ± 2.0	60.6 ± 1.3	42.4 ± 7.0
Tranylcypromine	100.0	100.0	100.0	100.0

[a] Figures are % inhibition $\pm$ 95% confidence limits using duplicate
assays of 3 rats.

DISCUSSION

The major thrust of this study was to investigate the toxicity
and action of the pesticide chlordimeform and some of its metabolites to rats and mice. Demethylchlordimeform, didemethylchlordimeform, 4'-chloro-o-formotoluidide, 4-chloro-o-toluidine, N-formyl
-5-chloroanthranilic acid, and 5-chloroanthranilic acid were isolated and identified in the urine of chlordimeform-treated rats by
us in previous studies (Knowles, 1976). In the present study we
used all of these compounds with the exception of the two anthran-
ilic acids.

Following intraperitoneal, subcutaneous, and intraventricular
treatment of rats toxicity decreased in the order didemethylchlordimeform > demethylchlordimeform > chlordimeform. This same
trend of formamidine toxicity also was observed following intraperitoneal treatment of mice. From the data on symptomology latent
periods prior to the appearance of overt symptoms of poisoning were
evident. Further, there existed a relationship between the latent
period interval and formamidine structure. Didemethylchlordimeform killed rats faster than did demethylchlordimeform which in
turn killed somewhat faster than chlordimeform. Thus it is

Table 6. Inhibition of Tryptamine Oxidative Deamination by Brain
Monoamine Oxidase Following Intraperitoneal Injection of Rats
with Chlordimeform (75 mg/kg), Demethylchlordimeform
(60 mg/kg), 4'-Chloro-o-formotoluidide (150 mg/kg),
Harmaline (40 mg/kg), and Tranylcypromine (30 mg/kg)

| Compound | % Inhibition at Indicated Hr Following Injection[a] | | | |
	1	2	4	8
Chlordimeform	14.2 ± 3.8	21.4 ± 5.2	18.9 ± 3.1	23.6 ± 3.7
Demethyl-chlordimeform	7.9 ± 2.8	2.4 ± 6.2	0	0
4'-Chloro-o-formotoluidide	28.7 ± 1.9	24.1 ± 3.4	32.1 ± 4.1	8.9 ± 4.2
Harmaline	75.8 ± 1.9	76.4 ± 1.2	66.1 ± 3.3	32.2 ± 16.9
Tranylcypromine	100.0	100.0	100.0	100.0

[a] Figures are % inhibition ± 95% confidence limits using duplicate
assays of 3 rats.

proposed that sequential oxidative N-demethylation of chlordimeform
resulted in the formation of two formamidines, demethylchlordimeform
and didemethylchlordimeform, that were faster acting and that possessed higher intrinsic toxicity when injected into rats than the
parent formamidine. Demethylchlordimeform and didemethylchlordimeform undoubtedly contributed to the toxic action of chlordimeform
in rats. The other two chlordimeform metabolites examined, 4'-
chloro-o-formotoluidide and 4-chloro-o-toluidine, were not as acute-
ly toxic to mice and rats as were chlordimeform, demethylchlordimeform, and didemethylchlordimeform. However, both compounds were
toxic at high dosages (400 to 500 mg/kg) and elicited anesthetic
effects. Also the ability of 4'-chloro-o-formotoluidide to inhibit
biogenic amine deamination will be mentioned later, and Knowles and
Aziz (1974) have reported that 4-chloro-o-toluidine interfered with
the binding of norepinephrine to rat cardiac receptors. Thus, these
two metabolites likely contributed to the action of chlordimeform.
It should be kept in mind that demethylchlordimeform, didemethylchlordimeform, 4'-chloro-o-formotoluidide, and 4-chloro-o-toluidine
are theoretical metabolites of other N'-(4-chloro-o-tolyl)-N-methyl
-N-substituted formamidines, such as BTS-23376 (Table 1), U-42558
(Table 1), and Hokupanon[R] or N'-(4-chloro-o-tolyl)-N-methyl-N-
methylthiomethyl formamidine.

Table 7. Brain Levels of Serotonin Following Subcutaneous
Injection of Rats with Chlordimeform (150 mg/kg), Demethylchlordimeform (100 mg/kg), 4'-Chloro-o-formotoluidide
(175 mg/kg), and Harmaline (40 mg/kg)[a]

| Compound | Serotonin Level (µg/g Brain Tissue) at Indicated Hr Following Injection | | | | | |
	0	1	2	4	8	24
Chlordimeform	0.31	0.49	0.41	0.47	0.44	0.44
Demethyl-chlordimeform	0.50	0.69	0.76	0.81	0.77	0.50
4'-Chloro-o-formotoluidide	0.18	0.26	0.21	0.27	0.28	0.26
Harmaline	0.68	13.91	10.90	3.45	1.47	0.74

[a] Three replicates were run at each time, and three controls were
run with each series.

Table 8. Brain Levels of Dopamine Following Subcutaneous
Injection of Rats with Demethylchlordimeform (100 mg/kg),
4'-Chloro-o-formotoluidide (175 mg/kg), and
Harmaline (40 mg/kg)[a]

| Compound | Dopamine Level (µg/g Brain Tissue) at Indicated Hr Following Injection | | | | | |
	0	1	2	4	8	24
Demethyl-chlordimeform	0.66	0.83	0.90	0.97	0.90	0.70
4'-Chloro-o-formotoluidide	0.78	0.98	1.05	0.90	1.03	0.83
Harmaline	0.93	2.18	1.98	1.09	1.15	0.93

[a] Three replicates were run at each time, and three controls were
run with each series.

Table 9. Influence of Chlordimeform and Related Compounds on Ethanol-Induced Sleep Time in Mice[a]

Compound	Time Prior to Treatment with Ethanol, Min	Sleep Time, Min
Control (n=51)		38.4 ± 3.8
Chlordimeform (50 mg/kg, n=32)	0	80.7 ± 7.5**
	30	111.2 ± 17.7**
	60	83.2 ± 4.2**
Demethylchlordimeform (50 mg/kg, n=23)	0	93.4 ± 12.9**
	30	73.8 ± 7.1**
	60	68.5 ± 16.2**
Didemethylchlordimeform (5 mg/kg, n=18)	0	14.1 ± 6.8**
	30	23.5 ± 10.2 (NS)
	60	25.0 ± 11.8 (NS)
4'-Chloro-o-formotoluidide (100 mg/kg, n=33)	0	55.9 ± 10.8**
	30	52.7 ± 7.9*
	60	84.9 ± 18.0**
Harmaline (50 mg/kg, n=17)	0	8.7 ± 4.7**
	30	12.0 ± 5.0**
	60	10.9 ± 1.8**
SKF-525A (50 mg/kg, n=18)	0	51.6 ± 11.9*
	30	48.8 ± 8.6 (NS)
	60	64.1 ± 12.7**
Triazole (500 mg/kg, n=6)	0	303.2 ± 43.9**

[a] Mice were injected intraperitoneally with 30% ethanol in saline at a dose of 0.017 ml/g. Sleep time modifiers were injected intraperitoneally at 60 min, 30 min, and 0 min prior to treatment with ethanol. Figures are sleep time in min ± 95% confidence limits.

NS = non-significant (0.05), * = significant (0.05), ** = highly significant (0.001).

$\underline{N}$'-(2,4-xylyl)-$\underline{N}$-methylformamidine (BTS-27271) also was more
toxic to mice than the $\underline{N},\underline{N}$-dimethyl derivative; 2,4-formoxylidide
and 2,4-xylidine were of low acute toxicity. BTS-27271, 2,4-
formoxylidide, and 2,4-xylidine are theoretical metabolites of
$\underline{N}$'-(2,4-xylyl)-$\underline{N}$-methyl-$\underline{N}$-substituted formamidines, such as amitraz
and U-42564 (Table 1). Thus these demethyl derivatives and sub-
stituted formanilides and anilines also might be involved in the
action of certain other formamidines.

Chlordimeform, the other formamidines, and related compounds
examined by us inhibited the oxidative deamination of tryptamine-^{14}C
by mouse brain homogenates. These data compared favorably with
with those reported by Benezet and Knowles (1976) for some of the
same compounds and rat brain preparations. In both cases 4'-
chloro-$\underline{o}$-formotoluidide was the most potent MAO inhibitor in vitro
and demethylchlordimeform was slightly more potent than was chlordimeform.

Rats treated with chlordimeform, demethylchlordimeform, and
4'-chloro-$\underline{o}$-formotoluidide showed a decreased capacity to deam-
inate tyramine and tryptamine. Thus, it was logical to suspect
that certain biogenic amines would accumulate in rat brain. In
fact Matsumura and Beeman (1976) reported that chlordimeform-
treated rats accumulated serotonin and norepinephrine. We have
confirmed this result with respect to serotonin and have extended
it to include dopamine. Also rats treated with demethylchlordimeform and 4'-chloro-$\underline{o}$-formotoluidide showed increased brain
levels of serotonin and dopamine. This increase in biogenic
amines resulting from treatment of rats with chlordimeform and
certain metabolites is possibly a consequence of MAO inhibition
and doubtlessly has physiological significance.

A most interesting effect shown by chlordimeform, demethylchlordimeform, and 4'-chloro-$\underline{o}$-formotoluidide was their ability
to increase ethanol-induced sleep in mice at moderately low doses
(50 to 100 mg/kg). The mechanism for this phenomenon is currently
not understood. At least two types of interaction must be considered. Chlordimeform and/or a metabolite(s) may be simply
prolonging the effects of ethanol, or they may be active sleep
inducers themselves. Chlordimeform and/or some of its metabolites
could increase the action of ethanol by slowing its degradation,
possibly by inhibiting an enzyme such as alcohol dehydrogenase.
This supposition receives support from the fact that triazole,
a known inhibitor of alcohol oxidation (Mannering and Parks,
1957), also increased ethanol-induced sleep. Further, a consequence of this inhibition might be an increase in levels of
endogenous sleep inducers, such as 5-hydroxytryptophol, which
could be derived from the 5-hydroxyindoleacetaldehyde formed from
serotonin (Feldstein and Kurcharski, 1971). Alternatively,
chlordimeform and/or certain metabolites may be active sleep

inducers, and the increased sleep time could be due to a synergistic interaction of one or more of these compounds with ethanol. This contention receives support from the toxicity experiments where it was observed that 4'-chloro-o-formotoluidide and 4-chloro-o-toluidine possessed marked anesthetic action.

The action of chlordimeform clearly is complex, and biochemical effects involving systems other than those mentioned here have been described (Hollingworth, 1976; Knowles, 1976; Matsumura and Beeman, 1976). It would appear that the toxic action of chlordimeform in rats and mice is a result of an attack upon several targets not only by the parent compound itself, but also by several of its metabolites.

ACKNOWLEDGMENT

This research was supported in part by a grant from the National Institutes of Health (1 R01 ES01316). Contribution from the Missouri Agricultural Experiment Station, Columbia; Journal Series No. 7553.

REFERENCES

Benezet, H. J., and Knowles, C. O. 1976. Inhibition of rat brain monoamine oxidase by formamidines and related compounds, Neuropharmacol. 15:369.

Chang, K.-M., and Knowles, C. O. 1977. Formamidine acaricides: toxicity and metabolism studies with twospotted spider mites, Tetranychus urticae Koch, J. Agr. Food Chem. In press.

Feldstein, A., and Kurcharski, J. M. 1971. Pyrazole and ethanol potentiation of tryptophol-induced sleep in mice, Life Sciences Part I. 10:961.

Hollingworth, R. M. 1976. Chemistry, biological activity, and uses of formamidine pesticides, Environ. Health Perspect. 14:57.

Knowles, C. O. 1976. Chemistry and toxicology of quinoxaline, organotin, organofluorine, and formamidine acaricides, Environ. Health Perspect. 14:93.

Knowles, C. O., and Aziz, S. A. 1974. Interaction of formamidines with components of the biogenic amine system, in: Mechanism of Pesticide Action (ACS Symposium Series No. 2) (G. K. Kohn, ed.), pp. 92-99, American Chemical Society, Washington, D. C.

Mannering, G. J., and Parks, R. E. 1957. Inhibition of methanol metabolism with 3-amino-1,2,4-triazole, Science 126:1241.

Matsumura, F., and Beeman, R. W. 1976. Biochemical and physio-
    logical effects of chlordimeform, Environ. Health Perspect.
    14:71.

Nagatsu, T. 1973. Biochemistry of Càtecholamines, University
    Park Press, Baltimore.

Noble, E. P., Wurtman, R. J., and Axelrod, J. 1967. A simple and
    rapid method for injecting H^3-norepinephrine into the lateral
    ventricle of the rat brain, Life Sciences 6:281.

Schlumpf, M., Lichtensteiger, W., Langemann, H., Waser, P. G., and
    Hefti, F. 1974. A fluorometric micromethod for the simul-
    taneous determination of serotonin, noradrenaline, and dopamine
    in milligram amounts of brain tissue, Biochem. Pharmacol. 23:
    2437.

Wurtman, R. J., and Axelrod, J. 1963. A sensitive and specific
    assay for the estimation of monoamine oxidase, Biochem.
    Pharmacol. 12:1439.

Section III

Neurotoxic Actions
of Arthropod Venoms

NEUROTOXIC ACTIONS OF ARTHROPOD VENOMS

INTRODUCTION

Thomas Smyth, Jr.

Department of Entomology, The Pennsylvania State
    University
University Park, PA   16802

Venoms are employed by many arthropods for defense or for
offense as in subduing prey for food or oviposition. Since fast
action is obviously helpful, it is not surprising that many
arthropod venoms contain neurotoxic constituents. Often the
venoms contain complex mixtures of substances which may contribute
both immediate and persisting actions or which have potency for a
wide spectrum of target organisms. Although many arthropods
produce secretions or possess spines that affect chemoreceptors or
cause pain, it is usual to restrict the term venom to substances
injected by a bite or sting. Since salivary glands are designed
to secrete enzymes and are under neural control, it is reasonable
that salivary neurotoxins are mainly proteins or neural transmitters.
Venoms associated with the sting apparatus are more complex and may
include components derived from pheromones or tanning reagents as
well as proteins. Neural transmitters and related small molecules
such as acetylcholine, serotonin and histamine have been identified
in several venoms; their actions are well known. The volatile
alkaloids of fire ant venoms that will be discussed by Schimdt
apparently act post-synaptically to dissociate transmitter
reception from ionic conductance change. Neurobiologists have
shown considerable interest in the protein neurotoxins as these
offer promise as probes of neural function. Protein neurotoxins of
the parasitic wasps discussed by Piek and Spanjer appear to block
synaptic transmission presynaptically. In contrast, the scorpion
venoms discussed by Zlotkin et al mainly excite presynaptically
and the spider venoms discussed by Smyth et al also act presynaptically to promote transmitter release. The latter may well be
derived from the ionophores of excitable membranes.

EFFECTS AND CHEMICAL CHARACTERIZATION OF SOME

PARALYSING VENOMS OF SOLITARY WASPS

T. Piek and W. Spanjer

Pharmacological Laboratory, University of Amsterdam

Polderweg 104, Amsterdam, The Netherlands

INTRODUCTION

The insect order of Hymenoptera can roughly be divided into two groups: (1) the ants, the bees and the social wasps, and (2) the solitary wasps. Members of the first group produce venoms, used by the insects for the defence. These venoms cause pain and local tissue damage in large vertebrates and are lethal to smaller animals. The solitary wasps, however, generally produce venoms, that are used to paralyse a prey (insect or spider), which serves as a host for the parasitizing larva of the wasp.

The paralysing effect of a sting by a solitary wasp was already known by the ancient Chinese. The Erh-Ya (Kuo Po, 276-324 A.D.) describes a green "worm" which was paralysed by a wasp. This knowledge has been overlooked by western science, and it was not before 1742 when Réaumur described an observation by Cossigni of a wasp stinging a cockroach, resulting in a loss of the cockroach's forces. Bartram (1744) described a mud-dauber wasp, disabling spiders but not killing them. Dufour (1841) however, believed that weevils collected by *Cerceris bupresticida* were dead, and that the wasp's venom contained a preservative. It fell to Fabre (1855) to conclusively settle these conflicting views. He observed that the weevils after attack by *C.bupresticida* were able to contract when stimulated by electric currents. Fabre's conclusion was that the prey of solitary Aculeata were paralysed and not dead. The above historical facts concern members of only one group of solitary wasps, *i.e.* the Aculeata, having an aculeus or sting, which is considered to be a fully modified ovipositor, which is no longer used for oviposition.

In his *"Souvenirs Entomologiques"* Fabre (1879-1910) presented the view that solitary Aculeata sting their victims in the central nervous system. He observed that the number of stings given by the

wasp was correlated with the number of main nerve ganglia in the
prey. From the work of many authors, which have confirmed Fabre's
view, here is only referred to Steiner (1962), who observed *Liris
nigra* to sting the cricket four times in the four big ganglia.

The second group of solitary wasps is that of the Terebrantia,
having an ovipositor (terebra or drill), which is also used as ductus
venatus. The available data on stinging behaviour of Terebrantia
indicate that these wasps do not sting into or in the direction of
the central nervous system.

CAUSES OF THE PARALYSIS

If the venoms of *Microbracon hebetor* (Say) (Terebrantia) and of
Philanthus triangulum F. (Aculeata) are injected into the haemolymph
either by a sting of the wasp or artificially with a needle they
do not affect the nervous system, the sensory system or the excitability and contractability of the muscle fibres (Beard, 1952;
Rathmayer, 1962; Piek, 1966a, 1966b; Piek *et al.*, 1971). Both venoms
inhibit the excitatory neuromuscular transmission (Piek and Engels,
1969; Piek *et al.*, 1971). The venom of *P.triangulum* in addition
blocks the inhibitory neuromuscular transmission (Piek *et al.*, 1971).
The venoms of *M.hebetor* and of *M.gelechiae* do not affect the peripheral inhibition (Piek and Mantel, 1970; Piek *et al.*,1974; Walther
and Rathmayer, 1974).

In insect muscle fibres the venoms of both *M.hebetor* and *P.
triangulum* cause a decrease in amplitude of the excitatory postsynaptic potential (**epsp**), and a decrease in frequency of the
miniature excitatory postsynaptic potentials (mepsp's), but the
amplitude of the miniature potentials remains unaltered (Fig. 1A,B;
Piek and Engels, 1969; Piek *et al.*, 1971; Piek and Njio, 1975).
Therefore, the ratio: epsp - amplitude over mepsp - amplitude decreases. This ratio is a measure for the quantum number of the epsp.
A decrease in the quantum number indicates a presynaptic effect.
The venom of *P.triangulum* also depresses the frequency but not the
amplitude of the inhibitory miniature postsynaptic potentials
(mipsp's) (Fig. 1A). The venom of *M.hebetor*, however, does not affect
either the frequency or the amplitude of the mipsp's (Fig. 1B).

Fig. 1 The effect of solitary wasp venoms on the frequency and the
median of amplitudes of miniature potentials recorded from insect
skeletal muscle fibres. (A) Effect of *Philanthus triangulum* venom
(3 B.U. per ml) on muscle fibres of *Schistocerca gregaria*. (B) Effect
of *Microbracon hebetor* venom (30,000 G.U. per ml) on a muscle fibre
of *Philosamia cynthia*. (After Piek and Mantel,1970, and Piek *et al.*,
1971). (For the definitions of B.U. and G.U. see legend of Fig. 2).
All frequencies and amplitudes are expressed as percentages of the
control values.

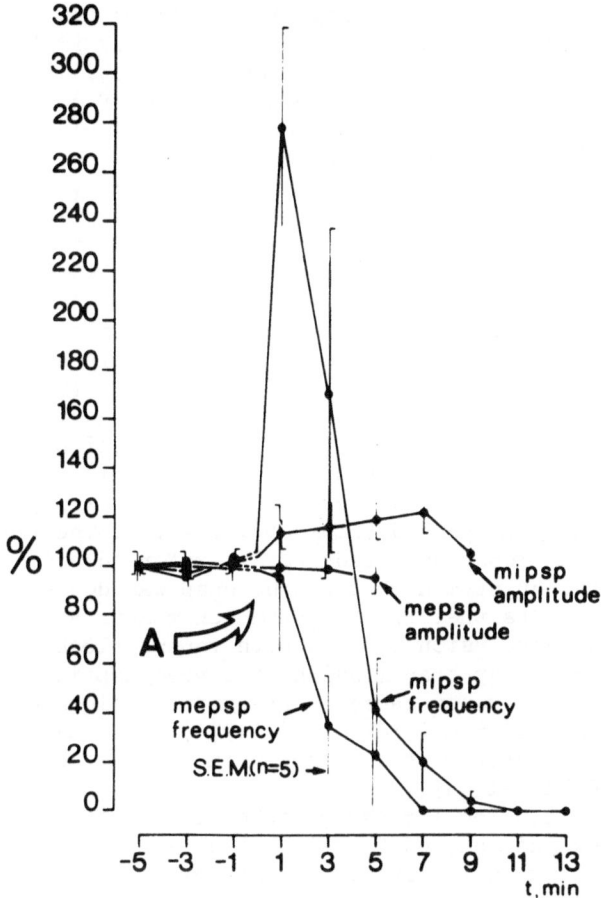

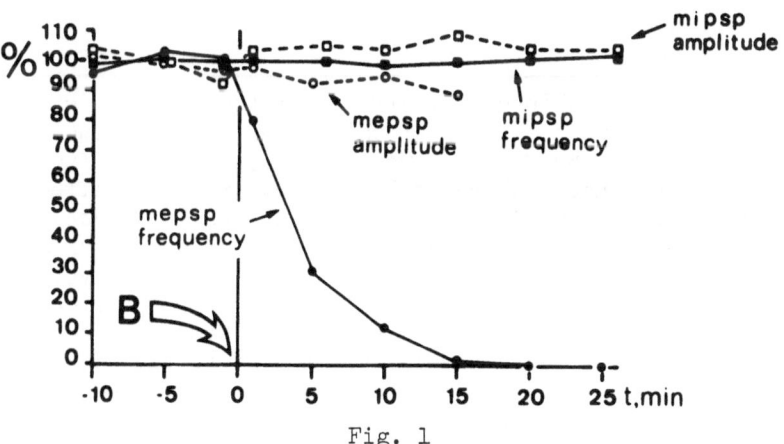

Fig. 1

The depression of the frequency of mepsp's by the venoms of
M. hebetor and *P. triangulum* does not automatically imply that the
depression of the epsp is also a presynaptic effect. For *M. hebetor*
venom a good correlation exists between the rate of decrease in
mepsp-frequency and the rate of decrease in epsp-amplitude (Fig.
2A). Therefore, it seems reasonable to assume that the depression
of the epsp-amplitude by *M.hebetor* venom is caused by the same
mechanism as the depression of the frequency of the mepsp's and
therefore is a presynaptic effect. In muscle fibres treated with
P.triangulum venom a similar correlation has not always been found.
Low concentrations of this venom (1 Bee Unit per ml) may cause a
decrease in the mepsp-frequency to nearly zero, while the epsp-
amplitude remains at a level, which is only slightly below the
control value (Fig. 2B). Therefore the effect of *P. triangulum*
venom on the epsp-amplitude is not directly coupled with its
effect on the mepsp-frequency. In experiments in which higher
concentrations of *P.triangulum* venom (3 B.U. per ml) were used the
epsp-amplitude showed a marked decrease, while the mepsp-amplitude
remained practically unchanged (Piek *et al.*, 1971). The ratio:
epsp-amplitude over mepsp-amplitude was therefore decreased. This
indicates that the quantum number of the epsp was decreased, and
this strongly suggests that *P.triangulum* venom acts at a presynaptic
site. The general conclusion is that both venoms block insect
excitatory neuromuscular transmission at a presynaptic site. In
addition *P.triangulum* venom causes a presynaptic block of inhibitory
neuromuscular transmission (Piek *et al.*, 1971), but does not block
the putative neurosecretory transmission in a locust skeletal
muscle (Piek and Mantel, 1977).

The above conclusion for the peripheral effect of *P.triangulum*
venom does not exclude an additional central effect. As a matter
of fact *P.triangulum* normally stings into or in the direction of
the thoracic ganglion mass of the honeybee. Therefore a central
effect might be probable.

Fig. 2   Time relationship of the effects of two solitary wasp
venoms on two different electrical phenomena in insect muscle
fibres. A: effect of 50 *Galleria* Units (G.U.) per ml perfusion
fluid on a flight muscle fibre of *Pieris brassicae*. B: effect of
1 Bee Unit (B.U.) (at t=0) per ml on a coxal muscle of *Schistocerca
gregaria*. The G.U. is defined as the activity of a *Microbracon*
venom preparation causing after 2 hr a 50 per cent paralysing effect
when injected into the haemolymph of 100 mg *Galleria mellonella*
larvae. The paralysing effect is expressed in scores, according to
the scoring system of Beard (1952) (see legend to Fig. 5) The B.U.
is defined as the activity of a *P.triangulum* preparation, injected
in equal amounts into 10 honeybee workers, causing 5 of these bees
to remain paralysed for at least 1 hr (Piek *et al.*, 1971).

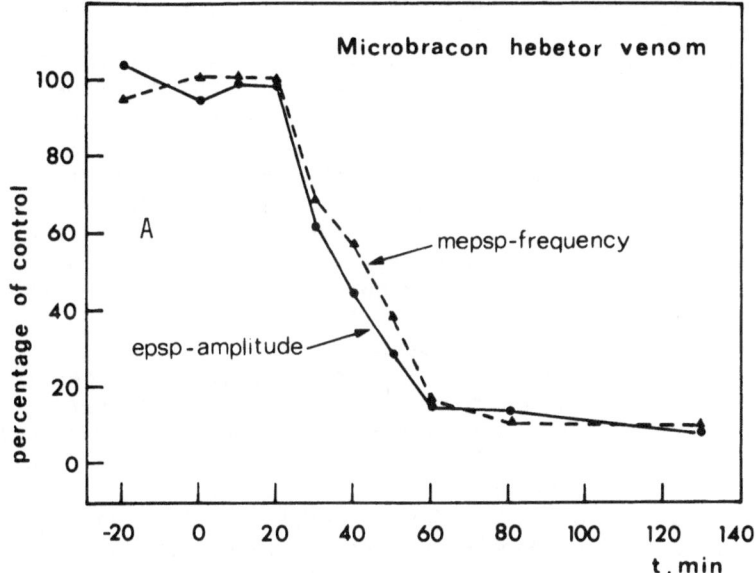

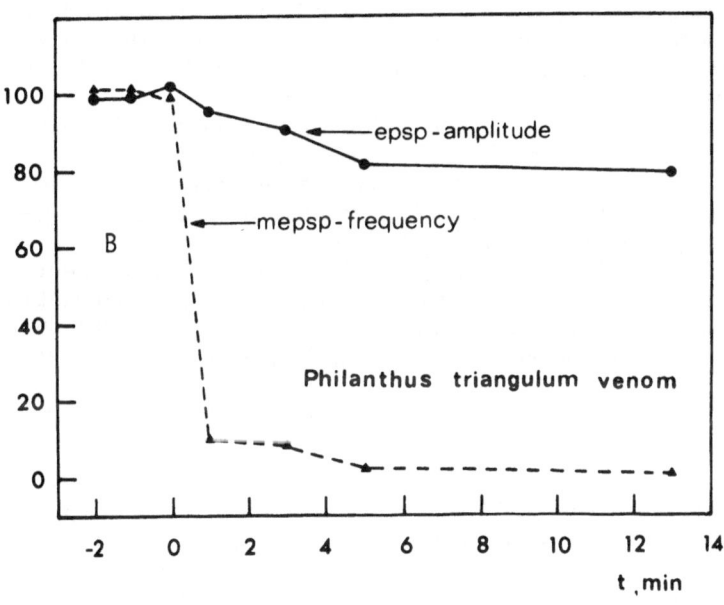

Fig. 2

FURTHER ANALYSIS OF THE PRESYNAPTIC EFFECT OF *P. TRIANGULUM* VENOM

From the study of the effect of *P. triangulum* venom on the electrical phenomena in insect muscle fibres, as described in the preceding section, it was concluded that the venom blocks the neuromuscular transmission presynaptically. An observation by Lepeletier de Saint-Fargeau (1841), that honeybee workers, which are paralysed after having been stung by *P. triangulum*, but show from time to time movements of the antennae, legs or tarsae, could not be explained if a complete peripheral paralysis existed. The following experiments will offer an explanation for the observation by Lepeletier de Saint-Fargeau.

Philanthus triangulum F., was collected in the South of France by Dr R.T. Simon Thomas, and stored in liquid nitrogen (Piek et al., 1971). The venom was obtained immediately prior to the experiments by extracting venom reservoirs with locust saline. This saline, which is also used for bathing the nerve muscle preparation, contains per liter 68 mmol NaCl, 5 mmol KCl, 3 mmol CaCl$_2$, 5 mmol MgCl$_2$, 6 mmol NaH$_2$PO$_4$, 4 mmol NaHCO$_3$ and 210 mmol glucose. The venom concentration is expressed in Bee Units (B.U.) per ml, (see legend to Fig. 2). Locusta migratoria R.& F. was reared in the laboratory. The nerve muscle preparation used was the extensor tibiae of the metathoracic leg, stimulated indirectly via nerve 5. The force of the isometric contractions was measured at the distal part of the tibia with a mechano-electrical transducer (Pixie) and recorded on a flat bed recorder (Siemens Kompensograph III). All experiments were repeated 4-5 times. Indirect stimulation of the jumping muscle via nerve 5 results in a twitch with a force varying from two to four gf. When stimulated once every ten sec the force can be maintained for four to five hr, showing in some preparations a gradual decrease with 5-15% between two and five hr.

Addition of the venom of *P. triangulum* in a concentration of 0.1 B.U. per ml did not cause a decrease of the contraction force at a stimulation frequency of 0.1 cps (Fig. 3A, left), but with 0.2 B.U. per ml the contraction force decreased (Fig. 3A, middle).

Fig. 3 Effects of different concentrations of the venom of *Philanthus triangulum* on the force of contraction of the musculus extensor tibiae of the rear leg of *Locusta migratoria* . Stimulation, every 10 sec indirectly via nerve 5 (fast contraction), is indicated by dotted bars. A. Effects of 0.1 and subsequently 0.2 B.U. per ml perfusion fluid. B. Effect of 0.3 B.U. per ml. C. Effect of 0.5 B.U. per ml. gf = gram force.
In the recovery period (washing) a single stimulus is sometimes followed by a short tetanic contraction (asterisks).

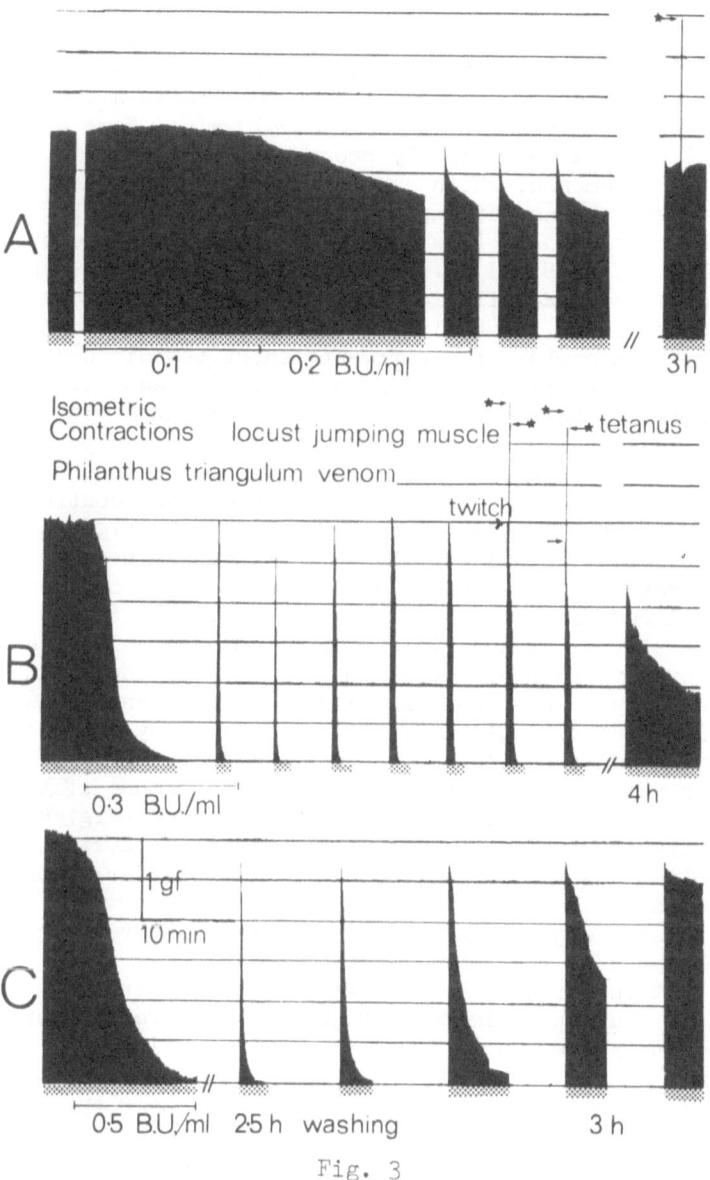

Fig. 3

Depending on the individual sensitivity of the locust used, venom
concentrations of 0.3 - 1.0 B.U. per ml are needed to paralyse the
nerve muscle preparation completely during stimulation at a
frequency of 0.1 cps (Figs. 3B, 3C).

After washing the preparation with locust saline and continued
stimulation, the effect of the venom persists for at least two hr.
When the preparation is not stimulated for 5-15 min, the first
stimulus given after the period of rest results in a contraction
with a force that often equals the control value. However, subsequent stimuli, cause a rapidly progressive decrease in contraction
force. This phenomenon, which can be repeated many times, is observed in preparations bathing in the venom solution (Fig. 3B) as
well as in preparations, in which the venom has been removed by
washing (Fig. 3, A, B and C). During prolonged washing, the original
contraction force gradually returns, in some preparations, however,
with a reduced force, probably due to the long duration of the
experiment. In a number of experiments short tetanic contractions
following a single stimulus are seen (Fig. 3, A and B).

Incompletely paralysed preparations stimulated with frequencies
higher than 0.1 cps show two different and competing phenomena:
exhaustion caused by the venom and facilitation caused by the increase in stimulation frequency. Fig. 4A shows the control situation. From 6 cps a distinct facilitation is visible. If venom now
is added (0.5 B.U. per ml) to the saline during a period of 5 min,
and the preparation is washed a depression of the contraction force
is seen at lower frequencies (Fig. 4B). At 0.1 cps the twitch
height gradually decreases. This exhaustion depends on the stimulation frequency. In the range from 0.1 to 3 cps the exhaustion is
more intensive at 3 cps than at 0.1 cps. At frequencies higher than
3 cps a distinct facilitation is visible, which may obscure the
progressive exhaustion. To show that the relatively high tetanus
over twitch ratio is not caused by a gradual restore of the preparation, the series of stimulus trains was repeated (Fig. 4C). To
show that the tetanus at 30 cps can be maintained during 2 sec the
top of the tetanus was recorded at an 8 times faster paper speed)
(Fig. 4C, inset).

The present experiments show that working nerve muscle preparations paralysed by the venom of *P. triangulum*, are able to exert a
full contraction force after a short period of rest (Fig. 3C). This
may indicate that the release mechanism of the transmitter has not
been affected by the venom. It is now clear how insects, which at
a first glance seem to be completely paralysed by the venom of *P.
triangulum*, from time to time can slowly move their antennae, their
legs or their tarsae. This phenomenon which was reported for the
first time for honeybees stung by *P. triangulum* (Lepeletier de
Saint-Fargeau, 1841) was also observed in *Halictus* bees stung by
P. denticollis (Claude-Joseph, 1928).

During high-frequency stimulation the release mechanism re-
quires a highly effective supply of transmitter substance. It is
likely that the rate of synthesis, reuptake and transport of

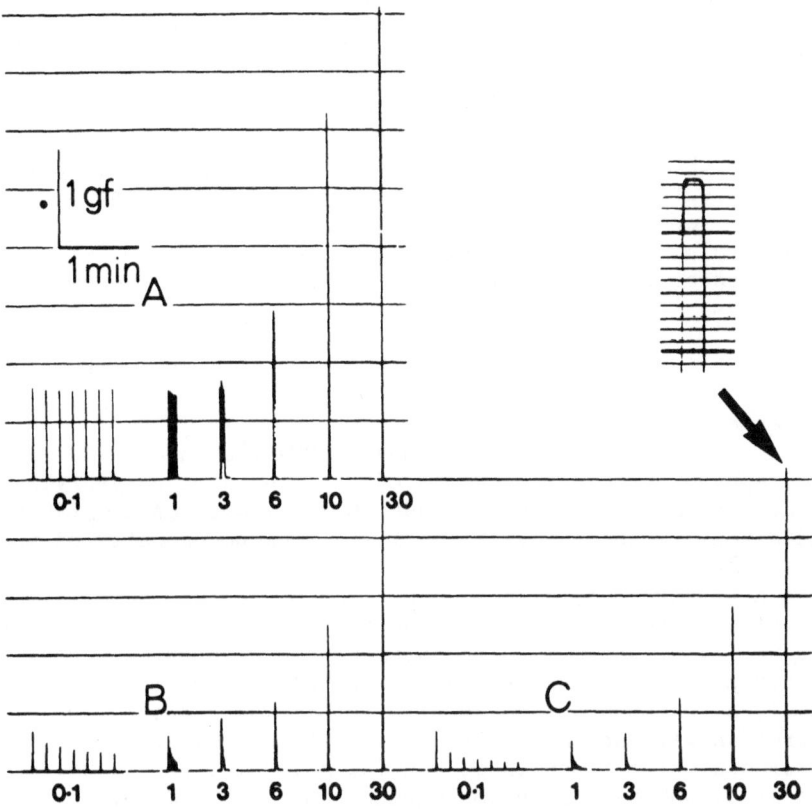

Fig. 4 Effects of 0.5 B.U. per ml of venom of *P.triangulum* on the force of the fast twitch and tetanus. A: before administration of venom; B: immediately after the beginning of washing of the preparation, pretreated during 5 min with the venom solution; C: after 50 min of washing. The intervals of the pulse trains are 5 min. Every pulse train consists of 7 pulses. Numbers indicate the frequency in cps of the trains of 7 pulses.
Inset: Top of the tetanic contraction, recorded with 8 times faster paper speed, indicating that the tetanic contraction can be fully maintained. gf = gram force.

transmitter substance in the nerve terminal increases with the
stimulation frequency, as has been demonstrated for postganglionic
cholinergic nerve terminals in the guinea-pig ileum (Paton, 1963).
During a pulse train, contractions in insect muscles show a
distinct facilitation (*cf.* Huddart, 1971). This is also the case
for the extensor muscle as shown in Fig. 4A, where the tetanus-
amplitude at stimulation at 30 cps is 5.6 times the twitch amplitude i.e. 80% of the sum of seven twitches. In Fig. 4B,C the tetanus-
forces at 30 cps are respectively 6.1 and 6.5 times the first twitch
and 180 and 290 per cent of the sum of the seven twitches at 0.1 cps.
It is obvious that this is only possible when a pronounced facilitation is present. This facilitation seems to compete with the
action of the venom. If this facilitation is caused by a stimulation
of the synthesis, the storage or the transport mechanism of transmitter substance, it is conceivable that *P.triangulum* venom inhibits one or a number of these processes.

PURIFICATION AND CHEMICAL CHARACTERIZATION OF SOLITARY WASP VENOM

(a) The venom of *Microbracon hebetor*

Using ion exchange chromatography on DEAE-Sephadex A-50, gel
chromatography on Sephadex G-100, electrophoresis on polyacrylamide
gel and gel chromatography on Sephadex G-75, Visser *et al.*, (1976)
isolated a toxin with paralysing activity from homogenates of whole
female *Microbracon hebetor* wasps.

This paralysing toxin showed the same biological activity as
extracts of isolated venom glands and of preparations obtained by
stimulating living wasps with trichloroethylene vapour (Drenth,
1974). This provides a strong indication that the purified toxin
is actually a component of the native venom. The toxin, a very
labile protein with an isoelectric point at pH 6.8, showed a single
band after disc electrophoresis, and its molecular weight was
assessed at 61,000 by gel chromatography and at 62,700 by the sedimentation equilibrium method using the analytical ultracentrifuge.

Using QAE-Sephadex A-50, Spanjer *et al.*, (1977) separated two
active preparations (called A and B) from a homogenate of female
M.hebetor wasps. The A-preparation formed a small part of the total
activity. Gel chromatography analysis indicated a molecular weight
for the activity in the A-preparation of about 42,000. The B-
preparation, providing about 85 per cent of the total recovered
biological activity showed a molecular weight for that activity
of about 57,000.

The two preparations have the same mode of action on the
neuromuscular transmission in a flight muscle of *Pieris brassicae*
(Spanjer *et al.*, 1977). The slopes of the log dose-effect curves
for the paralysis of *Galleria mellonella* larvae (Fig. 5), are
significantly different for the two preparations (Spanjer *et al.*,
1977). The slope for the B-preparation is the steepest (Fig. 5).

Compared with the sensitivity of *Galleria mellonella* for the
A- and the B-preparation, honeybee workers (*Apis mellifera*) are

more sensitive to the A-preparation than to the B-preparation.

This indicates that the two active principles present in the A- and B-preparation may show some differences in their biological spectrum.

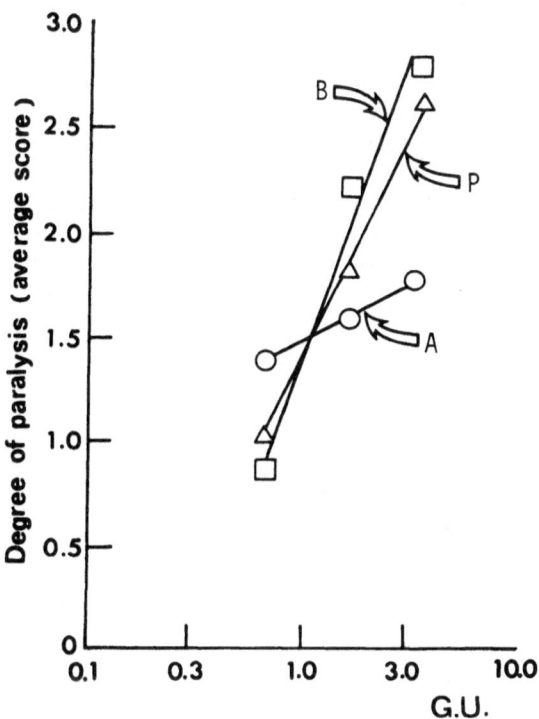

Fig. 5 Log-dose effect curves of the A- en B-preparation separated from a partly purified (P-) preparation of *M.hebetor* venom. The degree of paralysis (average score) is plotted against the number of *Galleria* units (*cf.* legend of Fig. 2). The scoring system is from Beard (1952), according to which unaffected *Galleria* larvae are scored '0', larvae showing uncoordinated movements are scored '1', incapacitated larvae are scored '2' and completely paralysed larvae are scored '3'.

(b) The venom of *Philanthus triangulum*

Crude venom preparations are obtained by extracting the collected venom gland with ice-cold water. After freeze drying 16 to 26 mg dry matter is obtained from 100 wasps. The paralysing potency of these crude preparations was not decreased by treatment with the enzymes carboxypeptidase A and leucine aminopeptidase.

    After gel chromatography of the crude preparation at 3°C on
Sephadex G-200 in distilled water, the low molecular weight fractions
containing the biological activity were chromatographed on Sephadex
G-25 in 0.2 mol/l ammonium acetate pH 4.75.

    When isolated fractions were tested only a small part of the
original biological activity was recovered. However, if the active
fractions were combined with neighbouring fractions the biological
activity was increased and the total activity was recovered completely.

    Using ion exchange chromatography on SE-Sephadex C-25 in 0.4
mol/l ammonium acetate pH 4.75 and a gradient up to 1 mol/l ammonium
acetate pH 4.75, at least three components could be separated. A
number of fractions were combined to form a β-, a γ- and a δ-section.
The β-section had no paralysing activity of its own. The δ-section
was biologically active but the dose-response curve was very flat.
The effect of the δ-section could be increased by combination with
the β-section, the increase being proportional to the quantity of
the β-section added (Fig. 6).

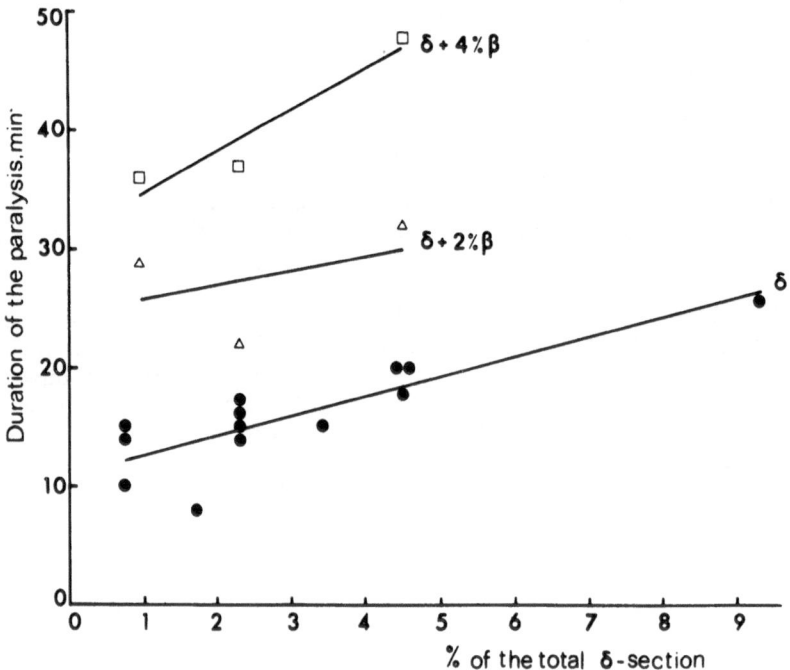

Fig. 6 Effect in honeybees (*Apis mellifera*) of partly purified
(after SE-Sephadex) *P.triangulum* venom. The δ-section alone (dots),
each dose combined with 2% of the β-section (triangles), and combined
with 4% of the β-section (squares). Calculated linear regression
lines.

    The γ-section had no paralysing activity in small quantities.
However, above a certain threshold value the γ-section suddenly
showed a considerable activity. Above the threshold value the
activity was further increased by addition of the β-section,
depending on the quantity of the β-section added. Moreover, if the
γ- and β-sections were combined the threshold value for the γ-
section was lowered (Fig. 7).

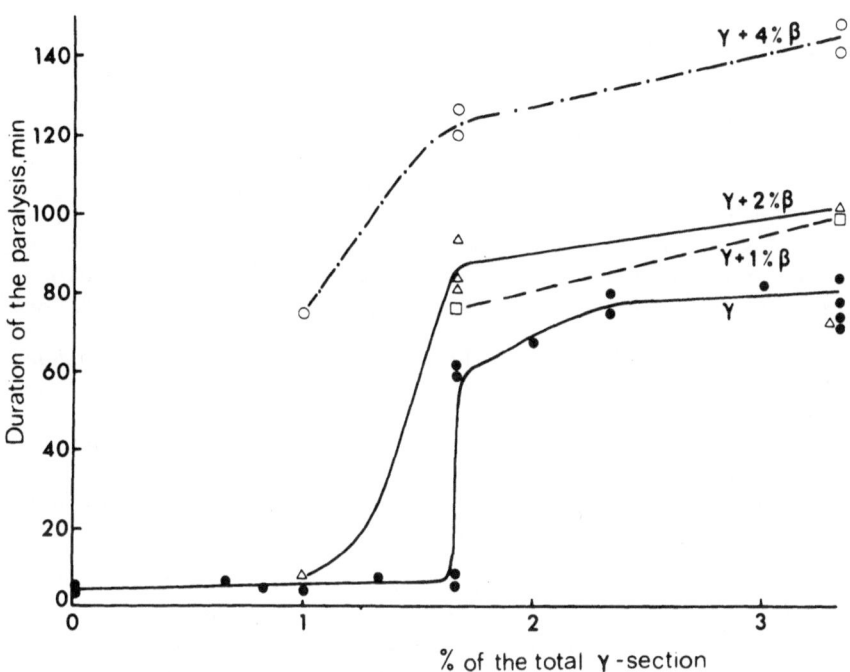

Fig. 7 Effect in honeybees of partly purified *P.triangulum* venom.
The γ-section alone (dots), each dose combined with 1% (squares),
2% (triangles) and 4% (open circles) of the β-section.

    Using thin layer chromatography on cellulose in butanol, acetic
acid, water in the ratio 4 : 1 : 2 (v/v), and spraying with ninhydrin
showed that the β-, γ- and δ-sections were inhomogeneous.
    The active components of the β- and δ-sections were isolated
using preparative thin layer chromatography. The active component(s)
of the γ-section could not be isolated. Apparently they change or
decompose on the cellulose layer in the presence of acetic acid.

The δ-component can be detected on the thin layer with reagents for phenol compounds. Using mass spectrometry with the field desorption technique (Laboratory for Organic Chemistry, University of Amsterdam) the β-component was shown to contain a sodium ion. The βH-component was prepared using an ion exchange technique. The βH-component and the δ-component seem to be isomers with a molecular weight of 390. The bruto formula for the δ-component is $C_{24}H_{38}O_4$ and there are no indications that nitrogen forms part of the molecule (Spanjer and De Haan, 1976).

DISCUSSION

This paper deals with some biological and chemical facts concerning two solitary wasp venoms, one from an aculeate wasp (*Philanthus triangulum*) and one from a terebrant wasp (*Microbracon hebetor*).

The majority of solitary wasps have attained an advanced degree of specialization both in structure and in behaviour. It therefore would not be very surprising if the venoms of solitary wasps would vary markedly in chemical composition and in biological action. The two venoms described apparently differ in chemical composition, but their biological effects are amazingly similar since both venoms block somatic neuromuscular transmission in insects at a presynaptic site.

Summarizing, the difference between the venoms of *Philanthus triangulum* (Aculeata) and of *Microbracon hebetor* (Terebrantia) are (a). *P.triangulum* probably stings, like other Aculeata, into the central nervous system; *M.hebetor* stings, like other Terebrantia, at different places. (b) *P.triangulum* venom is active in all insects and in spiders; *M.hebetor* venom, is only very active in Lepidoptera. (c) *P.triangulum* venom blocks the excitatory as well as the inhibitory neuromuscular transmission in insects; *M.hebetor* venom only blocks the excitatory system in insects. (d) *P.triangulum* venom contains active principles of low molecular weight; *M. hebetor* venom contains protein toxins with high molecular weights.

The question whether these differences are valid for the whole suborder of Aculeata and the whole suborder of Terebrantia can only be answered after venoms of several wasps, not only belonging to these two suborders, but also to different families, have been studied.

Acknowledgements- The authors thank Professor C. van der Meer for his stimulating interest, Mrs. A.B. van Marle-Marschall for help during the preparation of the manuscript, and Mr. P. Mantel, Mr. N. de Haan and Mr. R.L. Veenedaal for their skilful technical assistance.

REFERENCES

Bartram, J., 1744, An account of some very curious wasps nests made of clay in Pensilvania. *Phil.Trans.Roy.Soc.Lond.* <u>43</u>: 363.

Beard, R.L., 1952, The toxicology of *Habrobracon* venom: a study of a natural insecticide. *The Conn.Agric.Exp.St.New Haven Bull.* <u>562</u>: 1.

Claude-Joseph, F., 1928, Recherches biologiques sur les prédateurs du Chili. *Am.Sc.Nat.Zool.* <u>10</u>: 67.

Drenth, D., 1974, Stability of *Microbracon hebetor* (Say) venom preparations. *Toxicon* <u>12</u>: 541.

Dufour, L., 1841, Observations sur les métamorphoses du *Cerceris bupresticida* et sur l'industrie et l'instinct entomologique de cet Hyménoptère. *Ann.Sc.Nat.* <u>2</u> (15): 353.

Fabre, J.H., 1855, Observations sur les moeurs de *Cerceris* et sur la cause de la longue conservation des coléoptères, dont ils approvisionnent leurs larves. *Ann.Sci.nat.* <u>4</u>: 129.

Fabre, J.H., 1879-1910, *Souvenirs entomologiques*, Delagrave, Paris.

Huddart, H., 1971, Contraction of insect muscle. *Exp.in Physiol. and Biochem.* <u>4</u>: 219.

Kuo Po, 276-324 A.D., Erh-ya yin t'u Ying Sung Ch'ao-hui-t'u (dictionary of old terms with Sung illustrations).

Lepeletier de Saint-Fargeau, A., 1841, Histoire naturelle des insectes. Hyménoptères. p. 563, De Roret, Paris.

Paton, W.D., 1963, Cholinergic transmission and acetylcholine output. *Can.J.Biochem.Physiol.* <u>41</u>, 2637.

Piek, T., 1966a, Site of action of venom of *Microbracon hebetor* Say (Braconidae, Hymenoptera). *J.Insect Physiol.* <u>12</u>: 561.

Piek, T., 1966b, Site of action of the venom of the digger wasp *Philanthus triangulum* F. on the fast neuromuscular system of the locust. *Toxicon* <u>4</u>: 191.

Piek, T., and Engels, E., 1969, Action of the venom of *Microbracon hebetor* Say on larvae and adults of *Philosamia cynthia* Hübn. *Comp.Biochem.Physiol.* <u>28</u>: 603.

Piek, T., and Mantel, P., 1970, The effect of the venom of *Microbracon hebetor* (Say) on the hyperpolarizing potentials in a skeletal muscle of *Philosamia cynthia* Hübn. *Comp.gen.Pharmacol.* <u>1</u>: 87.

Piek, T., and Njio, K.D., 1975, Neuromuscular block in honeybees by the venom of the bee wolf wasp (*Philanthus triangulum* F.). *Toxicon* <u>13</u>: 199.

Piek, T., and Mantel, P., 1977, Myogenic contraction in locust muscle induced by proctolin and by *Philanthus triangulum* venom. *J.Insect Physiol.* (in press).

Piek, T., Mantel, P., and Engels, E., 1971, Neuromuscular block in insects caused by the venom of the digger wasp *Philanthus triangulum* F. *Comp.gen.Pharmacol.* <u>2</u>: 317.

Piek, T., Spanjer, W., Njio, K.D., Veenendaal, R.L., and Mantel, P., 1974, Paralysis caused by the venom of the wasp *Microbracon gelechiae. J.Insect Physiol.* <u>20</u>: 2307.

Rathmayer, W., 1962, Das Paralysierungsproblem beim Bienenwolf
    Philanthus triangulum F. (Hym.Sphec.). *Z.vergl.Physiol.* 45:
    413.
Réaumur, R.A. Ferchauld de, 1742, Mémoires pour servir à l'histoire
    des insectes. T.VI. Imprimerie Royale, Paris.
Spanjer, W., and de Haan, N., 1976, Isolation, some properties and
    characterization of paralysing components in the venom of the
    solitary wasp *Philanthus triangulum* F. *Abstr. 17th Dutch Fed.
    Meeting* 1976: 367.
Spanjer, W., Grosu, L., and Piek, T., 1977, Paralysis in insects
    by two different preparations from homogenate of the wasp
    Microbracon hebetor (Say). *Toxicon* (in press).
Steiner, A.L., 1962, Etude du comportement prédateur d'un
    Hyménoptère sphégien: "*Liris nigra*" V.d.L. (= "*Notogonia
    pompiliformis*" Pz.). Thesis, University of Paris.
Usherwood, P.N.R., and Cull-Candy, S.G., 1975, Pharmacology of
    somatic nerve muscle synapses. *In:* Insect muscle, P.N.R.
    Usherwood edit. Academic Press, London, New York, San Francisco.
Visser, B.J., Spanjer, W., de Klonia, H., Piek, T., van der Meer, C.,
    and van der Drift, A.C.M., 1976, Isolation and some biochemical
    properties of a paralysing toxin from the venom of the wasp
    Microbracon hebetor (Say). *Toxicon* 14: 357.
Walther, C., and Rathmayer, W., 1974, The effects of *Habrobracon*
    venom on excitatory neuromuscular transmission in insects.
    J.comp.Physiol. 89: 23.

CHEMISTRY, SPECIFICITY AND ACTION OF ARTHROPOD

TOXIC PROTEINS DERIVED FROM SCORPION VENOMS

E. Zlotkin[1,3], W. Rathmayer[2] and S. Lissitzky[3]

1) Department of Entomology, The Hebrew University of

Jerusalem, Israel; 2) Department of Biology, University of

Konstanz, Germany; 3) Department of Biochemistry, School

of Medicine, Marseille, France

INTRODUCTION

From an ecological point of view the usage of chemical means for
defense or food obtaining purposes may be considered as an efficient
and energy saving method. The venom apparatus of scorpions serves as
a perfect example of this principle. Scorpions feed on freshly killed
prey, consisting of arthropods and generally soft bodied insects.
However, as predators, scorpions appear to lack certain essential
anatomical and physiological qualities. They move relatively slowly,
are practically blind and have a rather undeveloped sense of smell.
Scorpions actually do not seek their food actively, but rather wait
for the prey to approach their lairs (Bearg, 1961; Stahnke, 1966).
Thus, a device for paralyzing the prey at the earliest moment of
contact is essential. This is achieved by the venom which is substantially employed for hunting and food obtaining. As we shall see
below, this function is associated with highly specified chemical
adaptations.

THE EFFECT OF SCORPION VENOMS TO ARTHROPODS

The symptoms of scorpion envenomation in arthropods mainly indicate a stimulatory effect on the skeletal musculature. In the
locust (adults Locusta), injected with 2-3 µg of the venom of L.
quinquestriatus, this is expressed in uncoordinated leg movements,
trembling of hindlegs and spasmodic contractions of the genital

227

valves (Kamon and Shulov, 1963). Similarly, injection of $2LD_{50}$ (23 μg per 100 mg of body weight) of A. australis scorpion venom into isopods (Armadillium vulgare, a terrestrial crustacean) causes a paralysis within 2-3 minutes preceded by irregular and uncoordinated movements of the legs and a curvature of the body due to a sustained contracture of the ventral body musculature (Fig. 1C, Zlotkin et al. 1972b). In blowfly larvae, injection of small amounts of different scorpion venoms (see Table 1) causes an immediate and sustained contraction of body musculature, expressed in drastic thickening and shortening of the body and accompanied by complete paralysis (Fig. 1A,B), the rate and duration of which are dosage dependent (Fig. 1C). This contraction paralysis of blowfly larvae was employed as a quick, convenient and sensitive bioassay for the evaluation of the paralytic potency of scorpion venoms. The paralytic potency of different scorpion venoms to blowfly larvae compared to their mice lethality is presented in Table 1 (Zlotkin et al. 1971a).

Table 1. The fifty percent lethal dose to mice (LD_{50}) and the contraction paralysis unit (CPU) to blowfly larvae of different scorpion venoms[a].

Scorpion venom	LD_{50} (μg/mouse) [b]	CPU (μg/larva) [c]
Leiurus quinquestriatus	5.1	0.22
Androctonus aeneas aeneas	6.2	0.05
Androctonus mauretanicus mauretanicus	6.3	0.47
Androctonus australis	7.0	0.29
Centruroides santa maria	7.7	3.82
Androctonus crassicauda	8.0	0.68
Tityus serrulatus	8.6	2.17
Buthiscus bicalcaratus	12.0	0.07
Centruroides limpidus tecomanus	13.7	0.22
Androctonus amoreuxi	15.0	0.36
Buthacus leptochelis	15.3	0.09
Buthus occitanus tunetanus	17.9	0.05
Buthacus arenicola	19.8	0.07
Buthus occitanus paris	83.0	0.03
Buthotux minax	85.0	0.30
Parabuthus transvaalicus	85.0	0.35

Remarks:
a) Taken from Zlotkin et al. (1971a). The venoms were obtained by electrical milking followed by lyophilization.
b) Subcutaneous injection into mice of both sexes weighing about 20 gms.
c) Tested on Sarcophaga falculata larvae weighing about 100 mg.

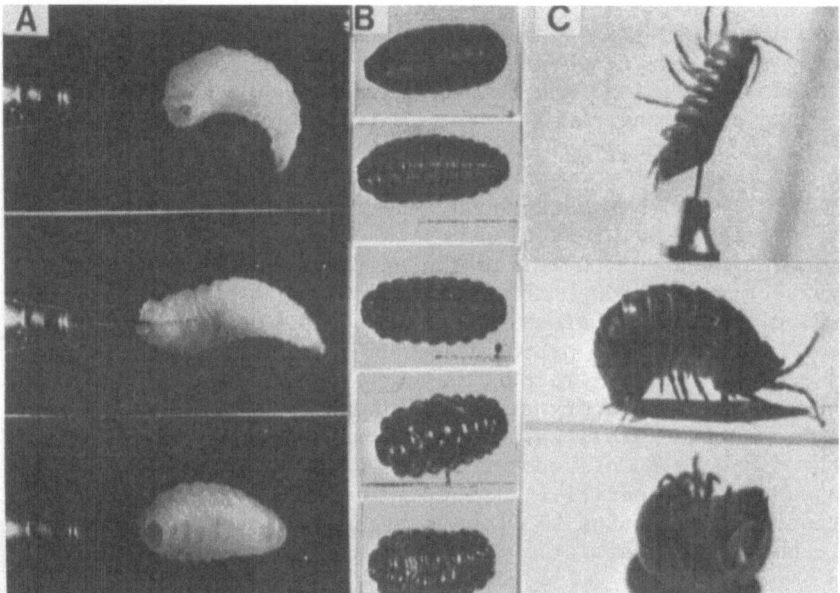

Fig. 1. Symptoms of scorpion venom paralysis of arthropods.
A. Testing scorpion venom on blowfly Sarcophaga falculata larvae.
Upper: Sarcophaga larva is placed on the needle connected to a
micrometrically operated syringe. The needle is inserted into the
ventral side of the last abdominal segment; the larva on the needle
prior to injection showing twisting movements. Middle: The larva
already responding while the venom solution is being injected; a
local contraction at the tip of the inserted needle can be seen.
Lower: Final contraction of the larva accompanied by complete im-
mobility.
B. The duration and rate of this larvae contraction paralysis are
dosage dependent. This figure shows contracted-deformed puparia of
Sarcophaga which have been injected as larvae with different amounts
of L. quinquestriatus scorpion venom 2 hr prior to puparium formation. From up to down: saline, 0.2, 0.4, 0.8 and 1.6 μg venom
injected respectively. The contracted shape of the larvae is fixed
by the sclerotization process in the article. The dependence of the
degree of contraction on the dosage is apparent. (Taken from Zlotkin
et al. 1971a).
C. The effect of the venom of A. australis on the terrestrial crustacean A. vulgare. Upper: 30 μg of venom are injected. The needle
is inserted through the intersegmental membrane between the thorax
and the abdomen from the dorsal side. Middle: After 25 sec the
animal stops; the body is curved while the legs exhibit irregular
and uncoordinated movements. Lower: After 35 sec a complete paralysis is obtained. The curvature of the body is increased and the
legs are contracted. The animal is unable to stand. The position
of the animal is inverted. It lies immobile on its curved dorsal
surface. (Taken from Zlotkin et al. 1972b).

The marked resistance of an intact nerve to scorpion venom, as previously shown in vertebrate preparations (Houssay, 1919; Del Pozo and Anguiano, 1947; Adam and Weiss, 1959; LaGrange and Russell, 1971), was also demonstrated by the application of concentrated solutions of L. quinquestriatus venom to the tympanic nerve (Zlotkin et al., 1970) as well as the ventral nerve cord of Locusta (Parnas et al., 1970). On this background, one may assume that the excitatory paralysis symptoms of scorpion envenomation in arthropods should represent a peripheral action on the skeletal musculature, either directly or through the neuromuscular junction. The latter point was clarified by Parnas et al. (1967,1970), with crustacean and insect neuromuscular preparations employing Centruroides and Leiurus scorpion venoms, respectively. It has been demonstrated that the muscle stimulatory effect of these venoms followed from a presynaptic action. This was expressed in the increase of quantal content and in the spontaneous contraction of the muscle which was correlated to the repetitive firing of the nerve. Both the axonal excitation and conduction block were assumed to result from the axonal membrane depolarization.

There is an apparent resemblance between the effects of scorpion venom to arthropods and those to mammals (Zlotkin et al., in press). This is expressed in the excitatory symptoms of envenomation and is emphasized when comparing the action of scorpion venom on the neuromuscular preparations of an insect and crustacean (Parnas and Russell, 1967; Parnas et al., 1970) to that of a mammal (Brazil et al., 1973; Zlotkin et al., in press). In all the above preparations, scorpion venom caused muscular stimulatory effects due to presynaptic excitation, especially at the level of the exposed nerve endings, resulting in the release of the corresponding transmitter. This similarity in action may lead to the assumption that the effect of scorpion venoms on mammals and arthropods is due to the same chemical factors in the crude venom.

TOXINS SPECIFICALLY ACTIVE TO ARTHROPODS

By the aid of the assay of the contraction paralysis of blowfly larvae (Fig. 1), it has been found that there was no correlation between larvae paralysis and mice lethal potencies of sixteen different Buthidae venoms (Zlotkin et al., 1971a, Table 1), hinting at the possibility that the two toxic activities may result from different factors. This assumption was strongly supported by the finding that the potent toxins I and II of A. australis, which are strongly lethal to mammals, previously isolated and purified according to biological criteria of mice lethality (Miranda et al., 1964ab; Rochat et al., 1967; Miranda et al., 1970), were completely inactive on larvae (Zlotkin et al., 1971b). The final proof of the diversity between factors affecting mammals and those paralyzing insects in scorpion venoms, was obtained by starch gel electrophoretical se-

paration of the venom of A. australis (Zlotkin et al., 1971b), and
six other Buthinae venoms (Fig. 2, Zlotkin et al., 1972a). It has
been found that three of the above venoms contain more than one
larvae contraction paralysis fraction. These fractions are not only
paralytic to fly larvae (Fig. 2) but are also lethal and readily inactivated by trypsin, thus demonstrating their protein nature
(Zlotkin et al., 1972a).

Basically, the same methodology previously employed for the
purification of the so-called mammal toxins (Miranda et al., 1970;
Zlotkin et al., in press) has also enabled the isolation and
purification of the insect toxin from the venom of the North African
scorpion Androctonus australis Hector. · Following a sequence of steps
composed of water-extraction, dialysis, recycling Sephadex G-50 gel
filtration and ion exchangers equilibrium chromatography by DEAE-
Sephadex A-50 followed by Amberlite CG-50 (Fig. 3), a final product,
267-fold purified and with a yield of 95% toxicity was obtained
(Zlotkin et al., 1971c). It is a single chained low molecular
weight protein composed of 67 amino acids and crosslinked by four
disulfide bridges (Fig. 3). Its amino acid composition and N-terminal primary sequence (compared to several other toxins obtained
from the same scorpion venom) are presented in Table 2 and Fig. 4,
respectively. On the basis of its composition, the insect toxin
resembles the mammal toxins by its total number of residues, the
presence of 8 half cystines (which were all found to participate in
disulfide bridging), the low amount of phenylalanine, histidine,
arginine, tryptophan and the absence of methionine. The N-terminal
sequences of these toxins, however, indicate a more obvious difference between the insect and the mammal toxins (see Fig. 4).

In contrast to the crude venom of A. australis, the insect toxin
and the so-called mammal toxins I and II, derived from the same
venom, were unable to affect an isopod (terrestrial crustacean, Armadillium vulgare) or a scorpion (Buthus occitanus), suggesting the
possibility that the activity of the crude venom on these arthropods
is due to discrete new toxins (Zlotkin et al., 1972b). Using a new
bioassay, based on paralysis of isopods (Fig. 1C) as well as column
chromatography by Sephadex G-50 gel filtration (Zlotkin et al., 1972b)
and ion exchange gradient chromatography on Amberlite CG 50 followed
by CM-Sephadex, a protein specifically toxic to isopods, called the
"crustacean" toxin, was isolated and purified from the venom of A.
australis (Fig. 3, Zlotkin et al., 1975). The pure toxin contained
about 20 percent of the crude venom's toxicity to isopods and was
250 times more active. The amino acid composition of the crustacean
toxin is presented in Table 2. Compared to the insect and mammal
toxins derived from the same venom, the crustacean toxin showed a
higher content of half cystines (indicating five disulfide bridges
instead of four) and also more Glu plus Gln than Asp plus Asn, which
is in contrast to all other toxins obtained until now from Buthinae
venoms (Zlotkin et al., in press).

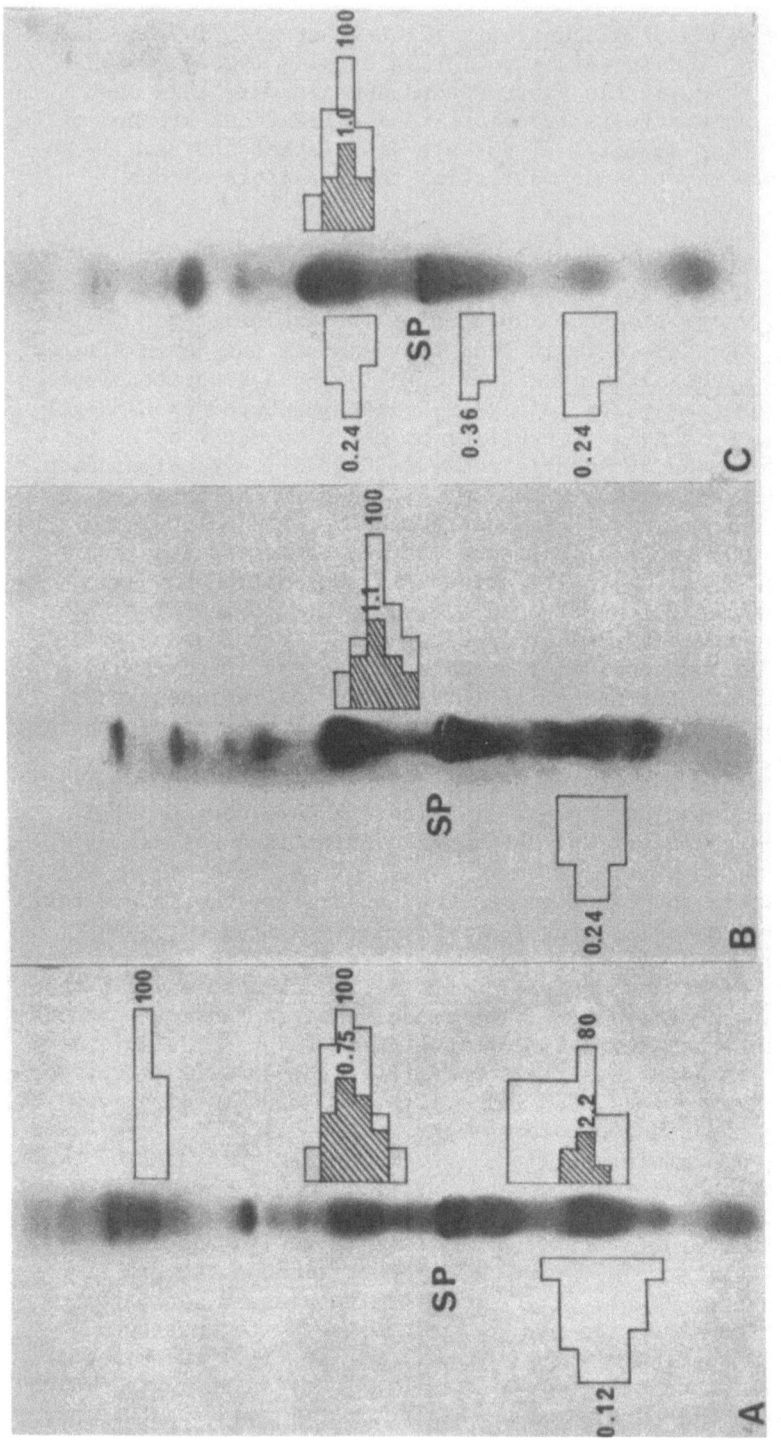

Fig. 2. Starch gel electropherograms of several Buthidae scorpion venoms indicating the diversity between mammal and insect toxic fractions. Ten mg of crude venom were dissolved in Tris-citric acid buffer pH 8.6 and applied in a slot of 23 cm in length. Empty areas on the left correspond to mice lethality. The shaded areas on the right indicate contraction-paralysis and the empty areas on the right indicate lethality of larvae. The numbers are related to maximal activities expressed: (1) for contraction-paralysis of larvae as the volume (μℓ) corresponding to one contraction-paralysis

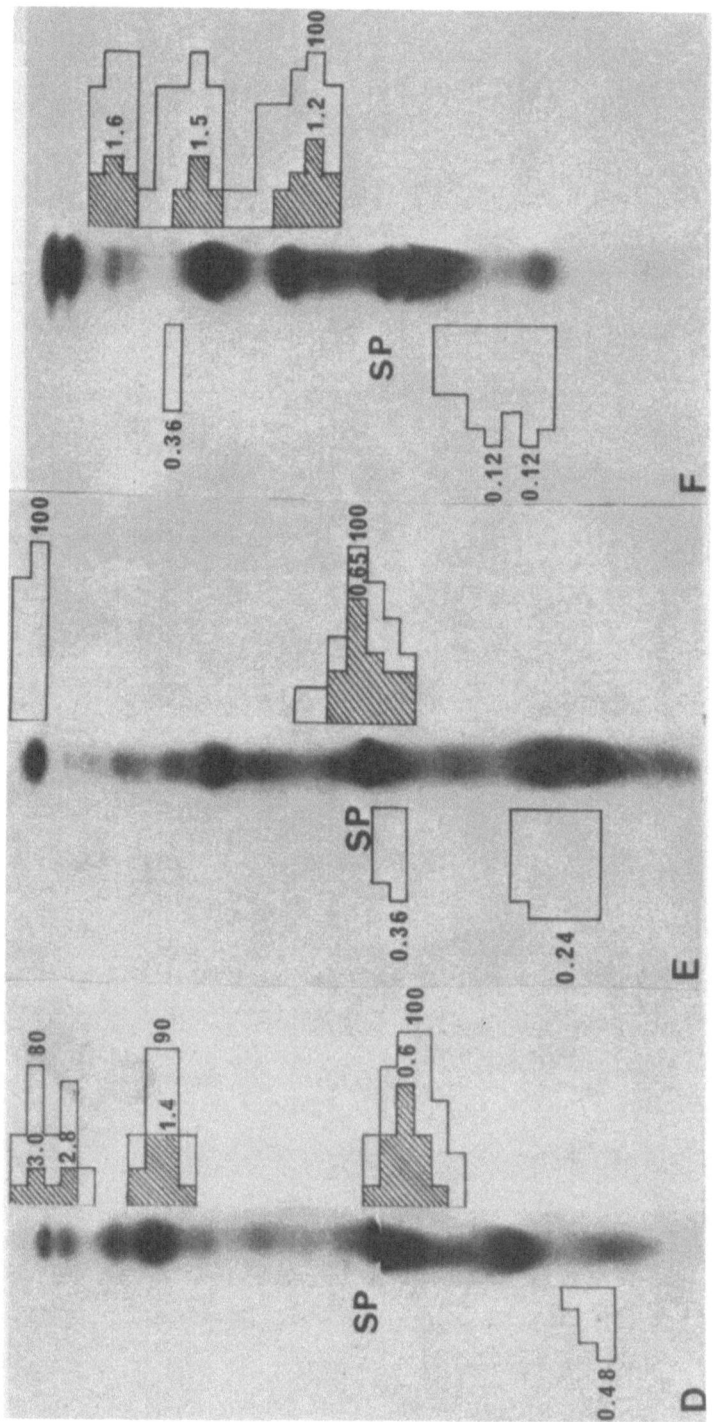

Fig. 2 (cont.)
unit (Zlotkin et al., 1971a); (2) for larvae lethality as percent death; (3) for mice lethality as the minimum volume of eluate (ml) causing death. SP = starting point; anode at top. The venoms of the following scorpions were used: A. Androctonus aeneas aeneas. B. Androctonus amoreuxi. C. Androctonus mauretanicus mauretanicus. D. Buthus occitanus paris. E. Buthus occitanus tunetanus. F. Leiurus quinquestriatus. (Taken from Zlotkin et al., 1972a).

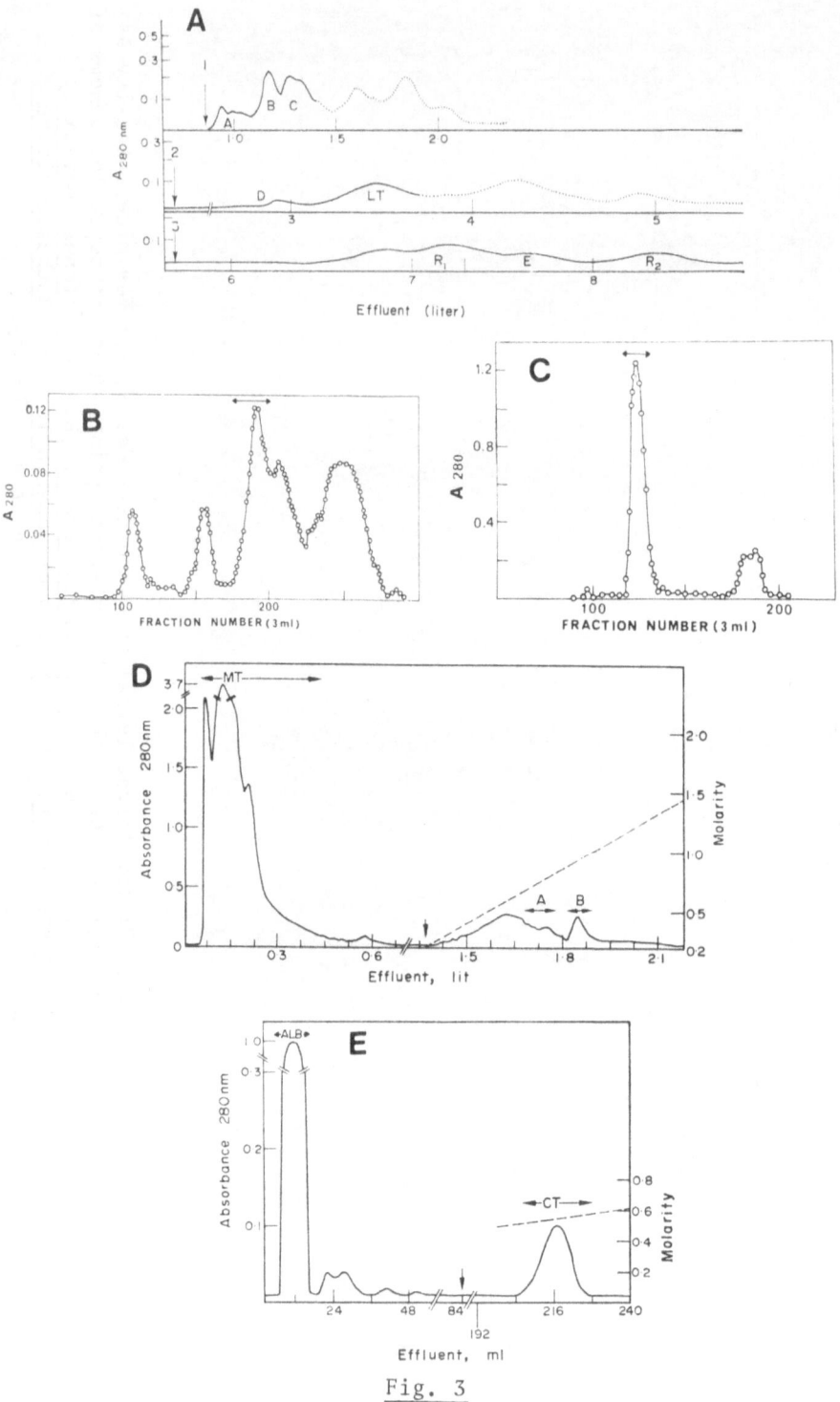

Fig. 3

Fig. 3. Isolation and purification of toxins specifically active to
arthropods from the venom of the scorpion Androctonus australis
Hector. A. Recycling gel filtration on Sephadex G. 50: Four columns of 3.2×100 cm in series in 0.1 M ammonium acetate buffer pH
8.5 - 8.6; flow rate 60 mℓ/hr. The mixture submitted to fractionation is the water extract of 2 g of crude venom, vertical arrows
and numbers correspond to the beginning of the consecutive cycles.
Fractions of the elution curves indicated by the full line are collected. The material marked by the dotted line is recycled. Toxicity to mice is located in fractions R1 and R2 (Miranda et al.,
1970), toxicity to fly larvae is located in fraction LT and toxicity
to isopods is located in fractions E and R2 (taken from Zlotkin et
al., 1972b).
B. Purification of the insect toxin: Chromatography on DEAE
Sephadex A-50 of the fly larvae toxic fraction (LT) obtained in A
from 0.5 g of crude venom. Column 2×200 cm in 0.1 M ammonium acetate buffer pH 8.50; flow rate 12 mℓ/hr. The horizontal arrow indicates the fraction toxic to fly larvae.
C. Chromatography on Amberlite CG 50 of the toxic fraction obtained in B from 0.5 g of venom. Column 2×200 cm in 0.2 M ammonium
acetate buffer pH 6.30; flow rate 12 mℓ/hr. The horizontal arrow
indicates the finally purified insect toxin fraction (taken from
Zlotkin et al., 1971c).
D. Purification of the crustacean toxin: Chromatography on Amberlite CG 50 of fraction R2 obtained in A from 10 g of crude venom.
Column 2.5×20 cm. Buffer: ammonium acetate, equilibrium conditions:
0.2 M pH 6.30; linear gradient conditions: up to 2.0 M and pH 7.3.
Flow rate 30 mℓ/hr. Fractions of 7.5 mℓ were collected. Dotted li
line - linear gradient of buffer concentration. Vertical arrow indicates the starting of gradient elution. M.T. fraction toxic to
mice, which corresponds to the mammal toxin II. A and B: fractions toxic to isopods.
E. Chromatography on CM-Sephadex of 2.9 OD_{280} units of fraction B
obtained in D and mixed with 29 mg of albumin prior to lyophilization
in order to preserve its activity. Column 1.4×12 cm. Buffer: ammonium acetate 0.2 M pH 7.3 followed by a linear gradient of concentration. Flow rate: 5 mℓ/hr in equilibrium conditions and 10
mℓ/hr in gradient elution. Fractions of 2.4 mℓ were collected.
Dotted line: linear gradient of buffer concentration. Vertical
arrow indicates the starting of gradient elution. ALB - albumin
fraction. CT: crustacean toxin (taken from Zlotkin et al., 1975).

Table 2.   The amino acid compositions of toxins derived from the
venom of the scorpion <u>Androctonus australis</u> Hector

Amino acid	Androctonus australis Hector					
	I^a	I'^b	II^a	III^a	IT^c	CT^d
Aspartic acid	9	9	8	8	11	6
Threonine	2	2	3	0	4	4
Serine	6	6	2	6	6	4
Glutamic acid	0	0	4	0	3	10
Proline	6	6	3	6	1	2
Glycine	6	6	7	6	4	4
Alanine	1	1	3	3	3	2
Half-cystine	8	8	8	8	8	10
Valine	5	4	4	6	3	4
Methionine	0	0	0	0	0	0
Isoleucine	2	3	1	3	2-3	2
Leucine	4	4	2	4	5-6	2
Tyrosine	3	3	7	3	5	4
Phenylalanine	1	1	1	1	1	0
Lysine	6	6	5	6	7	4
Histidine	1	1	2	2	1	0
Arginine	2	2	3	1	1	9
Tryptophan	1	1	1	1	1	2
Total	63	63	64	64	66-68	69

Remarks:
a) from Miranda et al., 1970.
b) determined from the sequence from Rochat et al., 1970.
c) the Insect Toxin from Zlotkin et al., 1971c.
d) the Crustacean Toxin from Zlotkin et al., 1975.

```
             10        20        30        40
IT   KKDGYAVDSS-GKAPECLL---SNYCNDZCKTVHYADKGY

I    KRDGYIVYPN-NCVYHCVPP-----CDGLCKKN-GGSSGS
I'   KRDGYIVYPN-NCVYHCIPP-----CDGLCKKN-GGSSGS
III  VRDGYIVNSK-NCVYHCVPP-----CDGLCKKN-GASSGS

II   VKDGYIVDDV-NCTYFCGR---NAYCNEECTKL-KGESG-
```

Fig. 4. The N-terminal primary sequence of the insect (IT) and the
mammal toxins purified from the venom of the scorpion <u>A. australis</u>.
The amino acids were placed in a manner to obtain maximum homology
(-: deletion) (taken from Zlotkin et al., in press).

Considering the symptomatology, potency and speed of action of the insect as well as crustacean toxins, it was assumed that both are basically neurotoxic. Some indirect evidence was recently obtained, suggesting that the specificity or selectivity in the action of these toxins is based on specific affinity to neural systems of the corresponding groups of animals. It has been found that the insect toxin is able to mimic the action of the crude venom in performing an excitatory block of the induced afferent transynaptic response at the sixth abdominal ganglion of the cockroach Periplaneta americana, in contrast to the complete inactivity of high doses of the mammal toxin II (D'Ajello et al., 1972). Similarly, an isopod toxic fraction obtained by Sephadex G-50 chromatography (Zlotkin et al., 1972b) was able to mimic the excitatory and blocking action of the crude venom on the crayfish stretch receptor organ, in contrast to the insect and mammal toxins which were inactive (Pansa et al., 1973).

These findings have established the conception claiming that scorpion venoms contain different toxins, selectively active to different groups of organisms, which may represent a chemical adaptation of scorpions to changes in food sources during evolution (Zlotkin, 1973).

NEUROPHYSIOLOGICAL STUDIES

The phenomenon of specificity and selectivity in the action of scorpion toxins, which was based mainly on simple bioassays, demanded a neurophysiological approach. The crude venom of the North African scorpion Androctonus australis Hector and its derived mammal toxins I and II, insect and crustacean toxins, were tested on mammal, insect, crustacean and arachnid nerve muscle preparations. The choice of such preparations was based on the consideration that they actually represent the true target organ for the paralytic action of scorpion venoms and their toxins.

Due to the accumulated background information concerning the action of scorpion venom on the guinea pig ileal smooth muscle preparation (Patterson, 1962; Diniz and Torres, 1968; Tazieff-Depierre et al., 1973a,1973b; Cunha-Melo et al., 1973), this preparation was chosen to represent a mammalian neuromuscular system. It has been found that the crustacean toxin induced a sustained prolonged contraction (Fig. 5A), in contrast to the rhythmic spasmodic ileal behavior caused by the crude venom and the mammal toxins (Fig. 5B). The excitatory effect of the crustacean toxin was completely inhibited by atropine, potentiated by eserine, tachyphylactic, blocked by tetrodotoxin and morphine and unaffected by hexamethonium (Tintpulver et al., 1976). It may be concluded that, like in the case of the crude venom and the mammal toxins (Zlotkin et al., in press),

the action of the crustacean toxin was due to a postganglionic presynaptic stimulation resulting in the release of a cholinergic
transmitter. Prolonged application of the crustacean toxin has
caused also a depressory postsynaptic action expressed in the reduced ileal response to several agonists. The insect toxin, however,
was inactive in the ileum smooth muscle preparation.

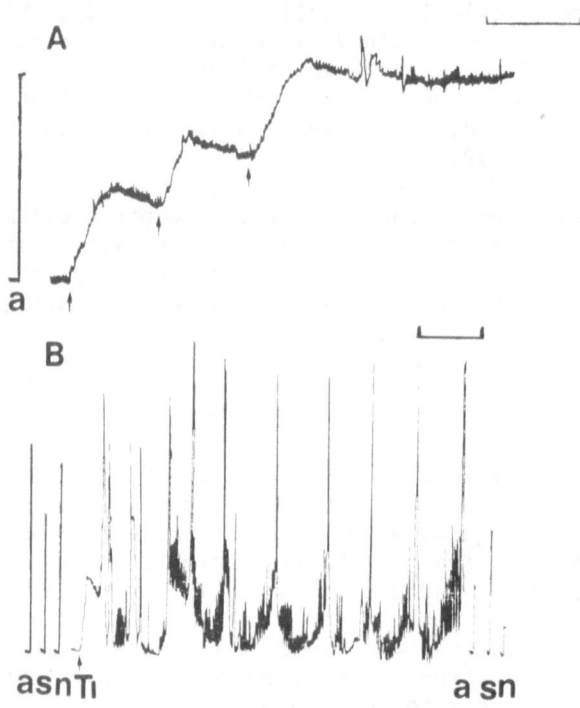

Fig. 5. The response of the ileal smooth muscle preparation to the
crustacean (A) and the mammal I (B) toxins.
A. The 'stepwise' ileal response to small repetitive doses of crustacean toxin. Acetylcholine (a) 15 ng/ml. The arrows point to the
application of 200 ng of crustacean toxin per ml. Time base 5 min.
B. The prolonged application of the toxin is (Tl, 500 ng/ml) followed by a depressed response of several agonists. Acetylcholine
(a) 5 ng/ml, serotonin (s) 100 ng/ml, nicotine (n) 1000 ng/ml. Time
base 10 min. (taken from Tintpulver et al., 1976).

Table 3. The relative activity of different scorpion toxins on several nerve muscle preparations(a as well as insect paralysis

Toxic material(b	Insect(c	Crustacean(d	Arachnid(e	Mammal(f	Insects(g paralysis
Crude venom	1	1	1	1	1
Insect toxin	115	No effect	No effect	No effect	25
Crustacean toxin	18	127	67	0.7	0.7
Mammal toxin I	7	27	11	1	5.7
Mammal toxin II	2	4	5	25	0.2

Remarks:
a) Based on a comparison of the average minimal doses causing an evoked repetitive muscular response. Numbers express the activity in terms of folds of that of the crude venom.
b) The different toxins were purified from the crude venom of the scorpion Androctonus australis Hector (Miranda et al., 1970; Zlotkin et al., 1971a,1975).
c) Locust leg extensor tibiae preparation (Walther et al., 1976).
d) The crayfish walking leg dactylus opener preparation (Rathmayer et al., 1977).
e) The claw closer muscle preparation in the leg of a mygalomorph spider (Ruhland et al., in press).
f) The guinea pig ileum smooth muscle preparation (Tintpulver et al., 1976).
g) Determined by injection into the body cavity of second and third instar locusts larvae.

   The above toxins were applied on the neuromuscular preparations
of an insect (the extensor tibiae muscle of Locusta hind leg, Walther et al., 1976), crustacean (the dactylus opener in the walking
leg of the crayfish Astacus leptodactylus, Rathmayer et al., 1977),
and arachnid (the claw closer muscle in the leg of the mygalomorph
spider Dugesiella hentzi, Ruhland et al., in press). For com-
plementary and comparative purposes, their effect on the crayfish
CNS axonal preparation (Rathmayer et al., 1977) as well as their
paralytic effect on locusts (Walther et al., 1976) were also tested.
In all the above preparations it has been found that muscular effects of the venom and the different toxins, expressed in the aug-
mentation of the recorded junction potentials, evoked repetitive
firing and spontaneous muscular repetitive firing, are due to excitatory presynaptic effects (Fig. 6). The pattern of axonal activities indicates that the various peripheral branches of the motor nerve are the primary target of the toxins. The relative activity of the different toxins on the different preparations is
summarized in Table 3.

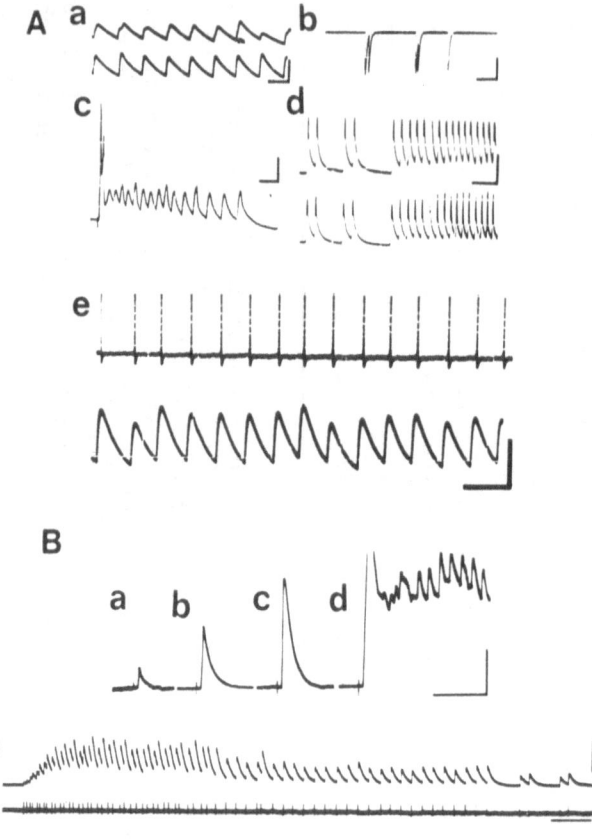

Fig. 6.

From the point of view of specificity and selectivity in the
action of the different toxins, the data presented in Table 3 may
indicate that: (1) The crustacean and the mammal toxins should be
considered as possessing only a relative affinity or specificity to
different organisms. The pharmacological diversity of these substances may represent either multiplicity of active sites or differential affinities to identical receptor sites in different organisms. It is noteworthy that the presence of a component such
as the crustacean toxin, which by itself is non-lethal to mammals
but is able to perform an excitatory action in mammalian systems,
may possess certain pharmacological as well as pharmaceutical advantages. (2) The discrepancy between the relative potencies of
the crustacean and the mammal II toxins on the locust nerve muscle
preparation, as compared to their extremely low ability to paralyze

Fig. 6. Neuromuscular effects of different scorpion toxins on
locust (A) and crayfish (B) preparations.
A.(a) Part of a train of spontaneous 'slow' ejps recorded synchronously from two different muscle fibres in the main muscle.
75 min after application of about 10 µg/mℓ crude venom. (b)
Spontaneous ijps from the accessory bundle. 50 min after application of 8 µg/mℓ crude venom. Preparation paralyzed by
Habrobracon-venom. (c) Single response of 'fast' and repetitive
response of 'slow' ejps in the main muscle on single synchronous
stimulation of the two motor axons. 60 min after application of
about 0.7 µg/mℓ crustacean toxin. (d) Start of spontaneous train
of 'slow' ejps synchronously recorded from the accessory bundle
(upper trace) and the main muscle (lower trace). 50 min after application of 0.15 µg/mℓ of insect toxin. (e) Spontaneous neuromuscular activity caused by insect toxin. Synchronous recording
from the 'slow' motor axon (upper trace; upward going signals positive) and a fibre in the main part of the extensor tibiae muscle
(lower trace). 65 min after application of approx. 0.4 µg/mℓ insect
toxin. Calibration bars: (a) 10 mV, 50 msec; (b) 5 mV, 500 msec;
(c) 10 mV, 50 msec; (d) 10 mV, 100 msec; (e) 50 msec; upper 0.5 mV,
lower 10 mV (taken from Walther et al., 1976).
B.(a-d) Effect of 0.026 µg/mℓ crustacean toxin on ejps evoked by
single stimuli. (a) control; (b) 25 sec, (c) 45 sec, and (d) 50
sec after toxin application. Calibration bars: 2 mV for (a); 10
mV for (b)-(d); 100 msec. (e) Correlation of ejps and activity of
the motor axons. Simultaneous intracellular recording of repetitive
ejps (upper trace) upon a single stimulus and extracellular recording
of action potentials (lower trace) from a branch of the motor axon
12 mm proximal of the muscle recording site; 0.2 µg/mℓ crustacean
toxin. Calibrations: 20 mV for upper, 400 µV for lower trace;
1 sec. (taken from Rathmayer et al., 1977).

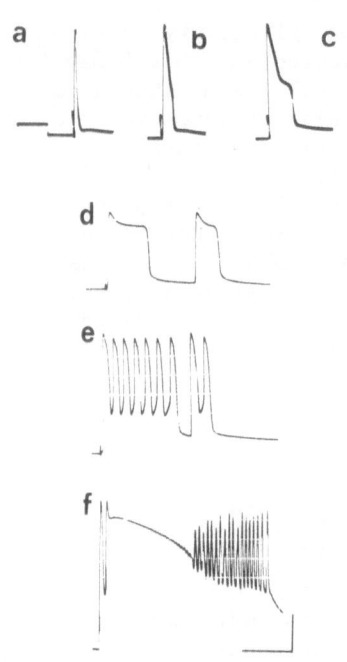

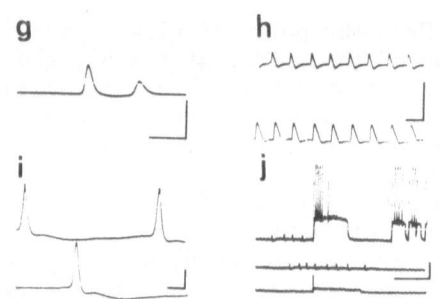

Fig. 7. Effects of toxins on nerve
action potentials.
(a-f) Various forms of repetitive
activity and prolongation of action
potentials induced by the crustacean
toxin and mammal toxin I in the isolated lateral giant axon from the
central nervous system of the cray-
fish.Astacus leptodactylus upon single stimuli. (a) control, (b) and
(c) 6 and 25 min after application
of 0.13 µg/mℓ of crustacean toxin.
(d) 45 min, (e) 80 min after ap-
plication of 1 µg/mℓ crustacean toxin. (f) Different preparation
treated with 3.6 µg/mℓ mammal toxin I after 25 min.(g-j) Quasi intracellular recordings from the motor nerve to the locust extensor tibiae muscle. (g) Control: from the 'slow' excitatory (first) and
the inhibitory axon, stimulated synchronously in a region remote of
the recording site. Recorded from the most distal part of the nerve
where the 'fast' axon is lacking. (h) Synchronous recordings from
both ends of the nerve, 80 min after application of approx. 8 µg/mℓ
mammal toxin I. Spontaneous activity of the 'slow' axon. Note prolonged decay phase of action potentials. (i) Successive recording
from the distal end of nerve. 45 min after application of approx.
2 µg/mℓ insect toxin. Spontaneous repetitive activity of the 'slow'
axon. Note late negative after potentials. (j) Successive recording from the nerve in the region of the main muscle. Spontaneous
activity 60 min after application of approx. 0.8 µg/mℓ crustacean
toxin. Preparation paralyzed by Habrobracon venom. Upper trace:
short train of small action potentials from the inhibitory axon,
followed by 'plateaus' plus superimposed bursts of large action potentials both originating in the 'slow' excitatory axon; inhibitory
train continuing on first plateau. Middle trace: train of action
potentials from inhibitory axon only. Lower trace: single action
potential and 'plateau' due to activity of the 'fast' excitatory
axon. Calibrations: calibration pulse in (a) 10 mV, 10 msec, ap-
plies also for (b) and (c). (d) 40 mV, 50 msec. (e) 25 mV, 50
msec. (f) 20 mV, 50 msec. (g) 1 mV, 2 msec. (h) 1 mV, 20 msec.
(i) 0.2 mV, 2 msec. (j) 0.2 mV, 200 msec. ((a)-(f) taken from
Rathmayer et al., 1977 and (g)-(j) taken from Walther et al., 1976).

the whole animal by injection (Table 3), may suggest that the specificity of the above toxins, at least partially, may be attributed
to their specific resistance or susceptibility to inactivation processes in the body. (3) There exists a close resemblance between
the response of the crayfish and the spider nerve-muscle preparation
to the different toxins (Table 3). This may indicate certain structural and functional similarities between the neuromuscular systems
of these two classes of arthropods, differentiating them from insects. (4) The insect toxin represents substances demonstrating a
high degree of selectivity being able to diversify between related
groups of arthropods. This may indicate certain differences in
the structure and function of their axonal membranes. The way the
insect toxin affects the axon might be quite different from that
previously reported for scorpion venoms or toxins (Fig. 7, Koppen-
hofer and Schmidt, 1968; Narahashi et al., 1972; Romey et al.,
1975). As such the insect toxin may serve as a pharmacological tool
in the investigation of insect neurons, and the molecular mechanism
of its action should be clarified.

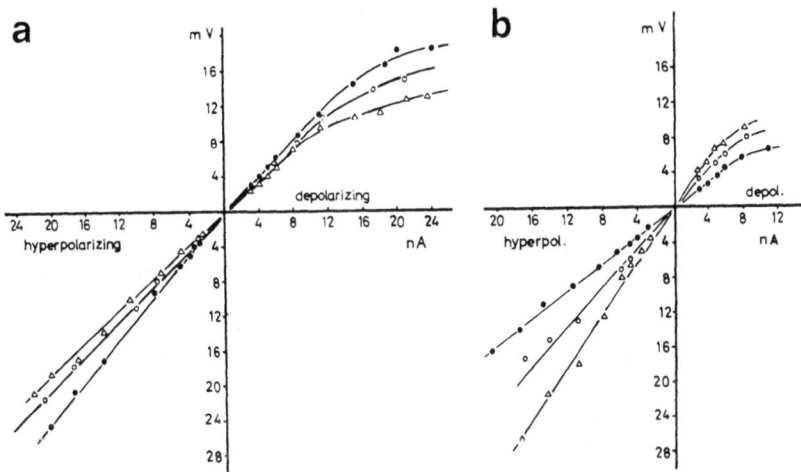

Fig. 8. Changes in current-voltage relationships induced in the
extensor tibiae muscle of a locust by insect toxin and crude venom.
(a) Insect toxin: Δ-Δ, before toxin; R_p -50 to -55 mV, $R_{Inp.}$ 9.6
$\times 10^5$ Ω. o-o, 20 min after application of 0.5 $\mu g/m\ell$; R_p -56 to -60
mV, $R_{Inp.}$ 10.4$\times 10^5$ Ω. •-•, 30 min after application of 0.5 $\mu g/m\ell$;
R_p -59 to -65 mV, $R_{Inp.}$ 12.5$\times 10^5$ Ω. (b) Crude venom Δ-Δ, before
venom; R_p -63 to -66 mV, $R_{Inp.}$ 15$\times 10^5$ Ω. o-o, 10 min after application of 37 $\mu g/m\ell$ venom; R_p -55 to -56 mV, $R_{Inp.}$ = 11.3$\times 10^5$ Ω. •-•,
30 min after application of 37 $\mu g/m\ell$; R_p -45 to -55 mV, $R_{Inp.}$ =
7.8$\times 10^5$ Ω (taken from Walther et al., 1976).

Apart from the differences in the potency of the different toxins on the different preparations (Table 3), there are some essential qualitative differences in their action:

(1) The most obvious phenomenon is the high selectivity of the insect toxin which was the most potent and only active on the insect neuromuscular preparation.

(2) The time course of nerve action potentials is affected by the crustacean and the mammal toxins which cause anomalous shapes and prolongations not caused by the insect toxin (Fig. 7).

(3) The insect toxin was the most potent in the induction of repetitive activity of the motor axon leading to long spontaneous trains (duration often exceeding 10 seconds) of junction potentials. The other toxins chiefly cause short bursts of action and junction potentials following single stimuli.

(4) The insect toxin increases the muscle membrane input resistance in contrast to the crude venom which at high doses causes a decrease (Fig. 8).

Acknowledgement: This work was supported by Grant No. 730 from the United States-Israel Binational Science Foundation (BSF), Jerusalem, Israel.

REFERENCES

Adam, K.R., and Weiss, C., 1959, Actions of scorpion venom on skeletal muscle, Brit. J. Pharmacol. 14:334.

Bearg, W.J., 1961, Scorpions: biology and effect of their venom, Agric.Exp. Sta. Univ. Arkansas Bull. Nb. 649.

Brazil, O.V., Neder, A.C., and Corrado,A.P., 1973, Effects and mechanism of action of Tityus serrulatus venom on skeletal muscle, Pharmac. Res. Comm. 5:137.

Cunha-Melo, J.R., Freire-Maia, L., Tafuri, W.L., Maria, T.A., 1973, Mechanism of action of purified scorpion toxin on the isolated rat intestine, Toxicon, 11:81.

D'ajello, V., Zlotkin, E., Miranda, F., Lissitzky, S., and Bettini, S., 1972, The effect of scorpion venom and pure toxin on the cockroach central nervous system, Toxicon 10:399.

Del Pozo, E.G., and Anguiano, L.G., 1947, Acciones del veneno de alacran sobre la actividad motora de musculo estriado, Rev. inst. salubridad y enfermedad trop. (Mex.) 8:231.

Diniz, C.R., Torres, J.M., 1968, Release of an acetylcholine-like substance from guinea pig ileum by scorpion venom, Toxicon, 5:277.

Houssay, B.A., 1919, Action physiologique du venin des scorpions (Buthus quinquestriatus and Tityus bahiensis), J. Physiol. et path. gén. 18:305.

Kamon, E., and Shulov, A., 1963, Estimation of locust resistance to scorpion venom, J. Insect Pathol. 5:206.

Koppenhöfer, E., and Schmidt, H., 1968, Incomplete sodium inactivation in nodes of ranvier treated with scorpion venom, Experientia 24:41.

La Grange, R.G., and Russell, F., 1971, Effects of Centruroides sculpturatus and C. gertschi venom on the mammalian nerve-muscle preparation: a possible mechanism of action, Proc. West. Pharmacol. Soc. 14:163.

Miranda, F., Rochat, H. and Lissitzky, S., 1964(a), Sur les neurotoxines de deux espèces de scorpions nord-africains. I. Purification des neurotoxines (scorpamines) d'Androctonus australis (L.) et de Buthus occitanus (Am.), Toxicon 2:51.

Miranda, F., Rochat, H., and Lissitzky, S., 1964(b), Sur les neurotoxines de deux espèces de scorpion nord-africains. II. Propriétés des neurotoxines (scorpamines) d'Androctonus australis (L.) et de Buthus occitanus (Am.), Toxicon 2:113.

Miranda, F., Kopeyan, C., Rochat, C., and Lissitzky, S., 1970, Purification of animal neurotoxins. Isolation and characterization of eleven neurotoxins from the venom of the scorpions Androctonus australis Hector, Buthus occitanus tunetanus and Leiurus quinquestriatus quinquestriatus, Eur. J. Biochem. 16:514.

Narahashi, T., Shapiro, B.I., Deguchi, T., Scuka, M., and Wang, Ch. M., 1972, Effects of scorpion venom on squid axon membranes, Amer. J. Physiol. 222:850.

Pansa, M.C., Migliori-Natalizi, G., and Bettini, S., 1973, Effect of scorpion venom and its fractions on the crayfish stretch receptor organ, Toxicon 11:283.

Parnas, I., and Russell, F.E., 1967, Effects of venoms on nerve, muscle and neuromuscular junction, in Animal Toxins (F.E. Russell and P.R. Saunders, eds.), pp. 401-415, Pergamon Press, Oxford.

Parnas, I., Avgar, D., and Shulov, V., 1970, Physiological effects of venom of Leirus quinquestriatus on neuromuscular systems of locust and crab, Toxicon 8:67.

Patterson, R.A., 1962, Pharmacologic action of scorpion venom on intestional smooth muscle, Toxicol. Appl. Pharmacol., 4:710.

Rathmayer, W., Walther, Ch., and Zlotkin, E., 1977 The effect of different toxins from scorpion venom on neuromuscular transmission and nerve action potentials in the crayfish, Comp. Biochem. Physiol. 56C:35.

Rochat, C., Rochat, H., Miranda, F., and Lissitzky, S., 1967, Purification and some properties of the neurotoxins of Androctonus australis Hector, Biochem. 6:578.

Rochat, H., Rochat, C., Miranda, F., Lissitzky, S., and Edman, P., 1970, The amino acid sequence of neurotoxin I of Androctonus australis Hector, Eur. J. Biochem. 17:262.

Romey, G., Chicheportiche, R., Lazdunski, M., Rochat, H., Miranda,
    F., and Lissitzky, S., 1975, Scorpion neurotoxin: a presynaptic
    toxin which affects both Na^+ and K^+ channels in axons, Biochem.
    Biophys. Res. Comm. 64:115.
Ruhland, M., Zlotkin, E., and Rathmayer, W., The effect of toxins
    from the venom of the scorpion Androctonus australis on a spider
    nerve muscle preparation, Toxicon, in press.
Stahnke, E.L., 1966, Some aspects of scorpion behavior, Bull. South.
    Calif. Acad. Sci. 65:65.
Tazieff-Depierre, F., Goudon, D., Andrillo, P., 1973(a), Influence du
    calcium sur la desensibilisation de l'iléon isolé de cobaye au
    venin de scorpion, C.R. Acad. Sci. Paris, D, 277:1089.

Tazieff-Depierre, F., Andrillon, P., 1973(b), Sécrétion d'acétyl-
    choline provoquée par le venin de scorpion dand l'iléon de cobaye
    et sa suppression par la tétrodotoxine, C.R. Acad. Sci. Paris, D,
    276:1631.
Tintpulver, M., Zerachia, T., and Zlotkin, E., 1976, The action of
    toxins derived from scorpion venom on the ileal smooth muscle
    preparation, Toxicon 14:371.
Walther, Ch., Zlotkin, E., Rathmayer, W., 1976, Action of different
    toxins from the scorpion Androctonus australis on the locust
    nerve-muscle preparation, J. Insect Physiol. 22:1187.
Zlotkin, E., Blodheim, S.A., and Shulov, A., 1970, Effect of the
    venom of the scorpion Leiurus quinquestriatus on the tympanic
    nerve of the locust Locusta migratoria migratorioides, Toxicon
    8:47.
Zlotkin, E., Fraenkel, G., Miranda, F., and Lissitzky, S., 1971(a),
    The effect of scorpion venom on blowfly larvae; a new method for
    the evaluation of scorpion venom potency, Toxicon 9:1.
Zlotkin, E., Miranda, F., Kupeyan, C., and Lissitzky, S., 1971(b),
    A new toxic protein in the venom of the scorpion Androctonus
    australis Hector, Toxicon 9:9.
Zlotkin, E., Rochat, H., Kupeyan, C., Miranda, F., and Lissitzky,
    S., 1971(c), Purification and properties of the insect toxin
    from the venom of the scorpion Androctonus australis Hector,
    Biochimie (Paris) 53:1073.
Zlotkin, E., Miranda, F., and Lissitzky, S., 1972(a), Proteins to-
    xic to mammals and insects in six scorpion venoms, Toxicon 10:
    207.
Zlotkin, E., Miranda, F., and Lissitzky, S., 1972(b), A toxic factor
    to crustacean in the venom of the scorpion Androctonus australis
    Hector, Toxicon 10:211.
Zlotkin, E., 1973, Chemistry of animal venoms, Experientia 29:1453.
Zlotkin, E., Martinez, G., Rochat, H., and Miranda, F., 1975, A
    protein toxic to crustacean from the venom of the scorpion An-
    droctonus australis, Insect Biochem. 5:243.
Zlotkin, E., Rochat, H., and Miranda, F., Chemistry and pharma-
    cology of Buthinae scorpion venoms, in The Handbook of Exper-
    imental Pharmacology: Arthropod Venoms (Ed. S. Bettini),
    Springer-in press.

ANT VENOMS: A STUDY OF VENOM DIVERSITY

Justin O. Schmidt

Department of Entomology

University of Georgia, Athens, GA   30602

INTRODUCTION

Ant venoms appear to represent an almost untapped reservoir of information capable of adding several exciting chapters to the story of toxinology. Ants share with some bees and wasps the distinction of being the only truly social group of venomous animals. This fact implies that most of the venomous individuals belong to an essentially sterile class of worker individuals, and that survival of the species depends on colony rather than individual survival. Unlike social bees and wasps, which use their stings solely for defense, ant stings are utilized for a variety of additional functions, including prey capture and the elaboration of trail, sex, aggregation, and alarm pheromones. In parallel with the evolutionary development of varied stinging behaviors were major changes in the venom composition and the sting apparatus itself. This plasticity in form, function, and composition associated with the sting apparatus may be correlated with the success of ants in dominating most of the terrestrial environments.

At present, a paucity of information exists pertaining to the proteinaceous ant venoms. This is partly because the few confirmed human deaths and serious envenomations resulting from ant stings have attracted little research interest. As a consequence, it is still generally believed that ant venoms, unlike those of snakes, scorpions, and spiders, are not especially toxic or antigenically active. The practical problem of obtaining ant venoms in reasonable quantities and purities for clinical and biochemical studies has also severely hampered research on these poison gland products. For example, ants generally possess 10 μg or less per individual of dried venom with the largest ants yielding perhaps 300 µg (as compared to many spiders, scorpions, and snakes which yield from 1 to 300 mg per individual). With an emerging awareness of the immunological responses to even small doses of venoms, there will, undoubtedly, be a great increase in studies of the pharmacological properties of ant venoms.

TAXONOMY AND MORPHOLOGY OF ANTS

The 7600+ worldwide species of ants comprise at least nine subfamilies within the family Formicidae (Bernard 1968). As a whole, the group has speciated explosively since the Cretaceous period (Wilson et al. 1967). The systematic relationships between ants and other Hymenoptera remain obscure: several conflicting theories have arisen to explain their evolutionary origin. The two main schools of thought believe that the ants originated either from a line of primitive solitary tiphiid wasps (Brown 1954, Wilson et al. 1967) or from solitary bethylid wasps (Malyshev 1968). However, based on measures of taxonomic distinctness, both groups of wasps appear to be unrelated to the ants. On the other hand, the Sierolomorphidae in the Vespiformes appear to be closer to the lineage from which the ants arose (Brothers 1975).

The morphological structures of ant sting apparatuses have been described in detail (Oeser 1961, Hermann and Blum 1966, 1968, Maschwitz and Kloft 1971). Figure 1 represents an example of a highly developed ant sting apparatus. It consists of a poison gland with its associated poison sac, a sting shaft formed from three parts, two of which are moveable, and the associated muscles and sclerites to drive the sting shaft. When an ant stings, it grasps a piece of tissue with its mandibles, arches its dorsum for leverage, and drives the sting downward. The moveable elements of the sting shaft, by their alternating backward and forward sliding movements, aid in sting penetration, in contrast to the fixed elements used for envenomation by scorpions, spiders, centipedes, and snakes. Several of the ant subfamilies have morphologically deviated from this general pattern presented. Two subfamilies, the Formicinae and the Dolichoderinae, have lost the major portion of the sting shaft as well as associated sclerites (Figure 2). The Formicinae have evolved, along with this change, a radically different type of venom, while the Dolichoderinae appear to have lost the function of the poison gland reservoir and have replaced it with the anal glands, organs which synthesize and secrete a variety of compounds including ketones, lactones, and aldehydes. The Dorylinae and some species of the Myrmicinae also possess a somewhat modified sting apparatus.

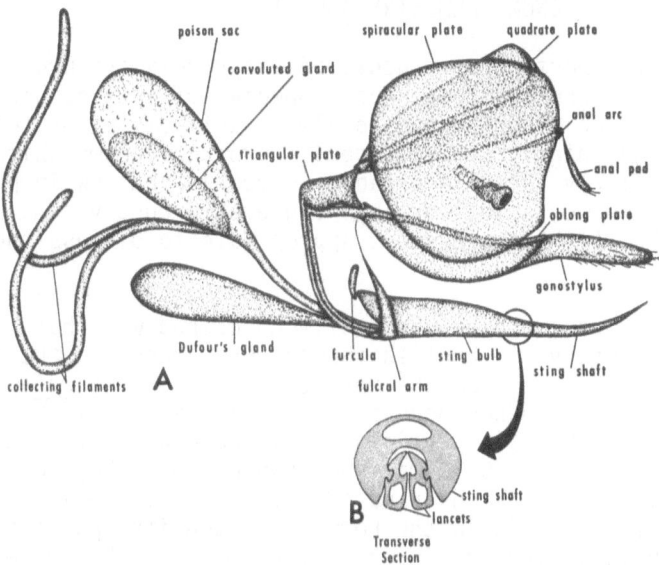

Figure 1.   A.   Poison apparatus of a typical stinging ant.
B.   Transverse section through sting.   (Redrawn from Hermann and
Blum 1968).

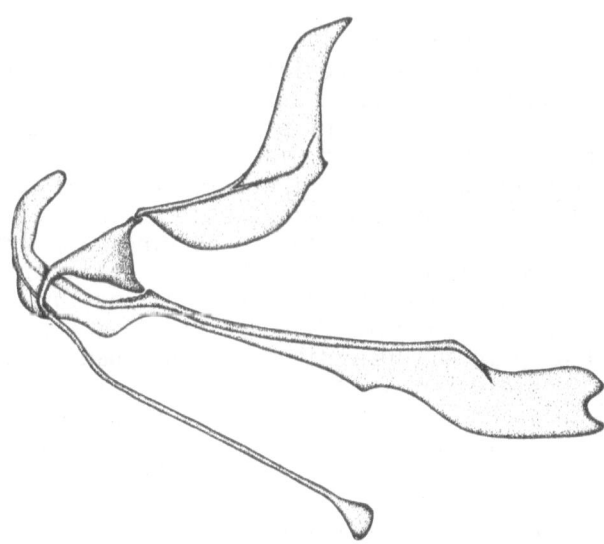

Figure 2.   Poison apparatus of a formicine ant.   (Redrawn from
Hermann and Blum 1968).

VENOM CHEMISTRY AND BIOCHEMISTRY

The most important components of ant venoms are proteins and fairly volatile organic compounds. Species of ants considered ancestral produce venoms composed almost entirely of proteins. On the other hand, highly derived species produce venoms which are rich in the fairly volatile organic compounds and low in proteins. To date the most detailed work has centered around venoms of this latter type. It therefore seems appropriate to discuss these first.

The first venom to be chemically described was that of an ant. In the 17th century the English chemist Wray reported the distillation of formic acid from the formicine ant Formica rufa. Since that time formic acid has been found in virtually all the species of ants in the subfamily Formicinae that have been studied (see Stumper 1922, 1952, 1960, Osman and Brander 1961, Regnier and Wilson 1968, Schreuder and Brand 1972). In fact, because of the ubiquity of formic acid in the Formicinae and its apparent absence from the venoms of species in other subfamilies, the presence of formic acid in an ant is considered a diagnostic subfamilial character. The venom of formicine ants may comprise up to 20% of the total weight of the ant, and formic acid may constitute as much as 60% or more of the venom (Osman and Brander 1961). The only compounds other than formic acid reported from the venoms of formicine ants are amino acids and small peptides which are only found in trace quantities (Osman and Brander 1961, Hermann and Blum 1968).

A veritable array of organic compounds are synthesized in the poison glands of various ant species in the subfamily Myrmicinae. The most thoroughly investigated ant venoms are produced by fire ants and consist predominantly of piperidine alkaloids. The alkaloids present in the red and the black forms of the imported fire ants, Solenopsis invicta and S. richteri, are illustrated in Figure 3. These alkaloids all contain alkyl side chains at the 6 position of the ring and, at the 2 position of the ring, a methyl group which may be either cis or trans to the side chain (Brand et al. 1972). The side chain may possess a site of unsaturation as well. The stings of the red imported fire ant, S. invicta, produce a much greater level of pain and necrosis in humans than do the stings of native North American fire ants (Brand et al. 1973). Moreover, the venom of this ant also contains a much higher percentage of unsaturated 13 and 15 carbon side chains trans to the ring than those of the other species of fire ants. Thus, the presence of longer side chains and especially the trans ring configurations appear to enhance venom toxicity by allowing greater exposure of both the unpaired electrons and the hydrogen atom of the amine nitrogen in the trans isomer. The increased polarity produced by the cis configuration of the double bond in the side chain may also contribute (Brand et al. 1972).

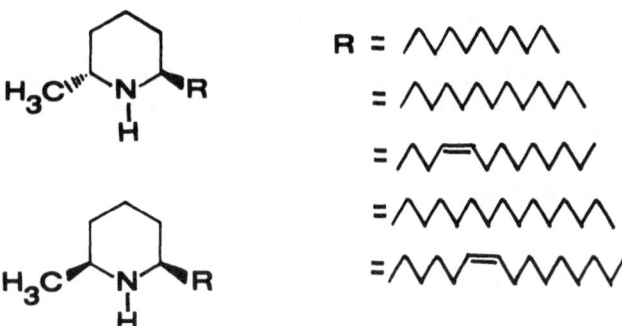

Figure 3.   Major components of <u>Solenopsis invicta</u> and <u>S. richteri</u> venoms.

In addition to the major piperidine alkaloids discussed above, cis- and trans-2-methyl-6-heptylpiperidine and cis- and trans-2-methyl-6-nonylpiperidine have been discovered in trace quantities in the venom of <u>S. richteri</u> by MacConnell <u>et al</u>. (1974). The compound 2-methyl-6-<u>n</u>-undecyl-$\Delta^{1,2}$-piperideine, presumed to be a precursor of piperidines was found in <u>S. xyloni</u> venom (Brand <u>et al</u>. 1972). In

	R	R'
I*	C_7H_{15}	C_2H_5
II	C_7H_{15}	C_4H_9
III	C_5H_{11}	C_4H_9
IV	C_7H_{15}	C_2H_5
V	C_5H_{11}	C_2H_5
VI	C_7H_{15}	C_2H_5
VII	C_5H_{11}	C_2H_5

*All alkyl groups are straight chained

Figure 4.   Pyrrolidines and pyrrolines present in the venom of <u>S. punctaticeps</u>.

addition to the piperidine derivatives, fire ant venom contains small
quantities of proteins (Brand et al. 1972, Buffkin and Russell 1972).
Recently Baer et al. (1977) isolated three antigenic peptides of
approximate molecular weights 2000, 5000 and 10,000 from the red
imported fire ant.

The African Solenopsis, S. punctaticeps, possesses an alkaloidal
composition different from those found in the New World fire ants
studied.   This ant, which belongs to a different subgenus than that
of the imported fire ants, produces dialkylpyrrolidines and -pyrro-
lines in the poison gland (Pedder et al. 1976).   These compounds,
illustrated in Figure 4, differ from those produced by the imported
fire ants in several important respects: the alkyl side chains are
much shorter, being seven carbons at maximum length, the methyl
group is replaced by an ethyl or butyl group, the number of carbons
in the ring is reduced by one, and the ring is frequently unsaturated.   These alkaloids also appear to be less pharmacologically
active than the fire ant piperidines.   A mild itching and erythema
are the only symptoms noted by stung humans (Pedder et al. 1976).

Several other myrmicine ant venoms contain the nitrogenous
compounds illustrated in Figure 5.   Monomorium pharaonis, commonly
called Pharoah's ant and frequently a pest in homes and hospitals,
produces 5-methyl-3-butyloctahydroindolizine, 2-(5'-hexenyl)-5-
pentylpyrrolidine, and the previously reported 2-pentyl-5-butyl-
pyrrolidine (Ritter et al. 1973, Talman et al. 1974, Ritter and
Persoons 1975).   These compounds, especially in mixture, induce
trail following behavior and may also be defensive compounds or
repellents to other insects.   The last compound is reported to act
as an aggregation pheromone for queens (Ritter and Persoons 1975).
Atta texana, the Texas leaf cutter ant, utilizes the venom component
methyl 4-methylpyrrole-2-carboxylate as one component of its trail
pheromone (Tumlinson et al. 1971).   Skatole is found in the venom of
the soldiers of Pheidole fallax (Law et al. 1965).

The major venom components of the myrmicine Myrmicaria natalensis are listed in Figure 6 (Grunager et al. 1960, Brand et al. 1974).
The exact role of these terpenes in this unusual venom is not known.
It is possible, however, that they function as topical toxins after
being smeared on the arthropod cuticle.

Behavioral investigations have demonstrated the presence of
volatile constituents in the venoms of species in several other
myrmicine ant genera.   Species in the genera Cyphomyrmex, Huberia,
Trachymyrmex, Acromyrmex, Tetramorium, Myrmica, Manica, Pogonomyrmex,
and Veromessor all possess trail pheromones which are found in the
venom reservoirs (Blum et al. 1964, Blum and Ross 1965, Blum 1966,
1974).   The presence of volatile sex pheromones has been demonstrated
in the venoms of Xenomyrmex floridanus (Hölldobler 1971),

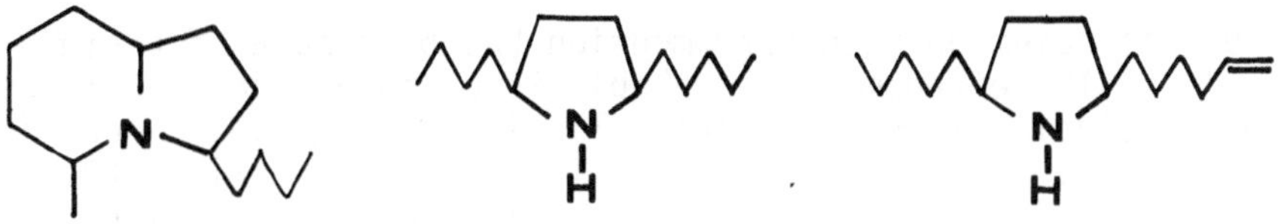

Monomorium pharaonis

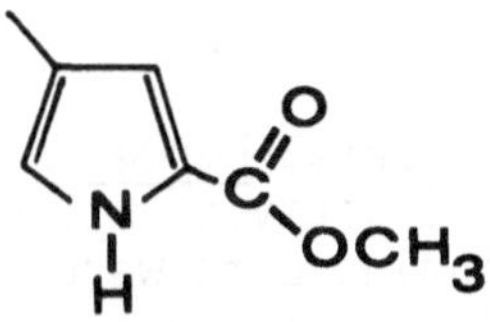

Atta texana 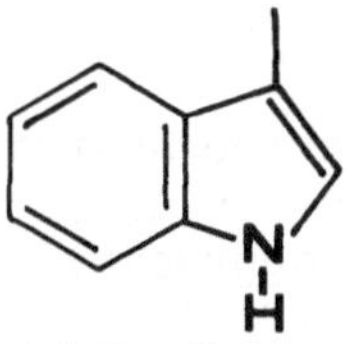   Pheidole fallax

Figure 5.   Nitrogenous compounds present in myrmicine ant venoms.

Harpagoxenus sublaevis (Bushinger 1972), and Formicoxenus nitidulus
(Bushinger 1976). Unfortunately, these pheromones have not been
chemically characterized nor have the venoms been biochemically
analyzed.

Ants of species in the genus Crematogaster possess spatulate
stings which function not as piercing organs, but rather as effective
topical applicators of the associated glandular exudate of unknown
chemical composition (Buren 1958). This secretion is apparently
very effective at penetrating arthropod cuticle and repelling many
potential predators.

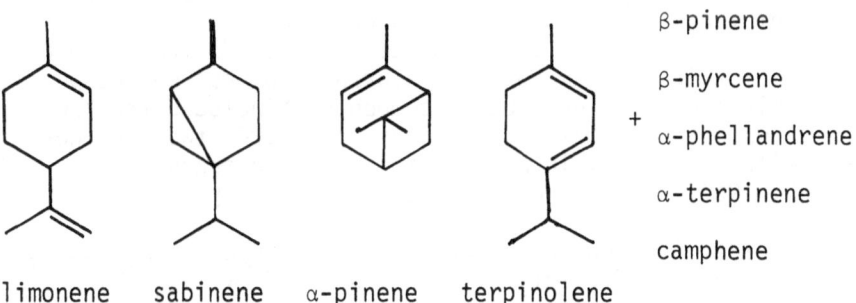

β-pinene

β-myrcene

+ α-phellandrene

α-terpinene

camphene

limonene   sabinene   α-pinene   terpinolene

Figure 6.   Monoterpenes present in Myrmicaria natalensis venom.

To this point only cursory mention has been made of protein-rich
ant venoms. These venoms are probably found in a majority of ant
species, including members of the following subfamilies: Ponerinae
(Hermann and Blum 1966), Myrmeciinae (De la Lande et al. 1963,
Cavill et al. 1964), Pseudomyrmecinae (Blum and Callahan 1963),
Dorylinae (Hermann and Blum 1967b), and some of the Myrmicinae
(Hermann and Blum 1967a, Jentsch 1969). Unfortunately, detailed
studies of proteinaceous ant venoms are rare. The three genera for
which the greatest amount of information is available -- Myrmecia,
Myrmica and Pogonomyrmex -- will be discussed separately.

The venoms of the Australian "bulldog" ants, Myrmecia pyriformis
and M. gulosa, possess great pharmacological activity. The venoms
from these large, aggressive, fiercely stinging ants were found to
contain histamine (De la Lande et al. 1963, Cavill et al. 1964),
phospholipase A (Lewis et al. 1968) and peptide fractions responsible
for smooth-muscle-stimulating (De la Lande et al. 1963, Cavill et
al. 1964), hemolytic (Cavill et al. 1964, Lewis and De la Lande
1967), and histamine-releasing (Thomas and De la Lande 1965) activities. 5-Hydroxytryptamine, acetylcholine (De la Lande et al.
1963), bradykinin-releasing activity (Lewis and De la Lande 1967),
proteases, cholinesterase and 5'nucleotidase (Cavill et al. 1964)
were not detected in these venoms. Venoms of both M. gulosa and M.
pyriformis were separated into seven proteinaceous components by
either paper electrophoresis (Cavill et al. 1964) or starch gel
electrophoresis (Wanstall and De la Lande 1974). However, the venom
of M. pyriformis failed to fractionate into distinct separate
components on 2 or 3 meter Sephadex G-50 columns (Wanstall and De la
Lande 1974). The authors were able to demonstrate that histamine-
releasing, smooth-muscle-stimulating and red-cell-lysing activities
were all produced by an apparent single peptide of molecular weight
11,000. Both phospholipase A and hyaluronidase exhibited molecular
weights greater than 23,800 (Wanstall and De la Lande 1974). The
pharmacological activities of four constituents of the venom were
not determined.

The venom of Myrmica ruginodis is proteinaceous and like
"bulldog" ant venom is capable of inducing pain in humans. This
venom, however, appears to differ in its composition from Myrmecia
venoms. It contains histamine and hyaluronidase, but no phospholipase or hemolyzing proteins. Other components included the "ant
fraction 2" which has a molecular weight of 14,900, two peptides
stainable with Ponceau S, 16 amino acids, and substances X_1, X_2 and
X_3 (Jentsch, 1969). Substances X_2 and X_3 may be peptides.

The venom of the New World harvester ant, Pogonomyrmex badius,
appears to be quite different from the venoms of Myrmica, Myrmecia
or any bee or wasp venom studied to date. This venom possesses at
least four different enzymes: hyaluronidase, phospholipase A, acid

phosphatase, and esterase. Protease was not found. Polyacrylamide
electrophoretic gels stained for esterase, indicating the presence of
three differently migrating enzymatic bands. General protein stains
revealed a minimum of nine separate proteins. In addition, the venom
contains histamine and numerous amino acids (Schmidt and Blum, unpublished). No 5-hydroxytryptamine was detected by paper chromatography or by the guinea pig-ileum assay (Schmidt and Pisano, unpublished).

PHARMACOLOGY AND MODE OF ACTION OF ANT VENOMS

Although the stings of many ants produce only minor symptoms in
humans, other ant venoms are highly active and painful. Formicine
ants are an example of ants whose venoms produce minor symptoms.'
These ants spray a mixture of formic acid from the venom reservoir
and the Dufour's gland products into mandible-abraded skin wounds,
thereby producing a burning sensation. More severe reactions are
caused by the alkaloid-rich venom of the imported fire ants -- a
sting by these ants produces pain, formation of an edematous flare,
and a wheal, followed by the formation of a purulent vesicle (Caro
et al. 1957). Stings of species causing the most severe reactions
are generally characterized by at least extreme local pain, erythema,
edema, and wheal formation. In addition to these symptoms, the
venom of Paraponera clavata causes pain and swelling in the axillary
lymph nodes (Hermann and Blum 1966). All of the above reactions
plus local sweating and piloerection are caused by the venoms of
Myrmica ruginodis (Jentsch 1969) and Pogonomyrmex spp. (McCook 1879,
Weber 1959, Williams and Williams 1964, Herman and Blum 1967a).

Systemic reactions in mice resulting from intravenous (iv)
lethal doses of Myrmica ruginodis venom include extreme sensitivity,
occasional paralysis of the hind quarters, clonic convulsions,
respiratory distress and death (Jentsch 1969). In contrast, intraperitoneal (ip) lethal doses of Myrmecia pyriformis venom induced
agitation and aggressiveness, usually followed by a quiescent period
before death. Muscular distress and spasms were rarely noted (Lewis
and De la Lande 1967). Pogonomyrmex barbatus venom in lethal ip
doses causes dragging and twisting of the abdomen, respiratory
distress, ataxia, extreme lethargy, and finally death by clonic
convulsions (Williams and Williams 1964); P. badius venom injected
iv also causes defecation and diarrhea (Personal observations).

Currently the lethal doses of ant venoms to mice are known for
species in only three genera. These data are included in Table I
along with similar data obtained for the venoms of spiders and
scorpions. Worthy of mention is the fact that some of the insect

Table I. Toxicities of highly active arthropod venoms.

	LD_{50} (mice) in mg/kg		Reference
Scorpions			
Centruroides sculpturatus	1.12	sc	Stahnke 1963
Tityus serrulatus	0.75	iv	Bücherl 1971a
Androctonus australis	0.42	sc	Zlotkin et al. 1971
Leiurus quinquestriatus	0.33	sc	Bücherl 1971a
Spiders			
Loxosceles similis	6.5	iv	Bücherl 1971b
Latrodectus m. mactans	1.3	ip	McCrone 1964
Phoneutria nigriventer	0.30	iv	Bücherl 1971b
Insects			
Apis mellifera	3-4	iv	Neumann and Habermann 1954
Vespa orientalis	2.5	ip	Edery et al. 1972
Vespula maculata	≈40	ip	Schmidt and Blum unpublished
Myrmica ruginodis	50-60	iv	Jentsch 1969
Myrmecia pyriformis	2-10	ip	Lewis and De la Lande 1967
Pogonomyrmex barbatus	1.29	ip	Williams and Williams 1965
Pogonomyrmex badius	0.42	ip	Schmidt and Blum unpublished

venoms are quite toxic and that the most toxic insect venom appears
to be from the ant P. badius. In fact, the toxicity of this venom
is comparable to that of the most toxic spiders and scorpions.

Comparison of P. badius venom toxicity to white mice by the
various routes (iv, ip, sc [subcutaneous]) revealed some striking
differences. LD_{50} values of 0.42 ip, ~1.2 iv, and 11.2 sc mg/kg
were obtained. Adminstrations of most animal venoms by iv or ip
versus sc routes results in LD_{50} ratios of 5-10:1 or less. P.
badius venom exhibits an ip:sc ratio of 27:1! Investigations are
currently underway to determine the exact explanations for this
ratio difference.

In addition to being generally toxic, ant venoms express a
variety of specific pharmacological activities. Perhaps the culmina-
tion of this expression of pharmacological activity is exhibited by
venom of the imported fire ants. These venoms are insecticidal
(Blum et al. 1958), antibacterial (Jouvanez et al. 1972), necrotic
(Caro et al. 1957), hemolytic (Androuny et al. 1959), allergenic
(Lockey 1974, Baer et al. 1977), and neurotoxic (Yeh et al. 1975).
Hemolytic activities are also found in the venoms of Myrmecia
(Cavill et al. 1964, Lewis and De la Lande 1967), and Eciton hamatum
(Hermann and Blum 1967b), and are most likely common to a great

many ant venoms.

Until recently, immunological studies of allergy to ant venoms were entirely lacking. Current evidence points directly to the ability of ant venoms to induce hypersensitivity and allergic responses (Lockey 1974, Pinnas 1975). In a brilliant piece of work, Baer et al. (1977) identified three proteins in trace quantities from fire ant venom and showed that they were directly responsible for causing the allergic reactions in human sera and in mammals.

The best studied example of ant venom neurotoxicity was undertaken with the cis- and trans-piperidine alkaloids identified as poison gland products of fire ants. These alkaloids, when applied to the frog nerve-sartorius muscle preparation, do not change the membrane potentials, but do irreversibly decrease the amplitude of spontaneous miniature end plate potentials, nerve-evoked end plate potentials, and the iontophoretically induced acetylcholine depolarizations (Yeh et al. 1975). Since d-tubocurarine pretreatment did not affect the blocking potential of the alkaloids and the alkaloids did not compete for the sites occupied by α-bungarotoxin, decamethonium, or carbamylcholine, the authors concluded that these alkaloids interfered with the coupling mechanism between acetylcholine-receptor binding and the ionic conductance increases.

The venoms of several other species of ants induce mammalian symptoms which strongly implicate neurotoxicity. Among these are the venoms of Paraponera clavata which may induce trembling, sweating and nauseous tendency (Hermann and Blum 1966), of Myrmica ruginodis which induces sweating and piloerection around the local sting site and causes death by clonic convulsions (Jentsch 1969), and of P. badius. The strong neurotoxicity to mice of this last venom is illustrated by its extreme toxicity (0.42 mg/kg ip), its ability to cause death by clonic convulsions, and by the lack of evidence of venom cytotoxicity near the lethal sc or ip injection sites. Moreover, P. badius venom induces local sweating and piloerection in stung humans implying peripheral as well as central neurotoxicity of the venom. The drastically reduced toxicity of this venom by the sc versus ip route of injection indicates that the connective tissues in the skin may either block the neurotoxins from gaining access to the blood stream or complex and render them inactive (see Higginbotham 1965). The swelling and tenderness of the lymph nodes following envenomation points to the lymphatic system as a major route for venom movement in the human body.

Recent studies utilizing insects as target organisms show that P. badius venom acts quite differently on mammalian and insect systems. The LD_{50} of P. badius venom for Galleria wax moth larvae is about 100 mg/kg -- a figure about 200 times larger than that

obtained for the ip LD$_{50}$ for mice. Death or paralysis of the
larvae usually occurs after at least 6 hours (Schmidt and Blum
unpublished). Thus, P. badius appears to possess at least one
neurotoxic component which is selectively toxic to mammals and not
to insects (see Frontali and Grasso (1964) and Zlotkin et al. (1977)
for examples of similar results from spiders and scorpions). The
presence of such a toxic component provides strong evidence for the
conclusion that this secretion is used primarily for defensive
purposes against large vertebrates rather than arthropods. Indeed,
since an average worker of P. badius contains only about 10 μg of
dried venom, in theory, the ant would have to use all its venom to
kill one 100 mg Galleria larva and would have to wait most of the
day for the larva to die after being stung!

SUMMARY

     Ant venoms exhibit greater variability in composition and
function than do venoms from any other group of arthropods. The
versatility of venom chemistry and role may be basic to the success
of ants as the dominant invertebrates in many of the world's habi-
tats. The insect venom most toxic to mammals, an ant product, is
of comparable toxicity to the most toxic scorpion and spider venoms.
Now that ant stings have been shown to be capable of causing ana-
phylaxis in humans, a much greater effort devoted to understanding
the biochemistry and pharmacology of these important and fascinating
venoms can be expected. Many of the more pharmacologically active
ant venoms produce neurotoxic symptoms in mammals. At present the
mode of neurotoxic action of ant venoms has been partially elucidated
only for two of the venom products produced by the red imported
fire ant. Several ant species which possess proteinaceous venoms
are also prime candidates for similar studies.

     At present there is no reason to expect ant venoms to be
biochemically similar in any but the most general aspects to the
venoms of other Hymenoptera or, for that matter, arachnids. Indeed,
the radically different evolutionary and ecological histories of
ants compared to those of bees and wasps and other arthropods would
seem to militate against the production of identical venoms in
these diverse groups. We have barely scratched the surface in the
field of ant toxinology, and already the most toxic and diverse
venoms found within insects have been discovered. Future research
should unveil even more exciting discoveries.

Acknowledgements: The author is most grateful to Murray S. Blum
of this department for helpful discussions and suggestions, and to
Debbie K. Schmidt and Jeffery R. Aldrich of the same University for
reviews of this manuscript.

REFERENCES

Androuny, G. A., Derbes, V. J., and Jung, R. C., 1959, Isolation of
    a hemolytic component of fire ant venom, Science 130: 449.
Baer, H., Liu, D. T., Hooton, M., Blum, M., James, F., Schmid, W. H.,
    1977, Fire ant allergy: isolation of three allergenic proteins
    from whole venom, J. Allergy clin. Immunol. (in press).
Bernard, F., 1968, Les fourmis (Hymenoptera Formicidae) d'Europe
    occidentale et septentrionale. Faune de l'Europe et du
    Bassin Mediterreen, no. 3, Masson et Cie, Paris.
Blum, M., 1966, The source and specificity of trail pheromones in
    Termitopone, Monomorium and Huberia, and their relation to
    those of some other ants, Proc. R. Ent. Soc. Lond. (A), 41:
    155.
Blum, M. S., 1974, Myrmicine trail pheromones: specificity, source,
    and significance, J. N. Y. Ent. Soc. 82: 141.
Blum, M., and Callahan, P. S., 1963, The venom glands of Pseudomyrmex
    pallidus (F. Smith), Psyche 70: 69.
Blum, M., and Ross, G. N., 1965, Chemical releasers of social
    behaviour V. Source, specificity, and properties of the odour
    trail pheromone of Tetramorium guineense (F.) (Formicidae:
    Myrmicinae), J. Insect Physiol. 11: 857.
Blum, M., Walker, J. R., Callahan, P. S., and Novak, A. F., 1958,
    Chemical, insecticidal, and antibiotic properties of fire ant
    venom, Science 128: 306.
Blum, M., Moser, J. X., and Cordero, A. O., 1964, Chemical releasers
    of social behavior. II. Source and specificity of the odor
    trail substances in four attine genera. (Hymenoptera: Formi
    cidae), Psyche 71: 1.
Brand, J. M., Blum, M. S., Fales, H. M., and MacConnell, J. G., 1972,
    Fire ant venoms: comparative analyses of alkaloidal components,
    Toxicon 10: 259.
Brand, J. M., Blum, M. S., Ross, H. H., 1973, Biochemical evolution
    in fire ant venoms, Insect Biochem. 3: 45.
Brand, J. M., Blum, M. S., Lloyd, H. A., and Fletcher, D. J. C.,
    1974, Monoterpene hydrocarbons in the poison gland secretion of
    the ant Myrmicaria natalensis (Hymenoptera: Formicidae), Ann.
    ent. Soc. Am. 67: 525.
Brothers, D. J., 1975, Phylogeny and classification of the aculeate
    Hymenoptera, with special reference to Mutillidae, Univ Kansas
    Sci. Bull. 50: 483.
Brown, W. L., Jr., 1954, Remarks on the internal phylogeny and
    subfamily classification of the family Formicidae, Insectes
    Sociaux 1: 21.
Buffkin, D. C., and Russell, F. E., 1972, Some chemical and pharmaco-
    logical properties of the venom of the imported red fire ant,
    Solenopsis saevissima richteri, Toxicon 10: 526.
Bücherl, W., 1971a, Classification, biology and venom extraction of
    scorpions, in: Venomous Animals and their Venoms, Vol. 3,

(W. Bücherl and E. E. Buckley, eds) pp. 317-349, Academic Press, New York.

Bücherl, W., 1971b, Spiders, in: Venomous Animals and their Venoms, Vol. 3, (W. Bücherl and E. E. Buckley, eds) pp. 197-277, Academic Press, New York.

Buren, W. F., 1958, A review of the species of Crematogaster, Sensu Stricto, in North America (Hymenoptera: Formicidae). Part 1., J. N. Y. Ent. Soc. 66: 118.

Buschinger, A., 1972, Giftdrüsensekret als Sexualpheromon bei der Ameise Harpogoxenus sublaevis, Naturwissenschaften 59: 313.

Buschinger, A., 1976, Giftdrüsensekret als Sexualpheromon bei der Gastameise Formicoxenus nitidulus (NYL) (Hym., Form.), Insectes Sociaux 23: 215.

Caro, M. R., Derbes, B. J., and Jung, R., 1957, Skin responses to the sting of the imported fire ant (Solenopsis saevissima), Arch. Dermatol. 75: 475.

Cavill, G. W. K., Robertson, P. L., and Whitfield, F. B., 1964, Venom and venom apparatus of the bull ant, Myrmecia gulosa (Fabr.), Science 146: 79.

De la Lande, I. S., Thomas, D. W., and Tyler, M. S., 1963, Pharmacological analysis of the venom of the "bulldog" ant Myrmecia forficata, in: Recent Advances in the Pharmacology of Toxins, Proc. 2nd. Int. Pharm. Meeting, Progue, Vol. 9, p. 71.

Edery, H., Ishay, J., Lass, I., and Gitter, S., 1972, Pharmacological activity of Oriental hornet (Vespa orientalis) venom, Toxicon 10: 13.

Frontali, N., and Grasso, A., 1964, Separation of three toxicologically different protein components from the venom of the spider Latrodectus tredecimguttatus, Arch. Biochem. Biophys. 106: 213.

Grünager, P., Quilico, A., and Pavan, M., 1960, Sul secreto del Formicidae Myrmicaria natalensis Fred. Accad. Nazion. Lincei 28: 293.

Hermann, H. R., and Blum, M. S., 1966, The morphology and histology of the hymenopterous poison apparatus. I. Paraponera clavata (Formicidae), Ann. ent. Soc. Am. 59: 397.

Hermann, H. R., and Blum, M. S., 1967a, The morphology and histology of the hymenopterous poison apparatus. II. Pogonomyrmex badius (Formicidae), Ann. ent. Soc. Am. 60: 661.

Hermann, H. R., and Blum, M. S., 1967b, The morphology and histology of the hymenopterous poison apparatus III. Eciton hamatum (Formicidae), Ann. ent. Soc. Am. 60: 1282.

Hermann, H. R., and Blum, M. S., 1968, The hymenopterous poison apparatus. VI. Campanotus pennsylvanicus (Hymenoptera: Formicidae), Psyche 75: 215.

Higginbotham, R. D., 1965, Mast cells and local resistance to Russell's viper venom. J. Immunol. 95: 867.

Hölldobler, B., 1971, Sex pheromone in the ant Xenomyrmex floridanus, J. Insect Physiol. 17: 1497.

Jentsch, J., 1969, A procedure for purification of Myrmica venom:

the isolation of the convulsive component, Proc. VI Congr.
IUSSI, Bern, p. 69.
Jouvanez, D. P., Blum, M. S., and MacConnell, J. G., 1972, Antibac-
terial activity of venom alkaloids from the imported fire ant,
Solenopsis invicta Buren, Antimicrob. Ag. Chemotherap. 2: 291.
Law, J. H., Wilson, E. O., and McCloskey, J. A., 1965, Biochemical
polymorphism in ants, Science 149: 544.
Lewis, J. C., and De la Lande, I. S., 1967, Pharmacological and
enzymic constituents of the venom of an Australian "bulldog"
ant Myrmecia pyriformis, Toxicon 4: 223.
Lewis, J. C., Day, A. J., and De la Lande, I. S., 1968, Phospholipase
A in the venom of the Australian bulldog ant Myrmecia pyrifor-
mis, Toxicon 6: 109.
Lockey, R. M., 1974, Systemic reactions to stinging ants, J.
Allergy clin. Immunol. 54. 132-146.
MacConnell, J. G., Williams, R. N., Brand, J. M., and Blum, M. S.,
1974, New alkaloids in the venoms of fire ants, Ann. ent.
Soc. Am. 67: 134.
Malyshev, S. I., 1968, Genesis of the Hymenoptera and the Phases
of their Evolution, Methuen, London.
Maschwitz, U. W. J., and Kloft, W., 1971, Morphology and function
of the venom apparatus of insects -- bees, wasps, ants, and
caterpillars, in: Venomous Animals and their Venoms, Vol. 3,
(W. Bücherl and E. E. Buckley, eds) pp 1-60, Academic Press,
New York.
McCook, H. C., 1879, The Natural History of the Agricultural Ant
of Texas, Lippincott's Press, Philadelphia.
McCrone, J. D., 1964, Comparative lethality of several Latrodectus
venoms, Toxicon 2: 201.
Neumann, W., and Habermann, E., 1954, Beiträge zur Characterisierung
der Wirkstoffe des Bienengiftes, Arch. exp. Path. Pharmakol.
222: 367.
Oeser, R., 1961, Vergleichend Morphologische Untersuchungen über
den Ovipositor der Hymenopteran, Mitt. Zool. Mus. Berlin 37: 1.
Osman, M. F. H., and Brander, J., 1961, Weitere Beiträge zur
Kenntnis der chemischen Zusammensetzung des Giftes von Amiesen
aus der Gattung Formica, Z. Naturforsch. 16b: 749.
Pedder, D. J., Fales, H. M., Jaouni, T., Blum, M., MacConnell,
J. G., and Crewe, R. M., 1976, Constituents of the venom of a
South African fire ant (Solenopsis punctaticeps), 2,5-dialkylpyr-
rolidines and -pyrrolines, identification and synthesis,
Tetrahedron 32: 2275.
Pinnas, J. L., Wang, T. M., Strunk, R. C., and Thompson, H. C.,
1975, Harvester ant hypersensitivity in vitro and in vivo
studies, J. Allerg. clin. Immunol. 55: 107.
Regnier, F. E., and Wilson, E. O., 1968, The alarm-defensive
system of the ant Acanthomyops claviger, J. Insect Physiol.
14: 953.
Ritter, F. J., and Persoons, C. J., 1975, Recent development in

insect pheromone research, in particular in the Netherlands,
Neth. J. Zool. 25: 261.

Ritter, F. J., Rotgans, I. E. M., Talman, E., Verwiel, P. E. J., and
Stein, F., 1973, 5-Methyl-3-butyl-octahydroindolizine, a novel
type of pheromone attractive to Pharoah's ants (Monomorium
pharaonis (L.)), Experimentia 29: 530.

Schreuder, G. D., and Brand, J. M., 1972, The chemistry of the
Dufour's gland and the poison gland secretions of Anoplolepis
custodiens (Hymenoptera: Formicidae), J. Georgia ent. Soc. 7:
188.

Stahnke, H. L., 1963, Some pharmacological and biochemical character-
istics of Centruroides sculpturatus Ewing scorpion venom, in:
Recent Advances in the Pharmacology of Toxins, Vol. 9, (H. W.
Raudonat and J. Vanecek, eds), pp. 63-70, MacMillan, New York.

Stumper, R., 1922, Nouvelles observations sur le venin des fourmis,
C. R. Acad. Sci. 174: 66.

Stumper, R. 1952, Données quantitatives sur la sécrétion d'acide
formique par les fourmis, C. R. Acad. Sci. 234: 149.

Stumper, R., 1960, Die Giftsekretion der Ameisen, Naturwissenschaften
47: 457.

Talman, E., Ritter, F. J., and Verwiel, P. E. J., 1974, Structure
elucidation of pheromones produced by the Pharoah's ant,
Monomorium pharaonis L. in: Proceedings International Symposium
on Mass Spectrometry in Biochemistry and Medicine, Milan, 1973,
Raven Press, New York.

Thomas, D. W., and Lewis, J. C., 1965, Histamine released by the ant,
Aust. J. exp. Biol. med. Sci. 43: 275.

Tumlinson, J. H., Silverstein, R. M., Moser, J. C., Brownleee, R. G.,
and Ruth, J. M., 1971, Identification of the trail pheromone of
a leaf-cutting ant, Atta texana, Nature 234: 348.

Wanstall, J. C., and De la Lande, I. S., 1974, Fractionation of
bulldog ant venom, Toxicon 12: 649.

Weber, N., 1959, The stings of the harvesting ant, Pogonomyrmex
occidentalis (Cresson), with a note on populations (Hymenoptera),
Ent. News 70: 85.

Williams, M. W., and Williams, C. S., 1964, Collection and toxicity
studies of ant venom, Proc. Soc. exp. Biol. Med. 116: 161.

Williams, M. W., and Williams, C. S., 1965, Toxicity of ant venom,
further studies of the venom from Pogonomyrmex barbatus, Proc.
Soc. exp. Biol. Med. 119: 344.

Wilson, E. O., Carpenter, F. M., and Brown, W. L., Jr., 1967, The
mesozoic ants, with the description of a new subfamily, Psyche
74: 1.

Wray, J., 1670, Some uncommon observations and experiments made with
an acid juyce to be found in ants. Phil. Trans. Roy. Soc. London
1670: 2063.

Yeh, J. Z., Narahashi, T., and Almon, R. L., 1975, Characterization
of neuromuscular blocking action of piperidine derivatives,
J. Pharmac. exp. Therap. 194: 373.

Zlotkin, E., Rochat, H., Kopeyan, C., Miranda, F., and Lissitzky, S.,
    1971, Purification and properties of the insect toxin from the
    venom of the scorpion Androctonus australis Hector, Biochimie
    53: 1073.
Zlotkin, E., Rathmayer, W., and Lissitzky S., 1978, Chemistry
    specificity and action of arthropod toxic proteins derived
    from scorpion venoms, in: Pesticide and Venom Neurotoxicity
    (D.L. Shankland, R.M. Hollingworth, and T. Smyth, Jr., eds.)
    Plenum Press, New York, pp. 227-246.

ACTIONS OF SOME NEUROTOXIC PROTEINS OF BLACK WIDOW SPIDER VENOM

T. Smyth, Jr., R. L. Ornberg and R. M. Meyer

Department of Entomology and Department of Biochemistry
  and Biophysics
The Pennsylvania State University, University Park,
  Pennsylvania, U.S.A.

INTRODUCTION

Black widow spiders are greatly feared although their bite is
seldom fatal to man. However, the toxins evoke muscle spasms and
excruciating pain which is resistant to the usual pain-reducing
drugs and lasts two to three days. These symptoms point to a
neurotoxic action and therefore have aroused the interest of
neurobiologists.

A flurry of recent studies has been concerned with two sorts
of questions: (i) the chemical nature and properties of the toxins
and (ii) their modes of action. This paper will consider these two
aspects of black widow spider venom (BWSV), with particular
reference to our own work with two protein fractions affecting
insects.

CHEMICAL NATURE OF THE TOXINS

D'Amour et al (1936) published a notably comprehensive report
on black widow spiders and their venom. They indicated that the
toxin is protein, based on its behavior in a number of extraction
procedures, destruction by proteinases, sensitivity to pH and
temperature, and the fact that it can evoke formation of antibodies.

By means of ion exchange gel chromatography Frontali and
Grasso (1964) were able to separate three toxicologically different
proteins all of high molecular weight. Two fractions paralyzed
houseflies, the third was toxic to guinea pigs. McCrone and Hatala
(1967) used polyacrylamide gel electrophoresis to separate seven
venom proteins. They reported that a protein with a molecular

weight of 5,000 was lethal to mice. In our laboratory Ornberg
(1974), Ornberg et al (1976) used discontinuous polyacrylamide gel
electrophoresis to separate venom proteins. More than twenty
protein bands could be distinguished and two of these proteins or
groups of proteins were toxic to cockroaches and flies on injection.
We elected to use American cockroaches for routine assay because
the assays are easy and inexpensive and because insects are the
normal prey of spiders which avoid contact with vertebrates, if
possible.

When the larger, slower moving protein is injected into assay
insects it may take some minutes or even hours to produce symptoms,
but insects showing symptoms seldom recover. Its molecular weight
was determined by analytical ultracentrifugation and SDS gel
electrophoresis to be about 125,000.

The smaller, faster electrophoresing fraction rapidly produces
paralysis in injected insects, but they generally recover with an
hour or so. We were unable to establish a firm value for the
molecular weight, but it is certainly low. Small amounts of a
protein with similar high mobility were seen when the larger toxic
protein was eluted and re-electrophoresed, but the amount obtained
was very small and toxicity was not demonstrated.

The toxic proteins did not stain with PAS glycoprotein stain
or Sudan black and therefore appear to have no sugar or lipid
components. Incubation with α and β-napthylacetate and α-naphthyl
acid phosphate at pH 5 and pH 9.5, and with azoalbumin gave negative
indications in tests for esterase, phosphatase and protease
activity.

Quite recently, Frontali et al (1976) have used two Sephadex
columns in series (and several additional techniques) to purify a
fraction that acts on frog neuromuscular junctions. They report
that it consists of at least four protein components with similar
molecular weights (about 130,000) which contain no sugar residues
and have little or no lipolytic or proteolytic activity. These
proteins are toxic to mice, but are different from the fractions
that act on houseflies, the crayfish stretch receptor and the
cockroach heart.

In summary, BWSV contains several toxic proteins that affect
different groups of animals selectively. So far, no enzymatic
activity has been associated with any of these. They appear not
to be glyco- or lipoproteins.

MODES OF ACTION –
TRANSMITTER RELEASE

Longenecker et al (1970), Clark et al (1970), and Okamoto et al (1971) reported that BWSV selectively destroys the cholinergic prejunctional motor nerve terminals in frog and cat skeletal muscles. This is indicated by massive discharge of transmitter quanta followed by transmitter depletion and permanent synaptic block. Electronmicroscopic examination showed the poisoned nerve terminals to be swollen and devoid of synaptic vesicles; their mitochondria also were swollen and distorted. These reports stimulated many neurobiologists to look at BWSV actions at other chemical synapses and in a variety of organisms. For example Kawai et al (1972) and Griffiths and Smyth (1973) applied BWSV to glutamergic and GABAergic neuromuscular junctions in the crayfish and cockroach, respectively; Cull-Candy et al (1973) studied glutamergic junctions in a locust; nor-epinephrine synapses in mammals were studied by Hamilton and Robinson (1973) and Pinto et al (1974), etc. All reported the same result, regardless of the nature of the vesicle-related transmitter or organism: BWSV evoked massive release of transmitter followed by permanent inactivation of synapses.

In cockroaches, this effect is caused by the larger of the two insect toxins mentioned in the previous section (Ornberg 1974). We have called this a "transmitter release component" (TRC). Its action will be discussed first.

We assume that the BWSV toxins react with the cell surface since the actions can be reversed by application of antivenin as demonstrated by Neri et al (1965) and Longenecker et al (1970). Just how such a reaction might cause transmitter release is not obvious because the normal process of quantal transmitter release is far from completely understood. However, there is a large volume of evidence indicating that release is dependent on the free calcium ion concentration within the nerve terminal. Changing the external calcium concentration has little effect on the time course of TRC action. To change the intracellular calcium levels Ornberg (1976) soaked the preparations in Ringer solutions containing 30 mm of citric, oxalic or malonic acid which are calcium chelators with varying effectiveness. With these he could set the level of spontaneous transmitter release, implying regulation of internal calcium. When BWSV was applied in the presence of these chelators it had relatively little effect, but its action appeared when the chelators were washed out. Thus, TRC action does appear to be dependent on the availability of intraterminal free calcium.

The turnover of calcium in many cells is related to the intracellular sodium level. Atwood et al (1975) have related synaptic facilitation to sodium accumulation. We found both spontaneous and TRC-induced transmitter release to be influenced by the extracellular sodium concentration. The sodium pump poison ouabain accelerated transmitter release and strongly synergized the TRC.

Since mitochondria are capable of sequestering calcium and are abundant in nerve terminals, we applied TRC to isolated lobster sarcosomes but it had no effect on this preparation.

In summary, our present hypothesis for the action of the TRC is that it combines with the surface of the nerve terminal, making it permeable to sodium ions. If sodium influx swamps the active sodium extrusion mechanism, the intraterminal concentration increases until calcium is released from internal binding sites, in turn promoting transmitter release. Concurrently, mitochondrial function is disrupted and they and the terminals swell.

OTHER ACTIONS

D'Amour et al (1936) reported that a methanol-precipitated fraction of BWSV reversibly paralyzed rats. As mentioned earlier, we found that a low molecular weight protein fraction reversibly paralyzed insects. This fraction did not evoke transmitter release, but Meyer (1975) found that it did reversibly block nerve impulse conduction in cockroach giant axons when the abdominal connectives were desheathed (but not through intact sheaths). Interestingly, the TRC protein could also reversibly block impulse conduction, leading him to speculate that the small paralytic protein might be a fragment of the larger TRC. Earlier, Gruener (1973) had reported that BWSV blocked impulse conduction in squid axons, and attributed this mainly to shortened kinetics of sodium and potassium activation and sodium inactivation. Ornberg (unpublished) has been unable to confirm these observations.

BWSV can inhibit firing of the crayfish stretch receptor according to Grasso and Paggi (1967) and they cite unpublished evidence that it depolarizes the membrane of the receptor cell. Such membrane depolarizations are usually associated with increased sodium conductance across a membrane.

CONCLUDING REMARKS

The great surprise and puzzle emerging is that there are several medium size proteins in BWSV that appear to have the same kind of transmitter releasing action but are specific for different groups of organisms. The significant primary action of the TRC we studied is to increase sodium permeability; presumably other TRCs act the same way. There is also the low molecular weight protein fraction that can produce reversible paralysis and nerve impulse block. This may also alter sodium (or small cation) permeability. These observations raise the possibility that the small protein functions as a toxophore, perhaps as a sodium ionophore in the membrane. It may be coupled with any of several larger protein units which serve as selectophores for different groups of target animals, binding tightly to nerve membranes and thus conferring relative irreversibility.

The selectivity of BWSV for prejunctional nerve terminals may reflect special chemical properties of these patches of cell membrane, but it could also be an artifact of the relative accessibility and small size of synaptic nerve endings.

REFERENCES

Atwood, H. L., Swenarchuk, L. E., and Gruenwald, C. R., 1975, Long term synaptic facilitation during sodium accumulation in nerve terminals, Brain Res. 100:198.

Clark, A. W., Mauro, A., Longenecker, H. E., Jr., and Hurlbut, W. P., 1970, Effects of black widow spider venom on the frog neuromuscular junction, Nature 225:703.

Cull-Candy, S. G., Neal, H. and Usherwood, P. N. R., 1973, Action of black widow spider venom on an aminergic synapse, Nature 241:353.

D'Amour, E. F., Becker, F. E., and van Riper, W., 1936, The black widow spider, Quart. Rev. Biol. 11:123.

Frontali, N., Ceccarelli, B., Borio, A., Mauro, A., Siekevitz, P., Tzeng, M.-C., and Hurlbut, W. P., 1976, Purification from black widow spider venom of a protein factor causing the depletion of synaptic vesicles at neuromuscular junctions, J. Cell Biol. 68:462.

Frontali, N., and Grasso, A., 1964, Separation of three different protein components from the venom of the spider Latrodectus mactans tredecimguttatus, Archs. Biochem. Biophys. 106:213.

Grasso, A. and Paggi, P., 1967, Effect of Latrodectus mactans tredecimguttatus venom on the crayfish stretch receptor neurone, Toxicon 5:1.

Griffiths, D. J. G., and Smyth, T., Jr., 1973, Action of black widow spider venom at insect neuromuscular synapses. Toxicon 11:369.

Gruener, R., 1973, Excitability blockade of the squid giant axon by the venom of Latrodectus mactans (black widow spider), Toxicon 11:155.

Hamilton, R. C., and Robinson, P. M., 1973, Disappearance of small vesicles from adrenergic nerve endings in the rat vas deferens caused by red back spider venom, J. Neurocytol. 2:465.

Kawai, N., Mauro, A., and Grundfest, H., 1972, Effect of black
    widow spider venom on the lobster neuromuscular junction.
    J. Gen. Physiol. 60:650.
Longenecker, H. E., Jr., Hurlbut, W. P., Mauro, A., and Clark,
    A. W., 1970, Effects of black widow spider venom on the frog
    neuromuscular junction, Nature 225:701.
McCrone, J. D., and Hatala, R. J., 1967, Isolation and character-
    ization of a lethal component from the venom of Latrodectus
    mactans mactans, in: Animal Toxins (F. E. Russell and P. R.
    Saunders, eds.), pp 29-34, Pergamon Press, Oxford.
Meyer, R. M., 1975, Demonstration of a nonsynaptic neurotoxic
    effect of black widow spider venom in vitro, M.S. Thesis in
    Biophysics, The Pennsylvania State University.
Neri, L., Bettini, S., and Frank, M., 1965, The effect of
    Latrodectus mactans tredecimguttatus venom on the endogenous
    activity of Periplaneta americana nerve cord, Toxicon 3:95.
Okamoto, M., Longenecker, H. E., Jr., Riker, W. F., Jr., and
    Songs, S. K., 1971, Destruction of mammalian motor nerve
    terminals by black widow spider venom. Science 172:733.
Ornberg, R. L., 1974, Isolation of a specific neurotoxic
    component from the venom of the black widow spider,
    Latrodectus mactans (Fab.), M.S. Thesis in Biophysics, The
    Pennsylvania State University.
Ornberg, R. L., 1976, The physiological mode of action of a
    neurotoxin isolated from the venom of the black widow spider,
    Latrodectus mactans (Fab.) Ph.D. Thesis in Biophysics, The
    Pennsylvania State University.
Ornberg, R. L., Smyth, T., Jr., and Benton, A. W., 1976, Isolation
    of a neurotoxin with a presynaptic action from the venom of
    the black widow spider (Latrodectus mactans, Fabr.) Toxicon
    14:329.
Pinto, J. E. B., Rothlin, R. P., and Dagrosa, E. E., 1974,
    Noradrenaline release by Latrodectus mactans venom in guinea
    pig atria, Toxicon 12:385.

Pesticide and Venom Neurotoxicity

Edited by D. L. Shankland
Mississippi State University

R. M. Hollingworth
Purdue University

and T. Smyth, Jr.
Pennsylvania State University

Of all organic insecticides, the most important have been those whose site of action lies within the nervous system. In this book, many of the world's leaders in the study of pesticide and venom neurotoxicity provide a dual examination of the nervous system as a physiological system and as a target for poisons — both natural and man-made — and consider how pesticides affect living organisms, both to man's advantage and to his detriment.

Devoted primarily to the consideration of invertebrate venoms, this book investigates potentially critical target sites and modes of action for chemicals in the nervous system. It examines comparative aspects which can lead to more selective and safer compounds, the mode of action and structure—activity relations of known neurotoxicants, and the development of model assay systems for screening purposes. Furthermore, several new classes of insecticides are presented for the first time, such as choline acetyltransferase inhibitors and the fast-acting nitromethylene insecticides. In addition, there are chapters concerning the chemistry and actions of venoms from scorpions, black widow spiders, solitary wasps, and a variety of ants. These venoms are not only of intrinsic biological and physiological interest, but they can also provide models for the development of novel chemicals for tomorrow's pest control.

Jacket design by Deborah England